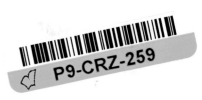

HEALTHY & HEARTY DIABETIC COOKING

SECOND EDITION

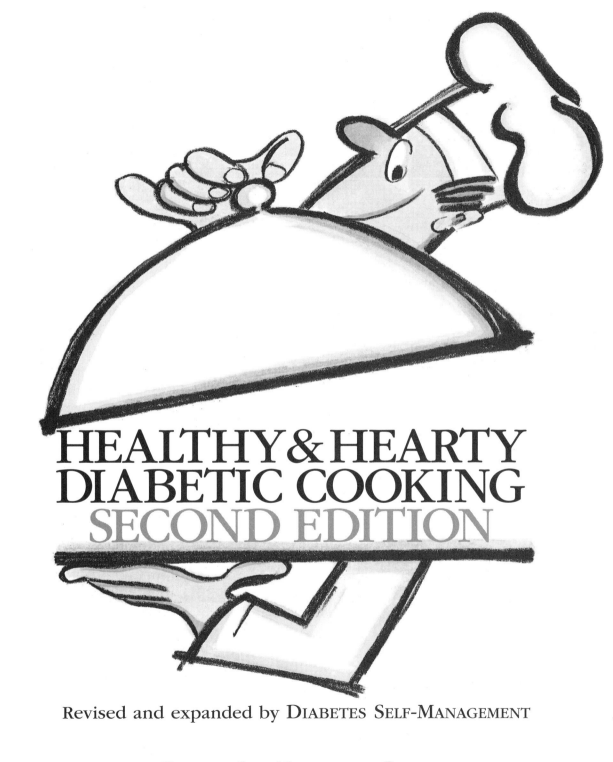

HEALTHY & HEARTY DIABETIC COOKING
SECOND EDITION

Revised and expanded by DIABETES SELF-MANAGEMENT

DIABETES SELF-MANAGEMENT BOOKS
New York

Published in cooperation with the Canadian Diabetes Association, Toronto, Ontario, Canada, publishers of the earlier version of this cookbook, *Choice Cooking* (copyright © 1982, Canadian Diabetes Association).

Exchange Lists for Meal Planning in the Appendix copyright © 1995 American Diabetes Association and the American Dietetic Association. Reprinted with permission.

Library of Congress Cataloging-in-Publication data

Healthy & hearty diabetic cooking.—
    2nd ed., rev., updated, and expanded.
        p.   cm.
        Includes Index.
        ISBN 0-9631701-6-3
        1. Diabetes—Diet therapy—Recipes. I. Title: Healthy and hearty diabetic cooking. II. Diabetes Self-Management Books.
    RC662.H43 2003
    641.5'6314—dc21   2003004852
                                  CIP

Project Editor: James Hazlett
Editorial Assistant: Tara Dairman
Design and Illustration: Richard Boland
Production Artist: Sean Boggs

Diabetes Self-Management Books is an imprint of R.A. Rapaport Publishing, Inc., 150 West 22nd Street, New York, NY 10011.

Printed in the United States of America.

10 9 8 7 6 5 4 3 2 1

Acknowledgements

Nobody ever put together a cookbook of this scope without a lot of help from a lot of people. Contrary to the adage of too many cooks spoiling the stew, the heavy involvement of many generous and talented people was a happy—and necessary—event. Their enthusiasm and professionalism have made this an excellent and indispensable cookbook for people who care about their health and enjoy good food. We are deeply grateful for the painstaking and thoughtful contributions made by the following individuals:

Technical Reviewers:
      Nancy Cooper, R.D., C.D.E.
      Lea Ann Holzmeister, R.D., C.D.E.
      Sue McLaughlin, R.D., C.D.E.

Nutrition Analysis and Exchange Calculations:
      Nancy C. Patterson, M.S., R.D., C.D.E.
      Madelyn L. Wheeler, M.S., R.D., F.A.D.A., C.D.E.

Recipe Editors:
      Bonnie Lee Black
      Robert J. Anthony

Contents

Foreword

Healthy & Hearty Diabetic Cooking is the United States version of the cookbook originally published by the Canadian Diabetes Association. In its first edition, this remarkable cookbook enjoyed tremendous popularity, with more than 175,000 copies sold in the United States.

To make this revised edition even more appealing and useful, we have added 75 new recipes and a brand new chapter, Snacks and Munchies. All of the nutrition information and food exchange values have been updated by experts in diabetes nutrition in order to meet the nutrition guidelines of both the American Diabetes Association and the American Dietetic Association. We have also included a new appendix describing the basics of carbohydrate counting for those who are using this new method to keep their blood glucose levels under control.

You will also notice the appearance of a new icon, like the one to the left, next to certain recipes. This symbol indicates "No Fuss" recipes that are simple to prepare and quick to get on the table. On those days when you are rushed to put together a meal—or just don't feel like spending a lot of time in the kitchen—look for these icons to make your life a little easier.

These new additions, along with all of the old favorites, are combined to make this the best edition of *Healthy & Hearty Diabetic Cooking* yet!

About the Recipes

Lea Ann Holzmeister, R.D., C.D.E.

This cookbook contains a wide variety of delicious recipes that can help you eat lightly and wisely every day. These recipes were developed for people of all ages and lifestyles and include dishes for everyday dining, as well as gourmet treats and a number of items with decidedly ethnic and regional flavors. Herbs, spices, and subtle flavorings have been emphasized to produce great-tasting dishes, while fat, sugar, and salt have been kept to a minimum.

ABOUT THE INGREDIENTS

All recipes in this cookbook have been designed to reduce your consumption of calories, refined sugar, saturated fat, cholesterol, and sodium. Some recipes have been modified by reducing the amount of certain ingredients, eliminating them completely, or substituting more acceptable ingredients. Generally, the following guidelines have been applied throughout the cookbook.

Milk: Skim milk is specified throughout. Other types of milk can be used, but substituting will increase the fat and cholesterol content of the recipes.

Meats: The leanest cuts of meat and ground meat available are specified in the recipes. Trim excess visible fat from meats before cooking to keep the fat content low. Also, drain the fat from meats while cooking. Lean ground turkey breast can be substituted for recipes containing ground beef.

Eggs: Whenever possible, we have substituted egg whites for whole eggs. When the recipes do include eggs, we have limited egg yolks in recipes to one-half per serving.

Cheese: When a low-fat version of a specific cheese is available, the recipe specifies the use of that cheese. For example, in most areas of the country low-fat Cheddar cheese is available. On the other hand, a low-fat version of Gouda or Edam cheese is not usually available. Since substituting in this case would take away from the character of the recipe, changes were not made. These particular recipes should be worked into your diet on an occasional basis.

Sour cream: "Light" sour cream is specified in most recipes whenever sour cream is used. However, nonfat sour cream or plain low-fat yogurt may also be substituted. While the taste and texture may change slightly, the results are still very appealing.

Fats and oils: Margarine is specified in the recipes instead of butter. When you buy margarine, look for a brand that lists a liquid oil as the first ingredient on the label. If a recipe calls for oil or margarine, choose those made from safflower, sunflower, corn, cottonseed, or soybean oil. To coat pans and muffin tins, we have specified nonstick spray or paper liners.

Broth: To reduce sodium content, low-sodium beef or chicken broth and bouillon are used in recipes that contain broth. To make your own beef or chicken broth, look in the chapter on soup recipes.

Flour: Unless otherwise specified, unsifted all-purpose flour is used throughout.

Sodium: Salt is listed as an optional ingredient for all recipes in which salt is used as a seasoning. However, salt is essential in yeast breads to ensure they rise properly, and it is a necessary ingredient in pickles and relish, where it is used as a preservative. For cooking vegetables, pasta, rice, and the like, use unsalted water. Instead of garlic salt and onion salt, use seasoning such as garlic powder and onion powder.

Most of the recipes contain less than 400 milligrams of sodium per serving. If your diet is limited in sodium, use the recipes with high sodium levels less often.

Sugar: Use of sugar in these recipes has been kept to a minimum, but sugar must be used in some recipes. For instance, without any sugar a cake could not hold its shape. When a recipe calls for the use of sugar, it usually represents a small portion of the recipe's total carbohydrate. For a food to be included in a diabetes meal plan on a regular basis, the food must have one teaspoon or less of added sugar per serving. Foods that contain more than one teaspoon of added sugar should be eaten in small portions, and only on occasional basis.

Alternative sweeteners: A variety of artificial sweeteners are available today. In the recipes in this book, we do not specify any particular brand, but you should be aware that there are differences among the various kinds available.

For instance, Equal sweetener (NutraSweet) can be used to sweeten foods and beverages that do not require heating. Equal loses its sweetness when exposed to heat, and it does not provide the bulk and structure required for baking. One teaspoon of Equal (one packet) is as sweet as two teaspoons of sugar.

3

Saccharin is another sweetener that can be used in recipes, including those that require heating, but it is best to add the sweetener toward the end of the cooking process or immediately afterward because saccharin tends to acquire a bitter aftertaste if it is exposed to high temperatures for a long time. The sweetening power of saccharin-containing sweeteners depends on which one you use, so be sure to read the label for this information.

Sweet One (Sunette) is yet another kind of sweetener; it is available in individual packets, can be used in cooking, and has no bitter aftertaste. Twelve packets of Sweet One carry the sweetening power of one cup of sugar.

ABOUT THE NUTRITION ANALYSIS

To help you put together a healthy diet, each recipe lists the food exchange value, carbohydrate choices, and nutrition information for a single serving. Please note that where optional ingredients are listed for recipes, a separate nutrient analysis has been provided. Sodium, for instance, is listed as an optional ingredient in many recipes in this book. The same is true of light sour cream. These additional analyses give you the freedom to tailor a menu to your individual needs.

To help you further in your meal planning, this cookbook lists the yield for each recipe. The total number of portions prepared from a recipe is important because exchange values are based on the number of servings yielded. For that reason, it is important to be accurate when you measure each ingredient. Most of the recipes yield four to six servings. A few that serve more are particularly suitable for plan-ahead meals that can be packaged, frozen, and reheated later. This is particularly useful if you have a busy lifestyle and use the microwave frequently.

Each recipe indicates the serving size and the corresponding nutrient content, exchange value, and carbohydrate choices. If the serving size specified is too large for your meal plan, you can divide the serving and the listed calculations to yield a more appropriate portion. When you want a larger portion, you can multiply nutrient information, exchange value, and carbohydrate choices to accommodate the portion you need. In either case, make sure you include this information in the calculation of your meal plan.

The food exchange values listed with the recipes are based on *Exchange Lists for Meal Planning* from the American Diabetes Association and the American Dietetic Association. The exchange system provides a convenient way of monitoring the nutrients and calories in your diet. (For more information on using the exchange lists for meal planning, see Appendix 1 beginning on page 367.) A newer system, carbohydrate counting, is based on the number of grams of carbohydrate in each recipe. Each recipe includes the number of carbohydrate choices in that recipe. (For more information on using carbohydrate counting for meal planning, see Appendix 2 beginning on page 383.)

This is a cookbook with a difference. The recipes will appeal to everyone who wants to eat well, be healthy, and enjoy food.

Microwaving—A Quick Course

Bonnie Lee Black

Over 80% of American kitchens today contain microwave ovens, but it's a safe bet that many of these are underutilized.

Most people use their microwave oven for the obvious jobs of defrosting and reheating, but not everybody sees this modern appliance for what it is: a quiet, quick, clean kitchen assistant, always ready to be put to work doing "real" cooking.

Your microwave oven "assistant" cannot do everything, and it does some things badly. But it does many things remarkably well; so well, in fact, you'll wonder how you ever did without it.

Here are the main points you need to know:

WHAT ARE MICROWAVES AND HOW DO THEY COOK FOOD?

Microwaves are a form of electromagnetic energy of very high frequency, vibrating millions of times per second. When this energy hits food in the microwave oven, it is absorbed, causing the molecules in the food to vibrate at the same frequency.

This vibration creates heat by the friction of the molecules rubbing against each other (the same way your hands get warm by rubbing them together). Contrary to what many people think, microwaved foods cook from the outside in—by microwave friction for the first 1½ inches or so, and by conduction thereafter.

ARE MICROWAVE OVENS SAFE?

The electromagnetic waves contained in a microwave oven are as safe as the electromagnetic waves of your radio and television. Microwave ovens, in fact, are said to be far safer, in terms of radiation, than television sets.

WHAT ARE THE ADVANTAGES OF MICROWAVE COOKING?

The first obvious advantage of the microwave oven is the speed with which it can produce meals; it takes one-fourth to one-fifth of normal cooking times. Because it cooks more quickly and doesn't need preheating, it also saves on fuel consumption.

Since the oven itself stays cool, it's an ideal way to cook in hot weather. And it's clean: It's easy to wipe down the interior of the oven and even easier to wash microwave-safe dishes (there are no messy pots and pans to scrub). It's so simple to operate that even a child can handle it safely.

Best of all, it's healthy. Because

foods cook in their own juices, more water-soluble vitamins are retained.

ARE THERE DISADVANTAGES TO MICROWAVE COOKING?

Essentially, microwave cooking is a wet-heat method of cooking (all those vibrating wet molecules cause steam). So, as a general rule, the microwave should not be used for dry-cooking assignments, such as baking and roasting, or for direct-heat methods, sauch as sautéing or broiling. For best results, use your conventional oven for baking cakes or pies and roasting meat, and use your broiler and sauté pans to achieve that beautiful browning.

In addition, because there are only so many microwaves to go around inside an oven, small quantities of food cook faster than large ones. In other words, large quantities of food cook more slowly in the microwave than they do by stovetop or conventional oven. Also, because of its speed, microwaving can quickly overcook food. It is therefore best to begin by underestimating the total cooking time and increasing the time in small increments until the food is cooked.

WHAT DOES THE MICROWAVE DO BEST?

Foods that contain water and/or fat and/or sugar microwave best. Most vegetables and fruits cook beautifully in the microwave. Casseroles, stews, rice, sauces, soups, and custards are also good choices. Fish cooks especially well.

HOW DO YOU DO IT?

The metal pots and baking pans used in conventional cooking are never used in microwave cooking because microwaves cannot penetrate metal to reach the food inside. Instead, use microwave-safe containers (which microwaves pass straight through) such as heat-tempered glass (Pyrex), glass-ceramics (Corning), ceramic, china (without metal trim), pottery, and microwavable plastic wrap and paper toweling.

Once you've chosen your cooking vessel, arrange the food—asparagus, for example—with the thicker portions placed toward the outside of the dish, and the thinner parts toward the inside (asparagus would be arranged spoke-fashion, with the thicker ends pointing outward).

Cover the plate with microwavable plastic wrap, such as Saran Wrap, leaving a small vent at one end, and microwave on High 3–4 minutes (depending on the quantity and size of asparagus). At three minutes, check for doneness by piercing a stalk with the tip of a knife. If crisp-tender at that point, remove the dish from the microwave oven and let stand for a minute or two before serving.

The main points to keep in mind are as follows:

■ Coverings retain heat and moisture. The recipe direction "cover tightly" means to cover with a casserole lid or plastic wrap that has been folded back on one corner. Foods that would normally be steamed, boiled, or braised are best cooked this way.

■ When foods can be arranged in a ring with an open center, they cook more evenly and quickly.

■ Foods with thick skins, such as potatoes or acorn squash, should be pierced with a sharp knife before cooking so that the steam that builds up inside will not cause the food to burst.

■ Foods that can be stirred, such as soups or stews, should be stirred once or twice to facilitate even cooking.

■ Some microwave ovens cook unevenly, so it is smart to rotate the dish a quarter- or half-turn during cooking.

■ Many foods continue to cook by heat conduction after they are removed from the microwave. This period, called "standing time," should be allowed for in the total cooking time.

■ Food cut into uniform pieces of 2 inches or less will microwave more quickly and evenly than single large chunks.

■ Refrigerator-cold foods will take longer to cook in the microwave than room-temperature foods.

■ Only use plastic wrap that is clearly labeled "Microwave Safe," which means it can safely withstand the oven's heat. Use plain white paper toweling not made from recycled paper. Wax paper and parchment paper are microwave-safe and good for looser coverings.

■ Do not attempt to deep-fry in the microwave oven.

■ Cooking time in the microwave oven is in direct relation to the amount of food being cooked: A small quantity will cook much faster than a large quantity. The larger the quantity being cooked, the less advantageous the microwave method will be.

■ Most recipes can be cooked on High, or 100% power.

How to Make Your Favorite Recipes Healthier

Nancy Cooper, R.D., C.D.E.

Many of the methods that were used to make the recipes in this cookbook healthy can be applied to your own recipes at home. With a little practice, you can turn any favorite recipe into a healthier dish.

One of the easiest ways to modify a recipe is to change the cooking technique. For example, baking or broiling a piece of meat or fish rather than frying it will significantly reduce the amount of fat you consume. Other ways to reduce fat in cooking include sautéing in broth, water, wine, or juice rather than oil, butter, or margarine; coating baking pans with vegetable cooking spray instead of butter or oil; and cooling soups and stews after cooking, which allows you to remove congealed fat from the surface.

Another way to modify a recipe is to reduce the amount of a particular ingredient, or to substitute a more acceptable ingredient. Sometimes an ingredient is a necessary part of the final product, such as sugar in a cake. Without any sugar a cake would not hold its shape, but the amount of sugar used in a cake recipe can certainly be reduced. In other recipes, certain ingredients may be added solely for taste or appearance and could easily be eliminated, especially if they are high in fat, sugar, or sodium. And finally, many ingredients can be substituted with something lower in fat, sugar, or salt content: for instance, skim milk can be substituted for whole milk, or leaner beef for a higher-fat type of beef. While you may notice slight changes in taste or texture, the results are still very appealing.

The following listing shows how you can make ingredient substitutions to make your favorite recipes healthier. The recipes that follow the listing show how you can put this knowledge to practical use; pay particular attention to the nutrient analysis at the bottom of both recipes.

RECIPE SUBSTITUTIONS TO REDUCE TOTAL FAT, SATURATED FAT, CHOLESTEROL, REFINED CARBOHYDRATE, AND SALT

For This	Substitute This
1 whole egg	¼ cup egg substitute or 2 egg whites or 1 egg white plus 1 teaspoon vegetable oil
butter	margarine
1 cup shortening or lard	¾ cup vegetable oil
½ cup shortening or lard	⅓ cup vegetable oil
whole milk	skim or 1% milk
cream	evaporated skim milk
1 cup sour cream	1 cup plain nonfat yogurt or 1 cup low-fat or nonfat cottage cheese blended with 2 tablespoons lemon juice until creamy
1 ounce regular cheese	1 ounce skim milk cheese or reduced fat cheese
cream cheese	light cream cheese
mayonnaise	reduced-calorie or fat-free mayonnaise
salad dressing	reduced-calorie, low-calorie, or fat-free salad dressing
oil-packed tuna or salmon	water-packed tuna or salmon
1 ounce baking chocolate (one square)	3 tablespoons cocoa powder plus 1 tablespoon vegetable oil
regular gelatin	sugar-free gelatin or fruit juice mixed with unflavored gelatin
1 can condensed cream soup	homemade white sauce (1 cup skim milk plus 2 tablespoons flour plus 2 tablespoons margarine)

10

For This	Substitute This
cream of celery soup	1 cup white sauce plus ¼ cup chopped celery
cream of chicken soup	1½ cups white sauce plus 1 chicken bouillon cube
cream of mushroom soup	1 cup white sauce plus 1 can drained mushrooms
1 ounce bacon (2 strips)	1 ounce Canadian bacon/lean ham
fat in baked recipes	use no more than 1–2 tablespoons oil per cup of flour; increase liquid slightly to add extra moistness
syrup-packed canned fruit	juice-packed canned fruit
2 tablespoons flour (as thickener)	1 tablespoon cornstarch or arrowroot
sugar in baked recipes	Reduce amount by up to ½ the original amount; use no more than ½ cup added sweetener (sugar, honey, molasses, etc.) per cup of flour. Add vanilla extract, cinnamon, and nutmeg to increase sweetness.
bouillon cubes or granules	low-sodium bouillon
garlic, onion, and celery salt	garlic, onion, and celery powder
baking powder	low-sodium baking powder
salt in recipes	reduce amount or eliminate; use spices and herbs

Beef Stroganoff—Original

1½ pounds stew meat
2 tablespoons butter
1 cup plus ½ cup beef bouillon
2 tablespoons ketchup
1 clove garlic, minced
1 teaspoon salt
½ cup sliced mushrooms
1 medium onion, chopped
3 tablespoons flour
1 cup sour cream
3 cups hot cooked noodles
2 tablespoons butter

1. Cook beef in 2 tablespoons butter over low heat in skillet until browned.
2. Stir 1 cup bouillon, ketchup, garlic, and salt into skillet. Cover and simmer until beef is tender, 1 to 1½ hours.
3. Stir in mushrooms and onion. Shake remaining ½ cup bouillon and flour in tightly covered container, stir into beef mixture.
4. Heat to boiling, stirring constantly. Boil 1 minute, remove from heat, and stir in sour cream. Toss cooked noodles with 2 tablespoons butter. Serve beef over noodles.

12

Yield: 6 servings
Serving size: ⅙ sauce over
½ cup noodles

Exchanges: 1½ starch
4 lean meat
3 fat
Carbohydrate choices: 1½

Nutrition per serving:
Calories: 472
Carbohydrate: . . . . 25 g
Protein: . . . . 36 g
Fat: . . . . 25 g
Saturated fat: . . . . 13 g
Cholesterol: . . . . 147 mg
Dietary fiber: . . . . 1 g
Sodium: . . . . 1,187 mg

Beef Stroganoff—Modified

1 pound stew meat
½ cup plus ½ cup low-sodium beef bouillon
2 tablespoons ketchup
1 clove garlic, minced
1 cup sliced mushrooms
1 medium onion, chopped
1½ tablespoons cornstarch
½ cup plain nonfat yogurt
½ cup light sour cream
4 cups hot cooked noodles

1. Cook beef in nonstick skillet over low heat until browned.
2. Stir ½ cup bouillon, ketchup, and garlic into skillet. Cover and simmer until beef is tender, 1 to 1½ hours.
3. Stir in mushrooms and onion. Stir together remaining ½ cup bouillon and cornstarch until blended. Add to beef mixture and stir.
4. Heat to boiling and boil 1 minute, stirring constantly. Remove from heat, stir in yogurt and light sour cream. Serve beef over cooked noodles.

13

Yield: 6 servings
Serving size: ⅙ sauce over
⅔ cup noodles

Exchanges: 2 starch
3 lean meat
Carbohydrate choices: 2

Nutrition per serving:
Calories: 331
Carbohydrate: . . . . 31 g
Protein: . . . . 27 g
Fat: . . . . 10 g
Saturated fat: . . . . 5 g
Cholesterol: . . . . 94 mg
Dietary fiber: . . . . 1 g
Sodium: . . . . 437 mg

A word about sugar substitutes: If you want to cook with a sugar substitute, it is best (if possible) to add the sweetener toward the end of the cooking process or immediately afterward. So when you make applesauce, for example, cook the fruit in water, remove it from heat, cool it slightly, and then add the sweetener. This is the standard recommendation when using sugar substitutes. Saccharin-containing sweeteners tend to turn bitter during baking. Equal sweetener will lose its sweetness when exposed to heat. Sweet One is a sweetening ingredient that is heat-stable and can be used in cooking and baking without any bitter aftertaste. In baking, it is a good idea to use recipes specifically developed for the sweetener for best results.

CALCULATING EXCHANGES

If you have a favorite recipe that you have modified and you make it often, you may want to know how many exchanges are in a single serving so you can fit it into your meal plan. This is easy to calculate. Just follow these steps:

1. List all the ingredients used in the recipe and their amounts.
2. Convert each ingredient into the number of appropriate exchanges it provides (refer to table beginning below).
3. Total each exchange group for the entire recipe. That is, add all the starch exchanges together, then all the meat exchanges, and so on.
4. Divide the exchange totals by the number of servings in the recipe. You can round off these numbers to the nearest one-half exchange (anything less than one-half does not need to be counted).

The following is a table of approximate exchange values of ingredients commonly used in cooking and baking.

EXCHANGES OF COMMONLY USED INGREDIENTS

Food	Amount	Carbohydrate (g)	Protein (g)	Fat (g)	Exchanges
STARCHES					
biscuit mix	½ cup	37	4	8	2½ starch, 1 fat
bread crumbs, dry	1 cup	65	11	4	4 starch
chow mein noodles	½ cup	17	3	8	1 starch, 1½ fat
cornmeal, uncooked	1 cup	117	11	5	7½ starch
cornstarch	2 tbsp	14	0	0	1 starch
cream soup, undiluted	1 can (10¾ oz)	22	5	19	1½ starch, 3½ fat

14

EXCHANGES OF COMMONLY USED INGREDIENTS *continued*

Food	Amount	Carbohydrate (g)	Protein (g)	Fat (g)	Exchanges
flour					
all-purpose	1 cup	87	11	1	6 starch
cake (sifted)	1 cup	79	8	1	5 starch
rye	1 cup	66	10	2	4½ starch
whole wheat	1 cup	80	16	2	5 starch
graham cracker crumbs	1 cup	90	8	14	6 starch, 2 fat
macaroni					
uncooked (3½ oz)	1 cup	79	7	trace	5 starch
cooked	1 cup	41	7	1	3 starch
noodles, egg					
uncooked (2½ oz)	1 cup	59	7	1	4 starch
cooked	1 cup	40	8	3	2½ starch
oatmeal, uncooked	1 cup	54	15	6	3½ starch, 1 fat
rice					
long-grain					
instant, uncooked	¼ cup	26	2	0	2 starch
instant, cooked	1 cup	40	4	0	2½ starch
white & brown					
uncooked	¼ cup	39	3	0	2½ starch
cooked	1 cup	36	3	1	2½ starch
wild, uncooked	¼ cup	21	4	0	1½ starch
spaghetti					
uncooked (3½ oz)	1 cup	79	7	trace	5 starch
cooked	1 cup	41	7	1	3 starch
wheat germ (1 oz)	¼ cup	13	9	3	1 starch, 1 lean meat

DAIRY PRODUCTS

Food	Amount	Carbohydrate (g)	Protein (g)	Fat (g)	Exchanges
butter or margarine	½ stick	0	0	49	10 fat
cheese					
Cheddar, shredded	1 cup	2	29	37	4 high-fat meat, 1 fat
cream	4 oz	3	8	40	1 high-fat meat, 6 fat
mozzarella, part-skim, shredded	1 cup	3	28	18	4 medium-fat meat
Parmesan, grated	¼ cup	1	8	6	1 medium-fat meat
cream					
half and half	½ cup	5	3	14	3 fat
heavy, unwhipped	¼ cup	2	1	22	4 fat
heavy, whipped	½ cup	2	1	22	4 fat
sour	½ cup	4	3	20	4 fat

15

EXCHANGES OF COMMONLY USED INGREDIENTS *continued*

Food	Amount	Carbohydrate (g)	Protein (g)	Fat (g)	Exchanges
egg, whole	1	0	6	6	1 medium-fat meat
egg yolk	1	0	3	5	1 fat
milk					
condensed, sweetened	⅓ cup	54	8	9	3½ carbohydrate, 2 fat
evaporated, skim	½ cup	14	9	0	1 skim milk
evaporated, whole	½ cup	12	8	10	1 skim milk, 2 fat
nonfat dry, instant	1 cup	31	21	0	2½ skim milk
yogurt, plain nonfat	1 cup	17	12	0	1 skim milk

FATS, OILS, CHOCOLATE, COCOA

Food	Amount	Carbohydrate (g)	Protein (g)	Fat (g)	Exchanges
chocolate, bitter	1 oz	7	4	16	½ carbohydrate, 3 fat
chocolate chips	1 cup	105	8	48	7 carbohydrate, 10 fat
chocolate-flavored syrup	2 tbsp	17	1	1	1 carbohydrate
carob powder	1 cup	113	6	2	7½ carbohydrate
cocoa powder	¼ cup	16	6	2	1 carbohydrate
mayonnaise	½ cup	1	1	88	17½ fat
mayonnaise-type salad dressing	½ cup	14	1	55	1 carbohydrate, 11 fat
shortening	½ cup	0	0	111	22 fat
vegetable oil	½ cup	0	0	111	22 fat

FRUITS AND VEGETABLES

Food	Amount	Carbohydrate (g)	Protein (g)	Fat (g)	Exchanges
barbecue sauce	3 tbsp	15	0	1	1 carbohydrate
ketchup	½ cup	30	2	1	2 carbohydrate
chili sauce	½ cup	30	2	1	2 carbohydrate
dates	1 cup	130	4	1	8½ fruit
raisins	½ cup	55	2	0	3½ fruit
tomatoes or tomato juice	1 cup	9	2	0	2 vegetable
tomato sauce or puree	1 cup	20	4	1	1 carbohydrate

SUGARS AND SYRUPS

Food	Amount	Carbohydrate (g)	Protein (g)	Fat (g)	Exchanges
corn syrup	1 cup	242	0	0	16 carbohydrate
gelatin, powdered regular	3-oz box	74	6	0	5 carbohydrate
honey	1 cup	264	1	0	17½ carbohydrate
molasses					
light	1 cup	213	0	0	14 fruit
dark	1 cup	180	0	0	12 fruit

Food	Amount	Carbohydrate (g)	Protein (g)	Fat (g)	Exchanges
sugar					
brown, packed	1 cup	212	0	0	14 carbohydrate
powdered, sifted	1 cup	100	0	0	6½ carbohydrate
powdered, unsifted	1 cup	119	0	0	8 carbohydrate
white	1 cup	199	0	0	13 carbohydrate

NUTS

Food	Amount	Carbohydrate (g)	Protein (g)	Fat (g)	Exchanges
almonds	½ cup	15	14	41	1 carbohydrate, 1 medium-fat meat, 6½ fat
cashews	1 cup	29	17	46	2 carbohydrate, 1 medium-fat meat, 7½ fat
coconut, shredded	1 cup	33	2	24	2 carbohydrate, 5 fat
peanuts	¼ cup	5	7	14	1 medium-fat meat, 2 fat
peanut butter	1 cup	34	76	137	2 carbohydrate, 10 medium-fat meat, 17 fat
pecans	1 cup	13	9	73	1 carbohydrate, 1 medium-fat meat, 13½ fat
sunflower seed kernels	½ cup	14	17	34	1 carbohydrate, 2 medium-fat meat, 5 fat
walnuts	1 cup	16	15	64	1 carbohydrate, 2 medium-fat meat, 10½ fat

MEATS

Food	Amount	Carbohydrate (g)	Protein (g)	Fat (g)	Exchanges
beef, lean, ground, raw	1 lb	0	79	66	11 medium-fat meat, 2 fat
chicken, canned	5½ oz	0	34	18	5 lean meat
salmon, pink, canned	16-oz can	0	93	27	13 lean meat
tuna					
water-packed	6½-oz can	0	53	3	7½ lean meat
oil-packed	6½-oz can	0	45	30	6 medium-fat meat

Here is an example of a recipe that has been converted into exchanges.

TUNA RICE CASSEROLE (8 servings, 1 cup each)

INGREDIENTS	EXCHANGES						
	Starch	Meat	Vegetable	Fruit	Milk	Fat	Free
1 cup wild rice	6						
¼ cup chopped onion							free
½ cup margarine						20	
¼ cup flour	1½						
chicken broth							free
1½ cups evaporated skim milk					3		
2 cans (6½ oz) tuna, water packed		15					
¼ cup diced pimento							free
2 tbsp parsley							free
½ tsp salt							free
½ tsp pepper							free
½ cups almonds, chopped	1	1½				6½	
Total exchanges	8½	16½	0	0	3	26½	
Total exchanges ÷ Total no. of servings	1	2	0	0	trace	3	

One cup of tuna rice casserole is 1 starch, 2 lean meat, and 3 fat.
(Or 1 starch, 2 medium-fat meat, and 2 fat.)

Calculating exchanges is really pretty simple once you know how. Use the form below to calculate exchange values for your own recipes. This kind of information can expand your culinary horizons and help you adhere to your meal plan.

Recipe Name _____

INGREDIENTS	EXCHANGES						
	Starch	Meat	Vegetable	Fruit	Milk	Fat	Free
Total exchanges							
Total exchanges ÷ Total no. of servings							

19

Glossary of Cooking Terms and Techniques

Bonnie Lee Black

Blanch: To dip foods briefly in a large pot of boiling water, then into cold water to stop the cooking process. Blanching is done to heighten color, loosen skins for peeling, or mellow flavors.

Broth (stock): The long-simmered, well-flavored liquid that results when meat, poultry, fish, or vegetables have been cooked with herbs and spices.

Cream: To beat an ingredient or combination of ingredients until the mixture is soft, smooth, and "creamy."

Combine: To mix two or more ingredients together until they do not separate.

Cut in: To mix a solid, cold fat (such as butter or shortening) with dry ingredients (such as a flour mixture) until the combination is in the form of small particles.

Degrease: To remove the fat from the top of a soup, sauce, stew, or stock by any of the following methods: (1) skimming the hot surface with a spoon; (2) allowing the food to chill and removing the resulting solidified fat from the surface; or (3) using a plastic degreaser constructed like a pitcher with a spout that allows the liquid to be poured from the bottom instead of the top (available in hardware stores).

Dice: To cut into small, equal-size cubes, approximately ¼ inch to ½ inch square.

Dredge: To lightly coat food, usually with flour or bread crumbs, before cooking.

Fold: To incorporate one ingredient into another by gently lifting and turning with a rubber spatula.

Fresh (ingredients): For superior flavor and the best results in cooking, always use the freshest possible ingredients. For example, use freshly ground black pepper over tinned, freshly squeezed lemon juice over bottled, and freshly minced parsley over dried.

Julienne: To cut fresh vegetables or other foods into thin strips of uniform length or width.

Knead: To develop gluten from wheat by manipulating dough on a floured surface. It is the gluten that gives dough its cohesiveness.

Mince: To chop into very fine, equal-size pieces, generally no larger than ¹⁄₁₆ inch square.

Nonreactive pan: A cooking pan that will not react with acid (that is, will not cause acidic food to have a metallic taste and be off-color). Stainless steel pans and pans with nonstick coating are nonreactive. Aluminum and iron, on the other hand, react with acid, giving food a metallic taste.

Peel and seed (tomatoes): To peel a tomato easily, core it, drop it into a pan of boiling water, count to 30, remove, and plunge it into a bowl of ice-cold water. To seed, cut the tomato in half crosswise and, holding one half like an inverted cup, gently squeeze out the seeds. They should drop out easily.

Pick over: To examine to ensure that the best are selected and to remove that which is unwanted.

Pipe: To decorate food by forcing a mixture through a pastry bag, usually fitted with a tip especially designed for decorating.

Poach: To cook gently in a simmering liquid.

Proof: To test yeast to ensure it is still active, dissolve the yeast in warm water, mix with a pinch of sugar or flour and allow it to stand in a warm place for 5–10 minutes; if active, the mixture will bubble and foam.

Puree: To finely grind food (by blender, food processor, or food mill) to a thin paste.

Reduce: To concentrate the flavor of a liquid, such as a stock or sauce, by cooking over high heat and allowing it to boil down to a desired concentration.

Roux: A mixture of equal amounts of fat and flour cooked over low heat at least 2 minutes (to eliminate a floury taste). The mixture is used as a base for thickening soups and sauces.

Sauté: To cook food briefly in a shallow pan using a small amount of fat, usually over high heat.

Simmer: To cook liquid over low heat, at just below the boiling point (205°–210°F), so that the surface barely moves.

Stir-fry: To fry quickly over high heat in a lightly oiled pan (or wok) while stirring continuously.

Stock: See *Broth.*

Whisk: A wire utensil used to whip (or whisk) sauces, dressings, toppings, etc. It is used with a swift, circular motion.

Zest: The outermost, colored part of the peel of citrus fruits. This term is also used to mean the removal of that portion of the peel; when zesting, be careful to avoid the white, bitter pith beneath the colored surface.

Chapter 1

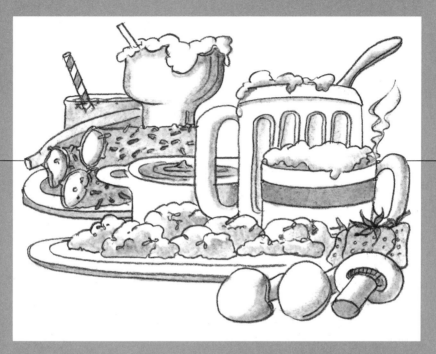

APPETIZERS AND BEVERAGES

*A*ppetizers can not only set the mood for the upcoming meal, they can also tide over hungry stomachs until the main course arrives. This chapter contains a little something for everyone.

If you need to whip up something that is both quick and healthy, try the Creamy Dill Dip. Do you want to wow your dinner guests? Serve them the unusual and tasty Cheese & Chutney Roll, or try a standard favorite such as the Classic Cheese Puffs. And if your party is an informal gathering of friends or family, set out a bowl of the Party Mix—you'll be surprised how quickly it disappears.

The appetizers in this chapter, like all the recipes in this book, are designed to be lower in fat, sodium, sugar, and calories than traditional recipes. Most of the recipes take very little time to prepare and can be made ahead of time for convenience.

The beverage recipes at the end of the chapter are not just delicious but perfect for people in a hurry. The Cantaloupe Cooler and breakfast shakes are great for those mornings when you might be running just a little late, while Chocolate Milk and Hot Chocolate will satisfy kids who need something right away.

Party mix

4 cups mini shredded wheat squares
2 cups puffed wheat cereal
2 cups Cheerios
2 cups thin pretzel sticks
1 cup unsalted, dry-roasted peanuts or mixed nuts
⅓ cup vegetable oil or melted margarine
1 tablespoon Worcestershire sauce
½ teaspoon garlic powder

1. Preheat oven to 250°F.
2. In a large bowl, combine shredded wheat squares, puffed wheat, Cheerios, pretzels, and nuts.
3. In a smaller bowl, whisk together oil (or melted margarine), Worcestershire, and garlic powder. Sprinkle over cereal mixture and toss well to coat lightly.
4. Spread mixture evenly on a large, shallow cake or roasting pan. Bake for 1 hour, stirring every 10–15 minutes, until all ingredients are toasted. (Or MICROWAVE on High, uncovered, in small batches, 3–4 minutes, stirring every 1–2 minutes.)

This snack mix is not only healthy, it also has a satisfying taste and crunch. Try it in place of potato chips and other high-fat snacks. Make it ahead of time and store in an airtight container.

Preparation time: 10 minutes
Baking time: 1 hour

Yield: 30 servings
Serving size: ⅓ cup

Exchanges: ½ starch
      1 fat
Carbohydrate choices: ½

Nutrition per serving:
Calories: 88
Carbohydrate: . . . . .10 g
Protein: . . . . .2 g
Fat: . . . . .4 g

Saturated fat: . . . . .1 g
Cholesterol: . . . . .0 mg
Dietary fiber: . . . . .1 g
Sodium: . . . . .88 mg

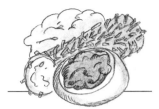

Creamy vegetable dip

This low-fat version of a classic recipe is great with either a vegetable platter or baked chips. Try it with the tortilla crisps from the Hummus and Tortilla Crisps recipe (see p. 45) in the next chapter.

1 cup low-fat cottage cheese
2 tablespoons ketchup
3 tablespoons light sour cream
(or plain nonfat yogurt)
8 drops Tabasco sauce
2 tablespoons chopped green onion or scallion

1. In a food processor or blender, combine the cottage cheese, ketchup, sour cream (or yogurt), and Tabasco sauce. Process until smooth, about 2 minutes.
2. Add the chopped onion and pulse until just blended. Pour mixture into a small bowl, cover, and refrigerate 1–2 hours before serving.

26

Preparation time: 10 minutes
Chilling time: 1–2 hours

Exchanges: 1 lean meat
Carbohydrate choices: 0

Yield: 6–7 servings
Serving size: 3 tablespoons

Nutrition per serving:

With sour cream		***With plain nonfat yogurt***	
Calories:	.50	Calories:	.40
Carbohydrate:	.3 g	Carbohydrate:	.3 g
Protein:	.5 g	Protein:	.6 g
Fat:	.2 g	Fat:	trace
Saturated fat:	.1 g	Saturated fat:	trace
Cholesterol:	.2 mg	Cholesterol:	.2 mg
Dietary fiber:	.0 g	Dietary fiber:	.0 g
Sodium:	.199 mg	Sodium:	.198 mg

Eggplant dip

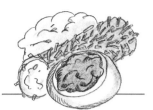

1 medium eggplant
3 medium green onions, finely chopped
1 large tomato, peeled, seeded, and chopped
1 clove garlic, minced
½ stalk celery, finely chopped
¼ cup chopped fresh parsley
1 tablespoon freshly squeezed lemon juice or vinegar
1 tablespoon vegetable oil
½ teaspoon salt (optional)
¼ teaspoon freshly ground black pepper

1. Preheat oven to 400°F.
2. Prick whole eggplant in several places with a fork. Place on a baking sheet and bake until soft, about 30 minutes. (Or MICROWAVE on High, uncovered, for 12 minutes.)
3. When cool enough to handle, cut eggplant in half and scoop flesh into a bowl (or the bowl of a food processor or blender). Discard eggplant skin. Chop eggplant flesh roughly (or pulse briefly). Add remaining ingredients and blend until just combined.
4. Cover and refrigerate for several hours to blend flavors.

A Mediterranean favorite, this low-calorie dip is the perfect appetizer for guests to snack on without filling up before the main course.

27

Preparation time: 45 minutes
Chilling time: 3–4 hours

Exchanges: free
Carbohydrate choices: 0

Yield: 16 servings
Serving size: 2 tablespoons

Nutrition per serving:
Calories: 14
Carbohydrate: . . . . .1 g
Protein: . . . . .trace
Fat: . . . . .1 g

Saturated fat: . . . . .trace
Cholesterol: . . . . .0 mg
Dietary fiber: . . . . .1 g
Sodium: . . . . .70 mg
(omitting salt) . . . . .3 mg

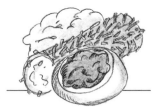

Substitute this dip for plain sour cream on baked potatoes. You'll be surprised at the reaction you'll get from your family.

Creamy dill dip

2 cups low-fat cottage cheese
½ cup low-fat sour cream (or plain nonfat yogurt)
2 tablespoons chopped dill pickle
1 tablespoon chopped fresh dill
**   or 1 teaspoon dried dillweed**
¼ teaspoon freshly ground black pepper

Place all ingredients in a food processor or blender. Process until smooth, about 1 minute.

28

Preparation time: 5 minutes

Yield: 10 servings
Serving size: 3 tablespoons

Exchanges: 1 lean meat
Carbohydrate choices: 0

Nutrition per serving:

With low-fat sour cream		**With plain nonfat yogurt**	
Calories:	.58	Calories:	.43
Carbohydrate:	.2 g	Carbohydrate:	.3 g
Protein:	.6 g	Protein:	.7 g
Fat:	.3 g	Fat:	.trace
Saturated fat:	.2 g	Saturated fat:	.trace
Cholesterol:	.6 mg	Cholesterol:	.2 mg
Dietary fiber:	.trace	Dietary fiber:	.trace
Sodium:	.203 mg	Sodium:	.198 mg

Stuffed mushrooms

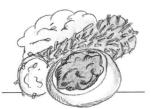

Nonfat cooking spray
12 medium-size white mushrooms
½ cup shredded Gruyère or Swiss cheese (2 ounces)
**¼ cup Seasoned Bread Crumbs (recipe, p. 363) or
commercial bread crumbs**
1 teaspoon water

1. Preheat oven to 400°F. Coat a baking sheet with
cooking spray.
2. Clean mushrooms. Remove the stems and reserve the
caps. Chop the stems (should measure about ⅓ cup).
3. In a medium bowl, cream the cheese with a fork until
soft; blend in bread crumbs, chopped mushroom stems,
and water. Working with your hands, form mixture into
12 balls.
4. Gently press one ball into each of the 12 mushroom
caps. Place on a greased baking sheet and bake 10–15
minutes, or until cheese mixture is hot and bubbling.
(Or MICROWAVE on High, uncovered, 2–3 minutes.)
Serve warm.

*These delicious hors
d'oeurves can be pre-
pared ahead of time for
easier entertaining. Just
cover and refrigerate the
uncooked, stuffed mush-
room caps up to 24
hours before you are
ready to bake them.*

29

Preparation time: 15 minutes
Baking time: 15 minutes

Exchanges: 1 lean meat
Carbohydrate choices: 0

Yield: 6 servings
Serving size: 2 mushrooms

Nutrition per serving:
Calories: 50
Carbohydrate: . . . . .2 g
Protein: . . . . .4 g
Fat: . . . . .3 g

Saturated fat: . . . . .2 g
Cholesterol: . . . . 11 mg
Dietary fiber: . . . .<1 g
Sodium: . . . . .20 mg

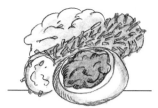

Crabmeat spread

A low-fat version of a traditional crab dip, this recipe is great for both parties and picnics. Serve it with crackers or crisp French bread.

½ cup low-fat cottage cheese (or part-skim ricotta)
1 tablespoon freshly squeezed lemon juice
1 tablespoon dry sherry
1 tablespoon ketchup
1 can (about 6 ounces) crabmeat, drained, picked over
2 tablespoons Cider Vinegar Dressing (recipe, p. 115) or commercial nonfat salad dressing
2 medium green onions, finely chopped
1 teaspoon freshly ground black pepper
1 teaspoon salt (optional)

1. Drain any excess liquid from the cottage (or ricotta) cheese. Place cheese, lemon juice, sherry, and ketchup in a blender or food processor. Process until smooth, about 2 minutes.

2. Add the crabmeat and dressing to the cheese mixture and pulse 3 to 4 times, just until combined. Stir in the onions, black pepper, and salt (optional), to taste. Chill at least 1 hour before serving to allow flavors to blend.

30

Preparation time: 15 minutes
Chilling time: 1 hour

Exchanges: 1 lean meat
Carbohydrate choices: 0

Yield: 5 servings
Serving size: ¼ cup

Nutrition per serving:

With cottage cheese	*With ricotta cheese*
Calories: 62	Calories: 79
Carbohydrate: . . . . .3 g	Carbohydrate: . . . . .3 g
Protein: . . . . .9 g	Protein: . . . . .9 g
Fat: . . . . .1 g	Fat: . . . . .2 g
Saturated fat: . . . . .trace	Saturated fat: . . . . .1 g
Cholesterol: . . . . .27 mg	Cholesterol: . . . . .33 mg
Dietary fiber: . . . .<1 g	Dietary fiber: . . . .<1 g
Sodium: . . . . .684 mg	Sodium: . . . . .630 mg
(omitting salt) . . . . . .258 mg	(omitting salt) . . . . . .204 mg

Salmon cream cheese spread

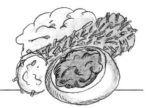

1 can (about 3 ounces) salmon, drained

¼ cup light cream cheese

¼ cup low-fat sour cream (or plain nonfat yogurt)

2 tablespoons chopped green onion or chives

1 tablespoon chopped fresh dill or
  1 teaspoon dried dillweed

1 teaspoon vinegar

¼ teaspoon freshly ground black pepper

½ teaspoon salt (optional)

Blend all of the ingredients together in a small bowl or food processor. Cover and chill until ready to serve.

NOTE: If crackers or bagels are served with this spread, remember to include them in your meal plan.

Cream cheese spreads are excellent for both snacks and smaller meals. Try this spread on cucumber slices or celery stalks as a party snack—or on a bagel for brunch.

31

Preparation time: 10 minutes

Yield: 6 servings
Serving size: 2 tablespoons

Exchanges: 1 lean meat
Carbohydrate choices: 0

Nutrition per serving:

With low-fat sour cream	**With plain nonfat yogurt**
Calories: 62	Calories: 50
Carbohydrate: . . . . .1 g	Carbohydrate: . . . . .1 g
Protein: . . . . .4 g	Protein: . . . . .5 g
Fat: . . . . .5 g	Fat: . . . . .3 g
Saturated fat: . . . . .3 g	Saturated fat: . . . . .2 g
Cholesterol: . . . . .19 mg	Cholesterol: . . . . .16 mg
Dietary fiber: . . . .<1 g	Dietary fiber: . . . .<1 g
Sodium: . . . . .237 mg	Sodium: . . . . .235 mg
(omitting salt) . . . . . . .58 mg	(omitting salt) . . . . . . .56 mg

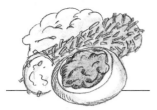

Strawberry-peach cream cheese spread

Be sure to let the cream cheese thaw on the counter for ten minutes, so that it is soft and spreadable when served. Also try this fruit sauce over ice cream or angel food cake for a wonderful dessert.

¼ cup strawberry 100% fruit spread
¼ cup peach 100% fruit spread
1½ teaspoons Amaretto
8 ounces (1 block) fat-free cream cheese

1. Combine strawberry fruit spread, peach fruit spread, and Amaretto in a bowl. Whisk well.
2. Place block of cream cheese on a serving plate. Spoon fruit topping over it. Serve with vanilla wafers.

32

Preparation time: 5 minutes

Yield: 24 servings
Serving size: 2 teaspoons

Exchanges: ½ carbohydrate
Carbohydrate choices: ½

Nutrition per serving:
Calories: 26
Carbohydrate: . . . . .5 g
Protein: . . . . .1 g
Fat: . . . . .0 g

Saturated fat: . . . . .0 g
Cholesterol: . . . . .1 mg
Dietary fiber: . . . . .0 g
Sodium: . . . . .45 mg

Gouda wafers

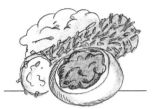

Nonfat cooking spray
½ cup whole wheat flour
¼ cup rice flour
½ teaspoon baking powder
¼ teaspoon salt (optional)
½ cup shredded Gouda cheese
1 tablespoon margarine
2 tablespoons sesame seeds
3–4 tablespoons iced water

These crunchy crackers are not only good snacks on their own, they are a great complement to soups. To give them an extra kick, use celery salt in place of regular salt—the sodium level stays the same, and the taste is fantastic!

1. Preheat oven to 400°F. Coat a baking sheet with cooking spray.
2. In a mixing bowl or food processor, combine the whole wheat and rice flours, baking powder, and salt (optional).
3. With a pastry blender or 2 knives, cut in the cheese and margarine (or pulse in a food processor) until the mixture resembles fine crumbs. Stir in the sesame seeds.
4. Add the water slowly, mixing until a stiff dough forms. Roll dough ⅛-inch thick on a lightly floured surface. Cut into 2-inch squares, place on baking sheet, and bake until golden brown, about 8–10 minutes. Cool on a rack. Store in an airtight container.

33

Preparation time: 20 minutes
Baking time: 10 minutes

Exchanges: ½ starch
Carbohydrate choices: ½

Yield: 36 wafers
Serving size: 3 wafers

Nutrition per serving:
Calories: 58
Carbohydrate: . . . . .5 g
Protein: . . . . .2 g
Fat: . . . . .2 g

Saturated fat: . . . . .1 g
Cholesterol: . . . . .5 mg
Dietary fiber: . . . . .1 g
Sodium: . . . . .108 mg
(omitting salt) . . . . . . .63 mg

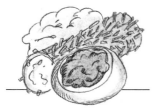

Chutneys come in a variety of flavors these days, and many are available at your local supermarket. Try different chutneys to give this appetizer distinctly different tastes.

Cheese & chutney roll

2 cups shredded Edam cheese
4 teaspoons chutney (or sweet pickle relish)
½ teaspoon curry powder
1 tablespoon skim milk
4 small green onions, finely chopped

Blend all but the green onions together in a bowl or food processor. Form mixture into a log about 1½ inches in diameter, and roll the log in the chopped green onions. Wrap and refrigerate until about 20 minutes before serving.

34

Preparation time: 15 minutes

Yield: 8 servings
Serving size: 2 tablespoons

Exchanges: 1 high-fat meat
Carbohydrate choices: 0

Nutrition per serving:
Calories: 106
Carbohydrate:. . . . . .2 g
Protein: . . . . .8 g
Fat: . . . . .7 g

Saturated fat: . . . . .5 g
Cholesterol: . . . . .25 mg
Dietary fiber: . . . .<1 g
Sodium: . . . . .300 mg

Cheese & chutney boats

VARIATION

Combine all the above ingredients, including the chopped green onions. Cut 2 medium zucchini in half lengthwise and scoop out the seedy pulp. Pack cheese mixture into hollows. Chill and serve sliced.

Preparation time: 20 minutes

Yield: 8 servings
Serving size: 2 tablespoons

Exchanges: 1 high-fat meat
Carbohydrate choices: 0

Nutrition per serving:
Calories: 110
Carbohydrate:. . . . . .2 g
Protein: . . . . .8 g
Fat: . . . . .7 g

Saturated fat: . . . . .5 g
Cholesterol: . . . . .25 mg
Dietary fiber: . . . .<1 g
Sodium: . . . . .302 m

Classic cheese puffs

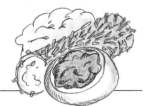

Nonfat cooking spray
1 cup water
¼ cup margarine
½ teaspoon salt (optional)
Pinch white pepper
1 cup all-purpose flour
4 large eggs (or 1 cup liquid egg substitute)
1 cup grated low-fat Swiss cheese
½ teaspoon dry mustard
1 teaspoon Dijon mustard
2 tablespoons light mayonnaise
3 tablespoons grated Parmesan cheese
Pinch paprika

These puffs are a hit at any party. This recipe may look time-consuming, but it's much easier than you might think. Make the puffs (except for the last step) the night before to make the next day's preparation a little easier.

1. Preheat oven to 400°F. Coat 2 baking sheets with cooking spray.
2. In a medium saucepan, combine the water and margarine; add the salt (optional) and pepper and bring to a rapid boil. Lower the heat to medium-low, add the flour all at once, and beat vigorously with a wooden spoon for several minutes, until the mixture forms a ball and no longer sticks to the sides of the pan. Remove the pan from heat and allow to cool about 5 minutes.
3. In the same pan (or in a food processor), add the eggs one at a time (or the egg substitute, ¼ cup at a time), off the heat, beating well after each addition. Beat (or process) the mixture until smooth and glossy, about 2 minutes.
4. Add the Swiss cheese and mustards and mix well. Using two teaspoons, drop the dough in small portions onto the cookie sheets. Bake until puffed and golden, about 20 minutes.
5. Just before serving, brush tops with mayonnaise and sprinkle with Parmesan. Return to oven and bake for 5 more minutes. Serve immediately.

35

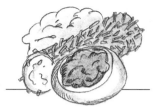

Preparation time: 10 minutes
Cooking time: 55 minutes

Yield: 36 puffs
Serving size: 3 puffs

Nutrition per serving:
With eggs
Calories: 151
Carbohydrate: . . . . .8 g
Protein: . . . . .6 g
Fat: . . . . .10 g
Saturated fat: . . . . .4 g
Cholesterol: . . . . .102 mg
Dietary fiber: . . . . .0 g
Sodium: . . . . .212 mg
(omitting salt) . . . . . .123 mg

Exchanges: ½ starch
1 medium-fat meat
1 fat
Carbohydrate choices: 1

With egg substitute
Calories: 131
Carbohydrate: . . . . .8 g
Protein: . . . . .6 g
Fat: . . . . .8 g
Saturated fat: . . . . .3 g
Cholesterol: . . . . .11 mg
Dietary fiber: . . . . .0 g
Sodium: . . . . .216 mg
(omitting salt) . . . . . .127 mg

Spicy cheese log

The Tabasco sauce and chili powder are what give this cheese log its uniquely spicy taste. If you like foods extra-hot and do not have to watch your sodium intake, feel free to add more Tabasco sauce than listed here— Tabasco and other hot sauces contain no calories but can be somewhat high in sodium.

1 cup shredded Edam cheese
½ cup low-fat cottage cheese, drained and mashed
¼ cup shredded low-fat Cheddar cheese
¼ cup grated Parmesan cheese
⅓ cup plus 1 tablespoon minced fresh parsley
¼ teaspoon garlic powder
¼ teaspoon paprika
⅛ teaspoon chili powder (or to taste)
3–4 drops Tabasco sauce (or to taste)

1. In a mixing bowl or food processor, combine the cheeses, 1 tablespoon of the parsley, and all of the remaining ingredients. Blend until smooth.
2. Form mixture into a log about 1½ inches in diameter, and roll the log in the remaining ⅓ cup parsley. Wrap and refrigerate for several hours. Allow to warm to room temperature before serving.

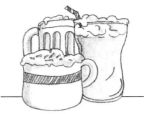

Preparation time: 15 minutes
Chilling time: 3–4 hours

Yield: 8 servings
Serving size: 2 tablespoons

Exchanges: 1 medium-fat meat
Carbohydrate choices: 0

Nutrition per serving:
Calories: 86
Carbohydrate: . . . . .1 g
Protein: . . . . .8 g
Fat: . . . . .5 g

Saturated fat: . . . . .3 g
Cholesterol: . . . . .18 mg
Dietary fiber: . . . . .0 g
Sodium: . . . . .263 mg

Chocolate milk

1 tablespoon Chocolate Sauce (recipe, p. 330)
1 cup skim milk

Stir the Chocolate Sauce into a glass of cold milk and enjoy.

Kids of all ages will love this cool and simple pick-me-up.

Preparation time: 1 minute

Yield: 1 serving
Serving size: 1 cup

Exchanges: 1 low-fat milk
Carbohydrate choices: 1

Nutrition per serving:
Calories: 91
Carbohydrate: . . . . .12 g
Protein: . . . . .9 g
Fat: . . . . .1 g

Saturated fat: . . . . .trace
Cholesterol: . . . . .trace
Dietary fiber: . . . .<1 g
Sodium: . . . . .126 mg

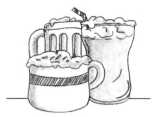

Breakfast shake

Skipping breakfast is never a good idea, but sometimes you can find yourself rushed in the morning. If you don't have the time to sit down to a full meal, this quick and nutritious shake can be a helpful substitute.

1 cup skim milk
¼ cup instant skim milk powder
1 medium banana
1 teaspoon vanilla extract
Artificial sweetener to taste

Combine all of the ingredients in a blender and blend at highest speed until thick and frothy. For an even thicker and frothier drink, add a few ice cubes to the blender.

38

Preparation time: 2 minutes

Yield: 1 serving
Serving size: 1½ cups

Nutrition per serving:
Calories: 258
Carbohydrate: . . . . .41 g
Protein: . . . . .21 g
Fat: . . . . .1 g

Exchanges: 1 fruit
          2 low-fat milk
Carbohydrate choices: 3

Saturated fat: . . . . .trace
Cholesterol: . . . . .10 mg
Dietary fiber: . . . . .1 g
Sodium: . . . . .288 mg

Chocolate shake

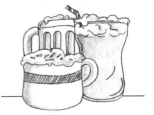

VARIATION

Add 1 tablespoon Chocolate Sauce (recipe, p. 330) to the above ingredients and proceed as above.

Preparation time: 2 minutes

Yield: 1 serving
Serving size: 1½ cups

Exchanges: 1 fruit
        2 low-fat milk
Carbohydrate choices: 3

Nutrition per serving:
Calories: 263
Carbohydrate: . . . . .42 g
Protein: . . . . .21 g
Fat: . . . . .1 g

Saturated fat: . . . . .1 g
Cholesterol: . . . . .10 mg
Dietary fiber: . . . . .2 g
Sodium: . . . . .288 mg

39

Strawberry shake

VARIATION

Add ½ cup fresh or frozen unsweetened strawberries to the basic recipe and proceed as above.

Preparation time: 2 minutes

Yield: 1 serving
Serving size: 1½ cups

Exchanges: 1½ fruit
        2 low-fat milk
Carbohydrate choices: 3

Nutrition per serving:
Calories: 281
Carbohydrate: . . . . .46 g
Protein: . . . . .22 g
Fat: . . . . .1 g

Saturated fat: . . . . .trace
Cholesterol: . . . . .10 mg
Dietary fiber: . . . . .3 g
Sodium: . . . . .289 mg

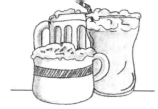

Hot chocolate

What can be more comforting on a cold day than a mug of hot chocolate?

1 tablespoon Chocolate Sauce (recipe, p. 330)
1 cup skim milk
Ground cinnamon (optional)

Heat the milk in a saucepan or in a microwave. Stir in the Chocolate Sauce and sprinkle with cinnamon.

Preparation time: 2 minutes
Yield: 1 serving
Serving size: 1 cup

Exchanges: 1 low-fat milk
Carbohydrate choices: 1

Nutrition per serving:
Calories: 91
Carbohydrate: . . . . .12 g
Protein: . . . . .9 g
Fat: . . . . .1 g

Saturated fat: . . . . .trace
Cholesterol: . . . . .trace
Dietary fiber: . . . .<1 g
Sodium: . . . . .126 mg

40

Instant Swiss mocha mix

With this homemade mix prepared ahead of time, it will take only seconds to make a great hot drink.

½ cup instant skim milk powder
2 tablespoons cocoa
1 tablespoon instant coffee

Blend all of the ingredients well. Keep in a tightly covered jar and shake well before using.

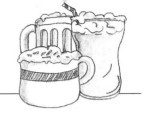

Preparation time: 2 minutes	Exchanges: ¼ low-fat milk
	Carbohydrate choices: 0
Yield: ½ cup mix	
Serving size: 2 tablespoons	

Nutrition per serving:

Calories:	27	Saturated fat:	..........0 g
Carbohydrate:	..........4 g	Cholesterol:	..........trace
Protein:	.............3 g	Dietary fiber:	..........0 g
Fat:	..................0 g	Sodium:	...........40 mg

Swiss mocha drink

2 tablespoons Instant Swiss Mocha Mix (recipe above)
1 cup boiling water
Artificial sweetener to taste

Place the mix in a coffee mug, add boiling water, and stir to dissolve. Sweeten to taste.

This is not only a great breakfast drink but a wonderful after-dinner drink for guests. Serve it with a pinch of cinnamon or a few drops of peppermint extract to enhance the flavor.

Preparation time: 4 minutes	Exchanges: ¼ low-fat milk
	Carbohydrate choices: 0
Yield: 1 serving	
Serving size: 1 cup	

Nutrition per serving:

Calories:	27	Saturated fat:	..........0 g
Carbohydrate:	..........4 g	Cholesterol:	..........trace
Protein:	.............3 g	Dietary fiber:	..........0 g
Fat:	..................0 g	Sodium:	...........40 mg

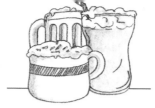

If you have to eat and run, this delicious cooler can tide you over until you are able to have a healthy midmorning snack.

Cantaloupe cooler

1 cup cubed cantaloupe
½ cup nonfat, no-sugar-added vanilla yogurt
¼ teaspoon lemon juice
1 packet NutraSweet
Dash cinnamon

Combine all the ingredients in a blender and blend until smooth.

42

Preparation time: 5 minutes

Yield: 1 serving
Serving size: 1½ cups

Nutrition per serving:
Calories: 108
Carbohydrate: . . . . .20 g
Protein: . . . . .6 g
Fat: . . . .<1 g

Exchanges: 1 fruit
       ½ low-fat milk
Carbohydrate choices: 1½

Saturated fat: . . . . .0 g
Cholesterol: . . . . .2 mg
Dietary fiber: . . . . .2 g
Sodium: . . . . .128 mg

Chapter 2

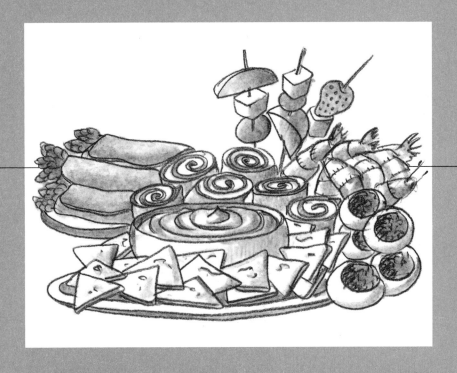

SNACKS AND MUNCHIES

*W*hether you're trying to keep your blood glucose levels under control, stave off between-meal hunger, or just satisfy a craving, snacking can be a good solution. And if the snacks you eat are as well balanced, nutritious, and tasty as the ones here, you will want to work snacks into your daily meal plan on a regular basis.

If it's a crunchy treat you're looking for, try the Parmesan Munch Mix. It's a lot more satisfying and a lot less fattening than potato chips. Got a craving for buffalo wings but worried about the cholesterol? Our Buffalo Chicken Bites will have you licking your fingers in no time. There is something here for everyone, and something to keep everyone both healthy and happy.

Hummus dip with tortilla crisps

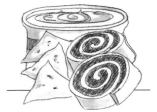

1 can (19 ounces) chickpeas (garbanzo beans),
   drained
1–2 cloves garlic, minced
½ cup nonfat plain yogurt
3 tablespoons lemon juice
½ teaspoon salt
½ teaspoon ground cumin
Dash hot pepper sauce
Pinch freshly ground pepper
4 eight-inch flour tortillas

The tortilla crisps in this recipe can be made ahead of time and used with many of the dips shown in Chapter 1. Or you can just snack on them alone.

1. In a food processor or blender, puree chickpeas with garlic until coarsely chopped. Add yogurt, lemon juice, and seasonings. Blend to smooth paste.
2. Remove mixture to a bowl, cover, and refrigerate for at least 2 hours to allow flavors to develop.
3. Cut each tortilla into 12 equal triangles. Place a single layer of tortilla wedges on a baking pan. Bake at 300°F for 15–20 minutes, or until the wedges are crisp and golden. Allow the crisps to cool; store in a tightly closed container.

45

Preparation time: 10 minutes
Baking time: 15–20 minutes
Chilling time: 2 hours

Yield: 2⅓ cups hummus and
   48 crisps

Serving size: ⅓ cup hummus
   with 6 crisps

Exchanges: 1 starch
Carbohydrate choices: 1

Nutrition per serving:
Calories: 95
Carbohydrate: . . . . .16 g
Protein: . . . . .5 g
Fat: . . . . .1 g
Saturated fat: . . . . .trace
Cholesterol: . . . . .0 mg
Dietary fiber: . . . . .3 g
Sodium: . . . . .178 mg

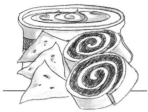

Pinto bean pinwheels

These bite-size Mexican treats will have everyone asking for more. Make sure to gently slice each tortilla, or you'll end up with more refried beans on the kitchen counter than in your pinwheels.

1 can (16 ounces) fat-free refried pinto beans
4 teaspoons taco seasoning mix
4 eight-inch flour tortillas
1 cup finely shredded mild Cheddar cheese
4 green onions
Salsa
Fat-free sour cream

1. Preheat oven to 350°F. Place refried beans and taco seasoning in bowl and stir until combined. Spread flour tortillas to the edges with bean mixture. Sprinkle evenly with cheese. Lay one green onion in the center of each tortilla. Roll up the tortillas jelly-roll style. Trim the rounded edges of each roll so the edges are straight.
2. Slice each roll into 6 slices using a sawing motion. Place pinwheels in a single layer in a 9" × 13" pan. Bake uncovered for 8–10 minutes, or until cheese is melted. Remove from oven and allow to cool slightly. Serve warm with salsa and fat-free sour cream, if desired.

46

Preparation time: 10 minutes
Baking time: 10 minutes

Yield: 24 pinwheels
Serving size: 2 pinwheels

Exchanges: 1 starch
    ½ fat
Carbohydrate choices: 1

Nutrition per serving:
Calories: 101
Carbohydrate: . . . . .14 g
Protein: . . . . .5 g
Fat: . . . . .2 g

Saturated fat: . . . .<1 g
Cholesterol: . . . . .10 mg
Dietary fiber: . . . . .1 g
Sodium: . . . . .330 mg

Hot and spicy mixed nuts

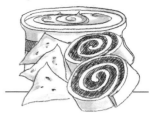

½ **cup whole almonds**
½ **cup pecan halves**
½ **cup walnut halves**
1 teaspoon canola oil
½ **teaspoon cumin**
½ **teaspoon curry powder**
⅛ **teaspoon cayenne pepper**
Dash white pepper

1. Preheat oven to 350°F. Toss the nuts with the oil in a large bowl. In a small bowl, combine the spices and mix well. Add spices to the nuts, stirring until nuts are covered evenly.
2. Spread the nuts on a baking sheet in a single layer. Bake the nuts for 10–12 minutes. Remove from oven and cool before serving.

At first glance this recipe might seem a little high in fat, but notice how low it is in saturated fat. Nuts are a valuable source of vitamins like folic acid, niacin, and vitamins E and B_6. They also contain omega-3 fatty acids, which play an important role in preventing heart disease and improving overall cholesterol.

47

Preparation time: 5 minutes
Baking time: 10–12 minutes

Exchanges: 2 fat
Carbohydrate choices: 0

Yield: 1½ cups
Serving size: ¼ cup

Nutrition per serving:
Calories: 96
Carbohydrate: . . . . .3 g
Protein: . . . . .2 g
Fat: . . . . .9 g

Saturated fat: . . . .<1 g
Cholesterol: . . . . .0 mg
Dietary fiber: . . . . .1 g
Sodium: . . . . .1 mg

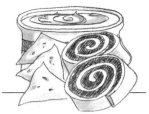

This healthy, protein-rich snack will be everybody's favorite on game day.

Buffalo chicken bites

Nonfat cooking spray
**1 pound cooked chicken breasts,
  cut into bite-size chunks**
½ cup hot (or Tabasco) sauce
3 tablespoons melted, reduced-calorie margarine
2 teaspoons dried parsley
¼ teaspoon garlic powder
Celery sticks
Fat-free ranch or blue cheese salad dressing

1. Preheat oven to 350°F. Coat a baking dish with cooking spray, and place chicken bites in baking dish. In a separate bowl, combine the hot sauce, margarine, parsley, and garlic powder. Pour evenly over chicken. (You can refrigerate the combined chicken and sauce until you are ready to heat and serve.)
2. Bake chicken for 20 minutes. Put a toothpick in each piece of chicken and place on a serving tray. Serve with celery sticks and salad dressing.

Preparation time: 5 minutes
Baking time: 20 minutes

Yield: 42 pieces
Serving size: 7 pieces

Exchanges: 3 lean meat
Carbohydrate choices: 0

Nutrition per serving:
Calories: 154
Carbohydrate: . . . . .1 g
Protein: . . . . .24 g
Fat: . . . . .6 g
Saturated fat: . . . . .1 g
Cholesterol: . . . . .48 mg
Dietary fiber: . . . .<1 g
Sodium: . . . . .209 mg

Rich broccoli and cheese dip

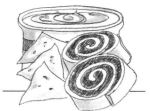

1 can (10¾ ounces) reduced-fat cream of
mushroom soup

8 ounces fat-free processed cheese loaf
(such as Velveeta), cut in cubes

1 can (14½ ounces) tomatoes with green chilies

1 teaspoon garlic powder

⅛ teaspoon black pepper

1 can (4 ounces) sliced mushrooms, drained

2 packages (10 ounces each) frozen chopped broccoli,
thawed and drained

1. In a large saucepan, combine soup, cheese, tomatoes
with green chilies, garlic powder, and black pepper.
Warm over medium heat, stirring frequently, until cheese
is melted and mixture is bubbly.

2. Mix in mushrooms and broccoli and continue to heat
for an additional 10 minutes or until mixture is bubbly
again. Serve with bagel crisps or low-fat snack crackers.

*This dip counts as a
free choice in your meal
planning, but be sure
to count the bagel crisps
or snack crackers you
use for dipping. To keep
calories low, use celery
or carrot sticks instead
of crackers.*

49

Preparation time: 5 minutes
Cooking time: 15 minutes

Exchanges: free
Carbohydrate choices: 0

Yield: 8 cups
Serving size: ¼ cup

Nutrition per serving:
Calories: 21
Carbohydrate: . . . . .2 g
Protein: . . . . .2 g
Fat: . . . .<1 g

Saturated fat: . . . .<1 g
Cholesterol: . . . . .1 mg
Dietary fiber: . . . . .1 g
Sodium: . . . . .221 mg

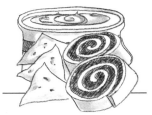

Try these pretzels with a small bowl of warm pizza sauce for dipping— it's delicious!

Cheesy soft pretzel twists

50

Nonfat cooking spray
1 cup (4 ounces) reduced-fat finely shredded Cheddar cheese
⅛ teaspoon garlic powder
½ teaspoon oregano
1 package (16 ounces) dry, yeast, hot roll mix plus ingredients to prepare
All-purpose flour (to prevent sticking)
1 tablespoon water
¼ teaspoon salt
2 teaspoons poppy seeds

1. Preheat oven to 375°F. Coat two baking sheets with cooking spray and set aside. In a small bowl, mix together cheese, garlic powder, and oregano; set aside.
2. Prepare hot roll mix dough according to package directions (the dough does not need to rise). On a clean, floured surface, using clean, floured hands, divide the dough into four equal portions (a sharp knife or pizza cutter works well to cut dough). Shape each portion into a ball. Take one dough ball at a time and divide it into four equal pieces (for a total of 16 pieces).
3. Roll each piece into an 8-inch rope. On a floured surface, pat each rope out until it is 1½ inches wide. Sprinkle each lightly with cheese mixture. Fold each rope over lengthwise and pat to seal. (You now have sixteen 8-inch dough ropes stuffed with cheese.) Place dough ropes on baking sheets and twist into pretzel shape.

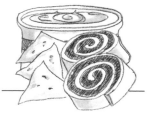

4. In a small bowl, whisk together egg white and water until frothy. Brush pretzels well with egg white mixture (this helps the pretzels brown during baking), sprinkle with salt and poppy seeds.

5. Bake for 14–16 minutes, or until golden brown (watch closely during last few minutes of baking). Transfer to a cooling rack. Store leftovers in an airtight container or zip-top bag in the refrigerator. Warm slightly before eating.

Preparation time: 45 minutes
Baking time: 14–16 minutes
             per pan

Yield: 16 pretzels
Serving size: 1 pretzel

Exchanges: 1½ starch
      ½ fat
Carbohydrate choices: 1½

Nutrition per serving:
Calories: 139
Carbohydrate: . . . . .22 g
Protein: . . . . .6 g
Fat: . . . . .3 g
Saturated fat: . . . . .1 g
Cholesterol: . . . . .4 mg
Dietary fiber: . . . .<1 g
Sodium: . . . . .297 mg

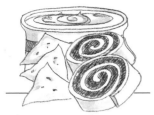

52

This mix can be prepared ahead of time and kept for last-minute snacking in front of the television.

Parmesan munch mix

1 bag (about 12 cups) popped low-fat butter-flavored microwave popcorn

3 cups rice square cereal (such as Rice Chex)

3 cups wheat square cereal (such as Wheat Chex)

1 bag (5½ ounces) or 3 cups Goldfish pretzel snack crackers (or substitute pretzel sticks)

3 cups reduced-fat baked cheese snack crackers (such as reduced-fat Cheez-Its)

1 stick reduced-calorie margarine, melted

½ teaspoon garlic powder

½ teaspoon seasoned salt

½ teaspoon onion salt

½ cup grated Parmesan cheese

1. Preheat oven to 300°F. In a large bowl, combine popcorn, rice square cereal, wheat square cereal, pretzels, and cheese crackers. In a small bowl, whisk together melted margarine, garlic powder, seasoned salt, and onion salt. Pour one-third of margarine mixture over cereal mixture and toss to coat. Repeat twice. Sprinkle with half the Parmesan cheese and toss to coat. Repeat.

2. Pour cereal into two 9" × 13" pans and bake for 30 minutes, stirring every 10 minutes. Cool to room temperature. Store in airtight container.

Preparation time: 15 minutes
Baking time: 30 minutes

Yield: 18 cups
Serving size: 1 cup

Exchanges: 1½ starch
1 fat
Carbohydrate choices: 1½

Nutrition per serving:
Calories: 162
Carbohydrate: . . . . .23 g
Protein: . . . . .4 g
Fat: . . . . .6 g

Saturated fat: . . . . .1 g
Cholesterol: . . . . .2 mg
Dietary fiber: . . . . .1 g
Sodium: . . . . .391 mg

Zesty munch mix

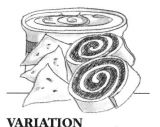

VARIATION

Nonfat cooking spray

4 cups pretzel sticks

3 cups oyster crackers

3 cups reduced-fat baked cheese snack crackers
(such as reduced-fat Cheez-Its)

5 cups wheat square cereal (such as Wheat Chex)

2 cups oat circle cereal (such as Cheerios)

¾ cup walnut pieces

2 envelopes (0.5 ounce each) butter-flavored mix
(such as Butter Buds)

¼ cup warm water

¼ cup Worcestershire sauce

2 tablespoons corn oil

½ teaspoon each onion powder, garlic powder,
curry powder, and seasoned salt

⅛ teaspoon cayenne pepper

53

1. Preheat oven to 300°F. Coat a large roasting pan or two
9" × 13" pans with cooking spray. Place pretzels, oyster
crackers, cheese crackers, wheat square cereal, oat circle
cereal, and walnut pieces in the pan(s). Set aside.
2. Place the remaining ingredients in a bowl and whisk
together. Pour over pretzel mixture and toss well to coat.
Bake for 40 minutes, stirring gently every 10–15 minutes.
Watch closely for the last 5–10 minutes to prevent burn-
ing. Pour out of the pans onto foil to cool.

Preparation time: 10 minutes
Baking time: 40 minutes

Yield: 17¾ cups
Serving size: 1 cup

Exchanges: 2 starch
      1 fat
Carbohydrate choices: 2

Nutrition per serving:
Calories: 215
Carbohydrate: . . . . .33 g
Protein: . . . . .5 g
Fat: . . . . .7 g

Saturated fat: . . . . .1 g
Cholesterol: . . . . .0 mg
Dietary fiber: . . . . .2 g
Sodium: . . . . .545 mg

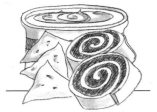

Here's a variation on the traditional shrimp cocktail that is great for parties. To save time, use precooked, frozen shrimp and let them thaw before beginning the recipe.

54

Chilled marinated shrimp

2 tablespoons corn or canola oil

2 tablespoons olive oil

2 tablespoons mild cayenne pepper (not Tabasco) sauce

1 clove garlic, minced

¼ teaspoon Old Bay seasoning

½ teaspoon dried basil

¼ teaspoon crushed, dried oregano

½ teaspoon dried parsley

½ teaspoon dried thyme

1 pound peeled and deveined cooked shrimp

Combine all ingredients except the shrimp in a small bowl and whisk together. Place shrimp in a zip-top bag, add marinade, and gently shake bag several times to coat shrimp. Refrigerate at least 8 hours to allow the flavors to blend; gently shake bag twice during marinating to recoat shrimp. Drain off excess marinade before serving.

Preparation time: 10 minutes
Chilling time: 8 hours

Yield: approximately 40 shrimp
Serving size: approximately
         10 shrimp

Nutrition per serving:
Calories: 157
Carbohydrate: . . . .<1 g
Protein: . . . . .23 g
Fat: . . . . .7 g

Exchanges: 3 very lean meat
         1 fat
Carbohydrate choices: 0

Saturated fat: . . . . .1 g
Cholesterol: . . . . .224 mg
Dietary fiber: . . . .<1 g
Sodium: . . . . .969 mg

Sun-dried tomato hummus wraps

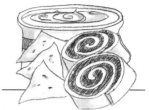

1 ounce (about ⅓ cup) sun-dried tomatoes
(about ¾ cup rehydrated)
1 can (19 ounces) garbanzo beans, rinsed and drained
2 tablespoons tahini (sesame seed paste)
¼ cup fresh lemon juice
3–4 tablespoons water
1 teaspoon salt
⅛ teaspoon cayenne pepper
½ teaspoon ground cumin
½ teaspoon chopped garlic
6 pieces (7½ inches each) wheat flatbread
12 ounces thinly sliced, smoked turkey breast
18 asparagus spears, trimmed and lightly steamed

This is one snack that can stand in for a meal. The garbanzo beans pack lots of protein and fiber into these small wraps.

1. Rehydrate tomatoes by placing them in a bowl, pouring boiling water over them to cover, and letting stand for 20 minutes.
2. Place tomatoes, beans, tahini, lemon juice, 3 tablespoons water, salt, cayenne pepper, cumin, and garlic in food processor or blender and process until smooth. Thin with an additional tablespoon of water, if necessary. Chill at least 2 hours to allow flavors to blend.
3. Warm flatbread according to package direction. Spread each piece of flatbread with ⅓ cup hummus and top with 2 ounces of turkey. Place 3 asparagus spears in the center of each, then wrap the bread around the asparagus. Serve on plate seam-side down.

Preparation time: 30 minutes
Chilling time: 2 hours

Yield: 6 wraps
Serving size: 1 wrap

Exchanges: 4½ carbohydrate
2 lean meat
2 fat
Carbohydrate choices: 4½

Nutrition per serving:
Calories: 536
Carbohydrate: . . . . .66 g
Protein: . . . . .28 g
Fat: . . . . .18 g

Saturated fat: . . . . .4 g
Cholesterol: . . . . .26 mg
Dietary fiber: . . . . .10 g
Sodium: . . . . .1,517 mg

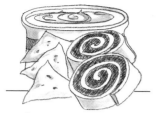

Ham and cheese roll-ups

Make sure you use soft, fresh bread in this twist on the classic ham-and-cheese. Otherwise, your sandwich will crumble into pieces when you try to roll it up.

1 slice fresh, soft whole wheat bread (trim hard crust if desired)
Mustard
1 slice (1 ounce) low-fat ham
1 slice (1 ounce) fat-free American cheese

Flatten bread with a rolling pin. Spread one side of bread lightly with mustard. Lay a slice of ham, then cheese on bread. Roll up jelly-roll style and eat.

Preparation time: 1 minute

Yield: 1 roll-up
Serving size: 1 roll-up

Nutrition per serving:
Calories: 126
Carbohydrate: . . . . .15 g
Protein: . . . . .12 g
Fat: . . . . .2 g

Exchanges: 1 starch
1½ very lean meat
Carbohydrate choices: 1

Saturated fat: . . . .<1 g
Cholesterol: . . . . .20 mg
Dietary fiber: . . . . .2 g
Sodium: . . . . .670 mg

Party pizza bites

Nonfat cooking spray
1 pound ground round
1 cup pizza sauce
1 can (12 ounces) plus 1 can (4.5 ounces) refrigerated
  biscuits (15 biscuits total)
4 ounces finely shredded light mozzarella cheese
¼ cup finely diced green pepper
¼ cup finely diced red pepper

1. Preheat oven to 375°F. Coat muffin tins with cooking spray and set aside. (Do not use paper or foil liners.)
2. Brown and drain ground round. Stir in pizza sauce. Set aside.
3. Place one biscuit in each of the 15 cups in the tins. Press the dough against the bottom and up the sides of each cup to form a dough cup. Fill the dough cups with meat sauce. Sprinkle with cheese, top with diced green and red peppers.
4. Bake for 20–25 minutes, or until biscuit edges are golden and cheese is melted. Using a spoon, loosen edges and remove from muffin tins promptly.

Who says these are just for parties? Kids and adults alike will love to snack on these mini pizza pockets.

Preparation time: 20 minutes
Baking time: 20–25 minutes

Yield: 15 pizza bites
Serving size: 1 pizza bite

Exchanges: 1 starch
　　　　　1 medium-fat meat
Carbohydrate choices: 1

Nutrition per serving:

Calories: 138	Saturated fat: . . . . .2 g
Carbohydrate: . . . . .12 g	Cholesterol: . . . . .19 mg
Protein: . . . . .9 g	Dietary fiber: . . . . .1 g
Fat: . . . . .6 g	Sodium: . . . . .258 mg

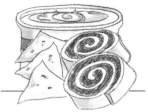

Pear and peanut butter breakfast stacks

Yet another breakfast-on-the-run, try this with the Cantaloupe Cooler (p. 42) for a complete and nutritious morning meal.

4 low-fat graham cracker squares
2 tablespoons reduced-fat peanut butter
½ fresh pear, seeded and thinly sliced
Cinnamon

Spread each graham cracker square with ½ tablespoon of peanut butter. Top two of the graham cracker squares with pear slices. Sprinkle lightly with cinnamon. Place the remaining graham cracker squares, peanut-butter-side down, on the pear slices. Serve.

58

Preparation time: 5 minutes

Yield: 1 serving
Serving: 1 serving

Nutrition per serving:
Calories: 296
Carbohydrate: . . . . .41 g
Protein: . . . . .9 g
Fat: . . . . .12 g

Exchanges: 2½ carbohydrates
1 high-fat meat
1 fat
Carbohydrate choices: 2½

Saturated fat: . . . . .2 g
Cholesterol: . . . . .0 mg
Dietary fiber: . . . . .5 g
Sodium: . . . . .275 mg

Turkey cheese-stuffed tomatoes

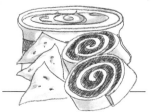

2 cups cherry tomatoes, washed and cut in half

6 ounces smoked or seasoned cooked turkey breast, minced

½ cup light vegetable flavored cream cheese

¼ cup Feta or blue cheese, crumbled

4 tablespoons chopped green onion

3 tablespoons chopped fresh basil

¼ teaspoon ground black pepper

⅛ teaspoon salt

Minced fresh basil, if desired

Scoop out pulp and seeds from tomato halves, drain upside down on paper towels. Combine turkey, cream cheese, Feta or blue cheese, green onion, basil, pepper, and salt in small bowl. Fill inside of tomatoes with turkey mixture. Garnish with minced basil, if desired.

These tasty tomato wedges make a great snack or an imaginative substitute for a dinner salad. A fat-free Italian dressing can add extra flavor to these tomatoes without adding extra calories.

59

Preparation time: 15 minutes

Yield: 9 servings
Serving size: 4 tomato halves

Exchanges: 1 vegetable
1 lean meat
Carbohydrate choices: 0

Nutrition per serving:
Calories: 85
Carbohydrate: . . . . .4 g
Protein: . . . . .7 g
Fat: . . . . .4 g

Saturated fat: . . . . .3 g
Cholesterol: . . . . .20 mg
Dietary fiber: . . . . .1 g
Sodium: . . . . .330 mg

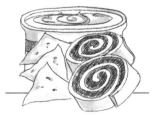

Curried honey vegetable dip

Honey and yogurt, a classic Mediterranean combination, give this dip a sweet and hearty taste.

½ cup light sour cream
¼ cup light mayonnaise
¼ cup nonfat plain yogurt
1 tablespoon honey
1 teaspoon curry powder
1 teaspoon grated orange peel
2 tablespoons finely chopped green onion
⅛ teaspoon salt
Assorted raw vegetables, cut into bite-sizes pieces

Combine all ingredients in a small bowl (except vegetables). Refrigerate 2–3 hours to blend flavors. Serve with raw vegetables.

60

Preparation time: 5 minutes
Chilling time: 2–3 hours

Exchanges: 1 fat
Carbohydrate choices: 0

Yield: 8 servings
Serving size: 2 tablespoons

Nutrition per serving:
Calories: 85
Carbohydrate: . . . . .5 g
Protein: . . . . .1 g
Fat: . . . . 6 g

Saturated fat: . . . . .2 g
Cholesterol: . . . . .5 mg
Dietary fiber: . . . . .0 g
Sodium: . . . . .160 mg

Tomato basil crostini

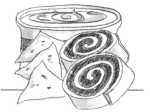

1 cup diced plum tomato
2 tablespoons finely chopped onion
1 clove garlic, finely minced
2 tablespoons finely shredded fresh basil
2 tablespoons shredded Parmesan cheese
1 tablespoon olive oil
⅛ teaspoon salt
⅛ teaspoon ground black pepper
12 slices (½-inch each) French baguette bread
Olive oil-flavored cooking spray

Crostini, an Italian favorite, make great appetizers. Experiment with different vegetables in the tomato topping for a wide variety of flavors.

Combine tomato, onion, garlic, basil, Parmesan cheese, olive oil, salt, and pepper in a small bowl; set aside. Place bread slices on a baking sheet in a single layer. Spray tops of bread slices lightly with cooking spray; broil approximately 30 seconds to 1 minute, or until bread starts to turn golden brown. Remove bread from oven and top each slice with about two teaspoons tomato mixture. Serve immediately.

61

Preparation time: 10 minutes
Cooking time: 1 minute

Exchanges: ½ starch
Carbohydrate choices: ½

Yield: 6 servings
Serving size: 2 slices

Nutrition per serving:
Calories: 65
Carbohydrate: . . . . .7 g
Protein: . . . . .2 g
Fat: . . . . .3 g

Saturated fat: . . . . .1 g
Cholesterol: . . . . <5 mg
Dietary fiber: . . . . .1 g
Sodium: . . . . .135 mg

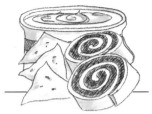

Shrimp lover's spread

This low-fat version of shrimp salad works great on crackers—or spread it on a pita for a nutritious lunch.

8 ounces light cream cheese
½ cup light mayonnaise
2 tablespoons chili sauce or seafood cocktail sauce
1 tablespoon lemon juice
2 tablespoons minced onion
⅛ teaspoon white pepper
½ pound chopped cooked shrimp
Crackers or sliced French bread

Combine cream cheese, mayonnaise, chili sauce, lemon juice, onion, and pepper in a small bowl; mix until well blended. Fold in shrimp. Refrigerate at least 3 hours. Serve with crackers or bread slices.

62

Preparation time: 10 minutes
Chilling time: 3 hours

Yield: 18 servings
Serving size: 2 tablespoons

Nutrition per serving:
Calories: 65
Carbohydrate: . . . . .2 g
Protein: . . . . .4 g
Fat: . . . . .4 g

Exchanges: ½ very lean meat
1 fat
Carbohydrate choices: 0

Saturated fat: . . . . .2 g
Cholesterol: . . . . .30 mg
Dietary fiber: . . . . .0 g
Sodium: . . . . .160 mg

Turkey vegetable spring rolls

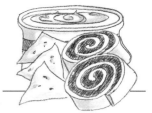

4 ounces seasoned or smoked cooked turkey breast, minced
½ cup shredded carrots
4 tablespoons chopped green onion
2 tablespoons minced fresh cilantro
1 tablespoon minced fresh mint
¼ cup chopped salted peanuts
8 rice paper spring roll wrappers
Sweet and sour sauce for dipping (optional)

Combine turkey, carrots, green onion, cilantro, mint, and peanuts in a small bowl. Lay rice paper wrappers on a flat surface. Place ⅛ of the turkey mixture in center of each rice paper. Fold rice paper over filling to make a triangle; then fold in left and right corners of triangle over filling. Roll up tightly, seal with water on the tip and place seam side down on a plate. Repeat procedure with each rice paper wrapper. Serve with dipping sauce, if desired.

Most rice paper wrappers come dried and brittle. Keep a shallow pan of cold water at hand and soak each wrapper for 15–30 seconds immediately before use. The wrapper should be pliable but not so limp that it will tear.

63

Preparation time: 15 minutes
Yield: 8 servings
Serving size: 1 roll

Exchanges: ½ starch
           ½ very lean meat
Carbohydrate choices: ½

Nutrition per serving:
Calories: 70
Carbohydrate: . . . . .7 g
Protein: . . . . .5 g
Fat: . . . . .3 g

Saturated fat: . . . . .0 g
Cholesterol: . . . . .5 mg
Dietary fiber: . . . .<1 g
Sodium: . . . . .200 mg

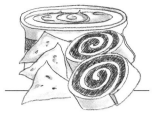

Fruit kabobs with orange ginger dip

No need to skewer these if you don't want to! Combine the fruit and the dip and turn this into a crunchy fruit salad.

1 carton (8 ounces) fat-free sour cream

1 tablespoon honey

1 tablespoon orange juice concentrate, thawed and undiluted

1 teaspoon grated fresh ginger root

1 medium pear, cored and sliced

1 medium apple, cored and sliced

1 medium orange, peeled, seeded, and sectioned

1 cup cubed pineapple

1 cup whole strawberries

1 cup grapes

In small bowl, stir together sour cream, honey, orange juice concentrate, and ginger root. Cover and refrigerate at least 2 hours. Wash and prepare remaining fruits. Alternately thread fruit pieces on wooden picks or skewers. Serve with chilled dip.

64

Preparation time: 15 minutes
Chilling time: 2 hours

Yield: 8 servings
Serving size: 2 tablespoons dip
    with ¾ cup fruit

Exchanges: 1½ fruit
Carbohydrate choices: 1½

Nutrition per serving:
Calories: 105
Carbohydrate: . . . . .24 g
Protein: . . . . .2 g
Fat: . . . .<1 g

Saturated fat: . . . . .0 g
Cholesterol: . . . . .0 mg
Dietary fiber: . . . . .2 g
Sodium: . . . . .25 mg

Chapter 3

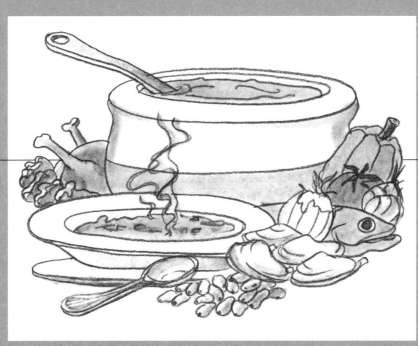

SOUPS

*S*oup is one of the most versatile foods. Not only can it be made ahead of time and reheated for a simple, nutritious, and light snack, it can also serve as the perfect complement to a satisfying meal. Whatever you are looking for, this chapter is sure to have a recipe perfect for you.

If you are looking for a warm bowl of something to take the sting out of a chilly day, try classics like the French Onion or Minestrone. Or if you want something cool to relieve the heat of a summer afternoon, try the Cold Cucumber Soup. Many of your favorite recipes are here, as well as some you might never have thought to try. Be adventurous! You won't be disappointed.

Also here are recipes for several homemade broths, which can be used in a number of other dishes in this book. Homemade broths, often called stocks by professional chefs, can lend a recipe fantastic flavor and make the difference between ho-hum fare and a happy feast. Try using them once and you will never go back to store-bought broths again.

French onion soup

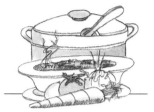

1 tablespoon margarine
1 large, mild onion, thinly sliced
2 teaspoons all-purpose flour
¼ cup dry white wine
4 cups low-sodium beef broth
½ teaspoon salt (optional)
¼ teaspoon freshly ground pepper
4 slices French bread, one inch thick
1 cup shredded low-fat Swiss cheese

Make sure to use mild onions in this classic soup or you'll over-whelm your guests with the taste. Bermuda and Spanish onions work well in this recipe.

1. Preheat oven to 325°F. In a heavy saucepan, melt the margarine and sliced onion. Cover and cook over low heat until the onion is tender, about 5–10 minutes.
2. Remove cover, increase heat to medium-high, and cook, stirring, until the onion is golden, about 15–20 minutes. Be careful not to brown or burn the onion.
3. Reduce the heat and stir in the flour and wine. Simmer, stirring, until thickened, about 2 minutes. Add the beef broth, bring to a boil, reduce heat, and simmer 5–10 minutes. Season to taste with salt (optional) and pepper.
4. Place bread in the oven for 5–7 minutes to dry. Put 4 ovenproof bowls on a baking sheet and divide the soup among the bowls. Place a slice of bread on top of each; allow the bread to soak up the soup, then cover with ¼ cup of shredded cheese per bowl. Bake 20–30 minutes, until the cheese is golden.

Preparation time: 15 minutes
Cooking time: 1¼ hours

Yield: 4 servings
Serving size: 1 cup

Exchanges: 1 starch
             1 medium-fat meat
Carbohydrate choices: 1

Nutrition per serving:
Calories: 185
Carbohydrate: . . . . .18 g
Protein: . . . . .12 g
Fat: . . . . .6 g

Saturated fat: . . . . .2 g
Cholesterol: . . . . .11 mg
Dietary fiber: . . . . .1 g
Sodium: . . . . .855 mg
(omitting salt) . . . . . . .588 mg

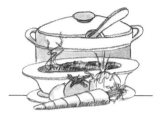

Minestrone soup

This hearty Italian classic is not only a veggie lover's delight, it's a good source of protein and fiber.

1 teaspoon vegetable oil
1 pound lean ground beef
1 cup chopped onion
1 cup chopped celery
1 cup chopped green pepper or zucchini
1 cup shredded cabbage
1 cup diced potato
1 cup sliced carrot
1 can (about 28 ounces) whole or crushed tomatoes
6 cups water
2 teaspoons salt (optional)
1 teaspoon Worcestershire sauce
¼ teaspoon freshly ground black pepper
2 whole bay leaves
1 can (about 14 ounces) red kidney beans
½ cup elbow macaroni, uncooked
⅓ cup grated Parmesan cheese (optional)

1. In a large, heavy pot, add the oil, and, over medium-high heat, brown the ground beef, stirring to break up clumps. Degrease.
2. Add the onion, celery, green pepper or zucchini, cabbage, potatoes, carrots, tomatoes, water, salt (optional), Worcestershire, pepper, and bay leaves. Stir well and bring to a boil. Reduce heat and simmer, covered, 1 hour.
3. Add the kidney beans and the macaroni and cook an additional 30 minutes, stirring occasionally. Ladle into soup bowls and sprinkle each with about 1 teaspoon grated Parmesan, if desired.

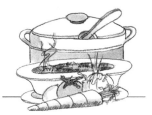

Preparation time: 20 minutes
Cooking time: 1¾ hours

Yield: 14 servings
Serving size: 1 cup

Exchanges: 1 starch
　　　　　　 1 medium-fat meat
Carbohydrate choices: 1

Nutrition per serving:

With Parmesan cheese	*Without Parmesan cheese*
Calories: 144	Calories: 135
Carbohydrate: . . . . .14 g	Carbohydrate: . . . . .14 g
Protein: . . . . .10 g	Protein: . . . . .9 g
Fat: . . . . .5 g	Fat: . . . . .5 g
Saturated fat: . . . . .2 g	Saturated fat: . . . . .2 g
Cholesterol: . . . . .22 mg	Cholesterol: . . . . .20 mg
Dietary fiber: . . . . .4 g	Dietary fiber: . . . . .4 g
Sodium: . . . . .525 mg	Sodium: . . . . .490 mg
(omitting salt) . . . . . .220 mg	(omitting salt) . . . . . .185 mg

Borscht

1 can (about 16 ounces) sliced beets

2 cans (about 10 ounces each) low-sodium beef broth

2 cups finely shredded cabbage

1 cup chopped celery

½ cup chopped onion

1 large bay leaf

1 teaspoon salt (optional)

¼ teaspoon freshly ground black pepper

2 tablespoons freshly squeezed lemon juice

½ cup low-fat sour cream (or plain nonfat yogurt)

1–2 tablespoons chopped fresh dill
　　or 1 teaspoon dried dillweed

This Russian soup is traditionally prepared without cabbage, but what a tasty addition it makes here!

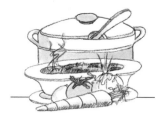

1. Drain the beets, reserving the juice. Add enough water to the beet juice to make 4 cups. Slice the beets into julienne strips.

2. In a large saucepan, combine the beef broth and beet liquid. Stir in the cabbage, celery, onion, bay leaf, salt (optional), and pepper. Bring to a boil, lower heat, and simmer, uncovered, about 30 minutes.

3. Remove the bay leaf. Stir in the lemon juice. Ladle the soup into bowls and top each with 1 tablespoon of sour cream (or yogurt) and a pinch of dill.

Preparation time: 20 minutes
Cooking time: 35 minutes

Yield: 10 servings
Serving size: 1 cup

Nutrition per serving:

With sour cream	**With nonfat yogurt**
Exchanges: 1 vegetable	Exchanges: 1 vegetable
½ fat	
Carbohydrate choices: ½	Carbohydrate choices: ½
Calories: 60	Calories: 42
Carbohydrate: . . . . .8 g	Carbohydrate: . . . . .8 g
Protein: . . . . .2 g	Protein: . . . . .2 g
Fat: . . . . .3 g	Fat: . . . . .0 g
Saturated fat: . . . . .2 g	Saturated fat: . . . . .0 g
Cholesterol: . . . . .5 mg	Cholesterol: . . . . .trace
Dietary fiber: . . . . .2 g	Dietary fiber: . . . . .2 g
Sodium: . . . . .465 mg	Sodium: . . . . .459 mg
(omitting salt) . . . . . . .199 mg	(omitting salt) . . . . . . .193 mg

Lemony mushroom soup

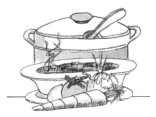

¾ pound fresh mushrooms, cleaned, ends trimmed, sliced

4 cups low-sodium chicken or beef broth

1 teaspoon low-sodium soy sauce

½ teaspoon grated lemon zest

¼ teaspoon freshly ground black pepper

1 tablespoon dry sherry

1. In a heavy, medium-sized saucepan, place mushrooms, broth, and soy sauce. Bring to a boil, reduce heat, and simmer for 20 minutes.

2. Stir in lemon zest and pepper; simmer 2 more minutes. Stir in sherry. Divide among 4 warm soup bowls and serve.

This soup is not only easy to make, it's also very low in calories. Not only that, but it contains no fat at all!

71

Preparation time: 15 minutes
Cooking time: 25 minutes

Exchanges: 1 vegetable
Carbohydrate choices: 0

Yield: 4 servings
Serving size: 1 cup

Nutrition per serving:
Calories: 45
Carbohydrate: . . . . .5 g
Protein: . . . . .5 g
Fat: . . . . .0 g

Saturated fat: . . . . .0 g
Cholesterol: . . . . .0 mg
Dietary fiber: . . . . .1 g
Sodium: . . . . .534 mg

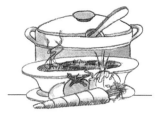

Cold cucumber soup

This is a great soup to accompany either a hot day or a spicy meal. The simplest way to seed a cucumber, as is required here, is to halve it lengthwise and use the tip of a spoon to scrape the seeds from the center of each half.

1 large cucumber, peeled, seeded, and sliced
1 cup low-sodium chicken broth
1 green onion, roughly chopped
1 tablespoon chopped fresh mint or
   1 teaspoon dried mint
1 teaspoon salt (optional)
1–2 cloves garlic
1 teaspoon freshly squeezed lemon juice
½ cup low-fat sour cream
1½ cups plain nonfat yogurt
Pinch ground white pepper

1. Set 4 slices of cucumber aside. In a blender or food processor, place remaining cucumber slices, broth, onion, mint, salt (optional), garlic, and lemon juice. Process until smooth, about 1 minute.
2. Add sour cream and yogurt and blend to combine. Season with pepper. Cover and refrigerate several hours before serving. Garnish each bowl with one of the reserved cucumber slices before serving.

Preparation time: 20 minutes
Chilling time: 3–4 hours

Yield: 4 servings
Serving size: 1 cup

Exchanges: 2 vegetable
          1 fat
Carbohydrate choices: ½

Nutrition per serving:
Calories: 119
Carbohydrate: . . . . .10 g
Protein: . . . . .7 g
Fat: . . . . .6 g

Saturated fat: . . . . .3 g
Cholesterol: . . . . .14 mg
Dietary fiber: . . . . .1 g
Sodium: . . . . .662 mg
(omitting salt) . . . . . . .129 mg

Lentil soup

1 cup split red lentils
6½ cups cold water
3 stalks celery
2 medium carrots, peeled and sliced
1 green pepper, seeded and chopped
2 cloves garlic, minced
⅓ cup chopped fresh parsley
2 teaspoons salt (optional)
¼ teaspoon freshly ground black pepper

1. Rinse lentils well and, in a large pot, combine with remaining ingredients.
2. Bring to a boil, reduce heat, and simmer, uncovered, until vegetables are tender, about 25–30 minutes. Ladle into soup bowls.

Because of the main ingredient, lentils, this soup is an excellent source of fiber for your diet.

73

Preparation time: 20 minutes
Cooking time: 35 minutes

Exchanges: 1 starch
Carbohydrate choices: 1

Yield: 8 servings
Serving size: 1 cup

Nutrition per serving:
Calories: 89
Carbohydrate: . . . . .16 g
Protein: . . . . .5 g
Fat: . . . . .trace

Saturated fat: . . . . .0 g
Cholesterol: . . . . .0 mg
Dietary fiber: . . . . .3 g
Sodium: . . . . .555 mg
(omitting salt) . . . . .22 mg

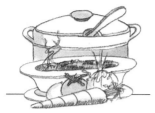

Tomato basil soup

To quickly peel a tomato, as required here, bring a pot of water to a boil and drop the tomato in for 30–45 seconds. Remove the tomato from the boiling water and immediately plunge it into a bowl of ice water. The peel should loosen and come off easily.

74

1 teaspoon vegetable oil
½ cup chopped carrots
⅓ cup chopped leek, white part only
1 large green onion, chopped
1 large clove garlic, minced
6 fresh, ripe tomatoes, peeled, seeded, and chopped, or 1 (28-ounce) can whole tomatoes, drained and chopped
4 cups low-sodium chicken broth (or water)
1 teaspoon salt (optional)
1 teaspoon dried basil leaves
1 bay leaf
¼ teaspoon dried leaf thyme
¼ teaspoon freshly ground black pepper
6 large fresh basil leaves, stacked, rolled, and sliced crosswise into thin julienne strips, for garnish

1. In a large, heavy saucepan, heat the oil; add the carrots, leek, onion, and garlic. Sauté, stirring often, for 2–3 minutes.

2. Add the tomatoes, chicken broth (or water), salt (optional), basil, bay leaf, thyme, and pepper. Cover and simmer 30 minutes.

3. Remove bay leaf. In 2-cup batches, puree soup in a blender or food processor until smooth. (For an even smoother consistency, strain through a sieve.) Ladle into 6 bowls. Garnish each with julienned basil.

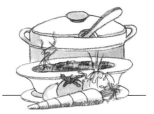

Preparation time: 20 minutes
Cooking time: 40 minutes

Exchanges: 2 vegetable
Carbohydrate choices: ½

Yield: 6 servings
Serving size: 1 cup

Nutrition per serving:
Calories: 61
Carbohydrate: . . . . .7 g
Protein: . . . . .2 g
Fat: . . . . .2 g

Saturated fat: . . . . .1 g
Cholesterol: . . . . .5 mg
Dietary fiber: . . . . .2 g
Sodium: . . . . .151 mg
(omitting salt) . . . . . . .88 mg

Creamy celery soup

2 cups Celery Sauce (recipe, p. 361)
1 cup skim milk
1 cup low-sodium chicken broth

In a medium saucepan over low heat, whisk together the sauce, milk, and broth. Heat to simmer, but do not boil. Ladle into soup bowls.

As long as you have the Celery Sauce prepared ahead of time, this will be the easiest soup you could ever make. Garnish it with sliced celery stalks for special occasions.

Preparation time: 5 minutes
Cooking time: 10 minutes

Exchanges: 1 carbohydrate
Carbohydrate choices: 1

Yield: 4 servings
Serving size: 1 cup

Nutrition per serving:
Calories: 80
Carbohydrate: . . . . .11 g
Protein: . . . . .4 g
Fat: . . . . .2 g

Saturated fat: . . . . .1 g
Cholesterol: . . . . .7 mg
Dietary fiber: . . . . .1 g
Sodium: . . . . .151 mg

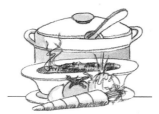

Creamy vegetable soup

The dark green tops of the leek, when cooked too long, can sometimes impart a bitter taste to soups and stews. Be sure to use only the white and very light green parts of the leek.

3 stalks celery, sliced
1 leek, cleaned, trimmed, and sliced (white and light green parts only)
1 carrot, peeled and chopped
1 white turnip, peeled and chopped
1 kohlrabi or ¼ cabbage, chopped
1 medium potato
½ cup frozen green peas
5 cups low-sodium chicken broth
1 tablespoon fresh cilantro or parsley, minced

1. In a large, heavy pot, combine all the ingredients except the cilantro or parsley. Bring to a boil, reduce the heat, and simmer until the vegetables are tender, about 20–30 minutes.
2. Stir in the cilantro or parsley. In 2-cup batches, blend the mixture in a blender or food processor until smooth. Refrigerate until ready to serve. May be served hot or chilled. Garnish with whole cilantro or parsley leaves, if desired.

76

Preparation time: 15 minutes
Cooking time: 40 minutes

Exchanges: 1 starch
Carbohydrate choices: 1

Yield: 5 servings
Serving size: 1 cup

Nutrition per serving:
Calories: 80
Carbohydrate: . . . . .12 g
Protein: . . . . .3 g
Fat: . . . . .2 g

Saturated fat: . . . . .1 g
Cholesterol: . . . . .7 mg
Dietary fiber: . . . . .3 g
Sodium: . . . . .138 mg

Cream of cauliflower soup

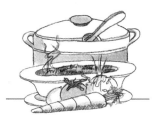

2 cups cauliflower florets
½ cup chopped celery
2 cups low-sodium chicken broth
1 cup evaporated skim milk
½ teaspoon salt (optional)
⅛ teaspoon white pepper
1 green onion, thinly sliced

This wonderful soup will look difficult to family and friends, but you will know what a snap it was to prepare. This basic recipe can be used with any vegetable — just substitute broccoli, asparagus, zucchini, or any other vegetable for cauliflower.

1. In a medium saucepan, combine the cauliflower, celery, and chicken broth. Bring to a boil, reduce heat, and simmer until the vegetables are tender, about 10–15 minutes.
2. In 2-cup batches, puree the mixture in a blender or food processor until smooth. Return to the saucepan and add the evaporated milk, salt (optional), and pepper. Heat over medium-low heat, stirring, until well warmed; do not boil. Ladle into bowls. Garnish with sliced green onions.

Preparation time: 10 minutes
Cooking time: 30 minutes

Yield: 4 servings
Serving size: 1 cup

Exchanges: ½ carbohydrate
Carbohydrate choices: ½

Nutrition per serving:
Calories: 69
Carbohydrate: . . . . .8 g
Protein: . . . . .6 g
Fat: . . . . .1 g

Saturated fat: . . . . .trace
Cholesterol: . . . . .6 mg
Dietary fiber: . . . .<1 g
Sodium: . . . . .417 mg
(omitting salt) . . . . . .150 mg

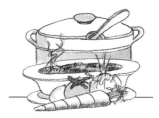

This slight variation on the traditional cream of potato recipe is both flavorful and simple to make.

Potato and leek soup

8 cups chicken or vegetable stock
6 medium potatoes, peeled and diced
6 stalks of celery, cut into 1-inch slices
3 medium leeks, trimmed and cut into 1-inch pieces
1 tablespoon margarine
¾ cup nonfat sour cream (optional)
Chopped fresh chives (optional)

1. In a large saucepan, place stock, potato, celery, and leek. Cover and cook over medium-high heat until vegetables are tender, about 20 minutes.
2. In 2-cup batches, puree the mixture in a blender or food processor until smooth. Return puree to saucepan, blending well. Place over medium heat, add margarine, and stir until melted. Ladle into 8 serving bowls and top each with 1 tablespoon sour cream and a sprinkling of chives for garnish, if desired.

Preparation time: 10 minutes
Cooking time: 25 minutes

Exchanges: 2 starch
Carbohydrate choices: 2

Yield: 12 cups
Serving size: 1½ cups

Nutrition per serving:
Calories: 172
Carbohydrate: . . . . .29 g
Protein: . . . . .8 g
Fat: . . . . .3 g

Saturated fat: . . . . .trace
Cholesterol: . . . . .3 mg
Dietary fiber: . . . . .3 g
Sodium: . . . . .833 mg

Squash and leek soup

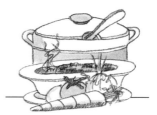

½ cup sliced leeks
1 teaspoon margarine
¼ teaspoon garlic salt
⅛ teaspoon white pepper
2 cups cooked winter squash
12 ounces evaporated skim milk
1 cup buttermilk
¼ teaspoon saffron threads

1. Place leeks, margarine, garlic salt, and pepper in a 2-quart casserole. Cover and microwave on High for 1–3 minutes, until margarine is melted and leeks are tender.
2. Add squash, skim milk, buttermilk, and saffron, and mix well. Cover and microwave for 6–8 minutes or until soup is hot, stirring twice during cooking time.

Using the microwave cuts the cooking time for this delicious soup by almost a third. Note that the recipe calls for saffron, which can be very expensive. You can use a cheaper, imitation saffron and still produce excellent results.

79

Preparation time: 10 minutes
Cooking time: 10 minutes

Yield: 5 servings
Serving size: 1 cup

Exchanges: 1 starch
          1 skim milk
Carbohydrate choices: 2

Nutrition per serving:
Calories: 149
Carbohydrate: . . . . .25 g
Protein: . . . . .9 g
Fat: . . . . .2 g

Saturated fat: . . . . .trace
Cholesterol: . . . . .5 mg
Dietary fiber: . . . . .3 g
Sodium: . . . . .261 mg

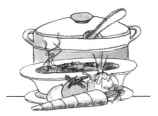

Beef broth

Beef broth takes a long time to cook, but the good news is that you don't have to do anything but let it sit on the stove until it's done. Try to get the larger, meatier neck bones from your butcher or supermarket—they will produce a much more flavorful broth.

80

2 pounds beef neck bones
4 quarts cold water
2 carrots, well washed, peeled, and roughly chopped
1 onion, peeled, stuck with 3 whole cloves
1 leek, washed and chopped
1 stalk celery, chopped
1 large clove garlic, peeled
1 bunch fresh parsley, stems only
1 large bay leaf
1 teaspoon dried leaf thyme
3 cups hot water

1. Place beef bones in a stockpot and cover with water. Bring to a boil, reduce heat, and simmer, skimming the surface occasionally, for 1 hour. Do not stir or the broth will become cloudy.
2. Add all of the remaining ingredients, plus 3 cups of hot water. Return to a boil, reduce heat, and simmer, uncovered, 4–5 more hours.
3. Strain the broth into a clean container and discard the solids. Degrease. Store in the refrigerator up to 3 days or in the freezer up to 3 months.

Preparation time: 15 minutes
Cooking time: 5–6 hours

Exchanges: free
Carbohydrate choices: 0

Yield: 8 servings
Serving size: 1 cup

Nutrition per serving:
Calories: 10
Carbohydrate: . . . . .trace
Protein: . . . . .trace
Fat: . . . . .trace

Saturated fat: . . . . .trace
Cholesterol: . . . . .0 mg
Dietary fiber: . . . . .0 g
Sodium: . . . . .25 mg

Brown beef broth

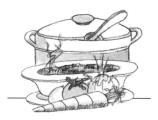

1. Preheat the oven to 350°F. Place the bones in a roasting pan and roast, uncovered, until browned, about 45 minutes. Add the vegetables and roast another 15 minutes.
2. Place the bones, vegetables, and any browned bits from the bottom of the roasting pan (use water to help dissolve them) in the stockpot. Add the 4 quarts of water and proceed from Step 2 in Beef Broth recipe.

VARIATION
Roasting the bones first will result in a much darker color and a somewhat sweeter flavor.

Chicken vegetable barley soup

Here is a comforting meal-in-a-bowl. Just add a salad and some fresh-baked bread, and supper's ready.

For the broth, or stock:
3 pounds chicken pieces
9 cups cold water
1 large stalk celery, with leaves, roughly chopped
1 onion, quartered
1 carrot, roughly chopped
1 bay leaf
1 large clove garlic, peeled

For the soup:
½ cup each chopped onion, chopped celery, chopped carrot, and chopped fresh parsley
½ cup uncooked barley
2 tablespoons freshly squeezed lemon juice
2 teaspoons salt (optional)
½ teaspoon freshly ground black pepper
¼ teaspoon celery seed
1½ cups cut fresh or frozen green beans

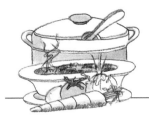

1. To make the stock: In a large stockpot, place all of the stock ingredients. Bring to a boil, reduce heat, and simmer, uncovered, until chicken is tender, about 1 hour.

2. Remove chicken pieces from stockpot. When cool enough to handle, slice meat from bones and set aside. Return chicken skin and bones to stock and continue cooking, uncovered, 1 more hour. Strain and degrease. (Can be made in advance; refrigerated up to 3 days, frozen up to 3 months.)

3. To make the soup: Add all of the ingredients, except the reserved chicken and the green beans, to the chicken stock. Bring to a boil, reduce heat, and simmer until vegetables are tender, about 20 minutes.

4. Add the green beans and continue cooking 10 more minutes. Cut the reserved chicken (about 12 ounces) into bite-size pieces and add to the soup in the last 5 minutes of cooking.

82

For the broth, or stock:
Preparation time: 10 minutes
Cooking time: 2 ¼ hours

For the soup:
Preparation time: 15 minutes
Cooking time: 40 minutes

Yield: 12 servings
Serving size: 1 cup

Nutrition per serving:
Calories: 110
Carbohydrate: . . . . .9 g
Protein: . . . . .12 g
Fat: . . . . .2 g

Exchanges: ½ carbohydrate
1 lean meat
Carbohydrate choices: ½

Saturated fat: . . . . .1 g
Cholesterol: . . . . .30 mg
Dietary fiber: . . . . .2 g
Sodium: . . . . .471 mg
(omitting salt) . . . . . . .116 mg

Chicken broth

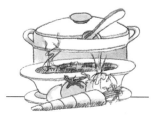

2 pounds chicken backs and necks
10 cups cold water
2 stalks celery, roughly chopped
1 medium onion, roughly chopped
1 large carrot, well washed and roughly chopped
1 large clove garlic, peeled
1 large bay leaf
8 whole black peppercorns
1 bunch parsley, stems only
1 teaspoon dried leaf thyme

1. Rinse chicken parts under cold water. In a stockpot, place the chicken and all of the remaining ingredients. Bring to a boil, reduce heat, and simmer 2–2½ hours, skimming the surface occasionally.
2. Strain the stock into a clean container and discard the solids. Degrease the stock, if needed. Refrigerate up to 3 days or freeze up to 3 months.

Homemade chicken broth should be called "liquid gold" because of its invaluable role in a variety of recipes. For quick use, try freezing the broth in an ice cube tray—then you can grab a "cube" of broth whenever you need it.

83

Preparation time: 10 minutes
Cooking time: 2–2½ hours

Exchanges: free
Carbohydrate choices: 0

Yield: 8 servings
Serving size: 1 cup

Nutrition per serving:
Calories: 18
Carbohydrate: . . . . .trace
Protein: . . . . .trace
Fat: . . . . .trace
Saturated fat: . . . . .trace
Cholesterol: . . . . .trace
Dietary fiber: . . . . .trace
Sodium: . . . . .110 mg

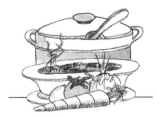

Tortilla soup

The crunch of crisp tor-tillas in this spicy soup will surprise and delight you. Feel free to increase or decrease the amount of chilies you use—it won't affect the nutri-tion values of the recipe.

2 teaspoons vegetable oil

1 onion, thinly sliced

1 large clove garlic, minced

2 tomatoes, peeled, seeded, and chopped (or 1 cup drained canned tomatoes, chopped)

¼ teaspoon freshly ground black pepper

5 cups low-sodium chicken broth

1 teaspoon salt (optional)

½ cup finely chopped celery

½ cup finely chopped carrot

2 tablespoons crushed, dried chilies, seeds and veins removed

2 six-inch Whole Wheat Flour Tortillas (recipe, p. 365), or commercial whole wheat tortillas, sliced into bite-size pieces and oven toasted

½ cup (about 4 slices) crumbled, crisp bacon (or turkey bacon)

½ cup shredded farmer cheese

1. In a medium saucepan, add the oil, onion, and garlic, and cook over medium-high heat, stirring, until the onion is translucent, about 5 minutes.
2. Add the tomatoes and pepper and cook an additional 10–15 minutes. Stir in the broth and salt (optional). Bring to a boil, lower heat, and simmer 15 minutes.
3. Add the celery, carrot, and 1 tablespoon of the crushed chilies. Simmer 10 minutes longer.
4. Divide the toasted tortilla chips among 6 soup bowls. Ladle soup over chips. Sprinkle each with bacon, cheese, and the remaining tablespoon of chilies.

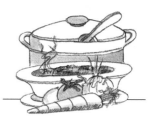

Preparation time: 20 minutes
Cooking time: 50 minutes

Yield: 6 servings
Serving size: 1 cup

Exchanges: 1 carbohydrate
         1 high-fat meat
Carbohydrate choices: 1

Nutrition per serving:

With bacon

Calories:	164
Carbohydrate:	. . . . .12 g
Protein:	. . . . .8 g
Fat:	. . . . .9 g
Saturated fat:	. . . . .3 g
Cholesterol:	. . . . .22 mg
Dietary fiber:	. . . . .2 g
Sodium:	. . . . .728 mg
(omitting salt)	. . . . . .373 mg

With turkey bacon

Calories:	160
Carbohydrate:	. . . . .12 g
Protein:	. . . . .8 g
Fat:	. . . . .8 g
Saturated fat:	. . . . .2 g
Cholesterol:	. . . . .16 mg
Dietary fiber:	. . . . .2 g
Sodium:	. . . . .707 mg
(omitting salt)	. . . . . .352 mg

Chicken tortilla soup

Add 6 ounces cubed, cooked chicken to the Tortilla Soup recipe in the last 5 minutes of cooking.

VARIATION

Yield: 6 servings
Serving size: 1 cup

Exchanges: 1 carbohydrate
         2 medium-fat meat
Carbohydrate choices: 1

Nutrition per serving:

With chicken and bacon

Calories:	211
Carbohydrate:	. . . . .12 g
Protein:	. . . . .17 g
Fat:	. . . . .10 g
Saturated fat:	. . . . .3 g
Cholesterol:	. . . . .46 mg
Dietary fiber:	. . . . .2 g
Sodium:	. . . . .749 mg
(omitting salt)	. . . . . .394 mg

**With chicken
and turkey bacon**

Calories:	207
Carbohydrate:	. . . . .12 g
Protein:	. . . . .17 g
Fat:	. . . . .9 g
Saturated fat:	. . . . .3 g
Cholesterol:	. . . . .40 mg
Dietary fiber:	. . . . .2 g
Sodium:	. . . . .728 mg
(omitting salt)	. . . . . .373 mg

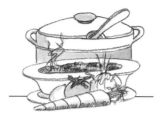

Clam chowder

This New England style clam chowder is not only quick to make, it's also lighter and less fattening than traditional chowders that use heavy cream.

1 can (about 5 ounces) clams
1 cup diced potato
½ cup chopped celery
½ cup chopped onion
½ teaspoon salt (optional)
¼ teaspoon white pepper
4 cups skim milk
1 tablespoon margarine
2 tablespoons instant skim milk powder

1. In a large, heavy saucepan, combine the clams (including the juice from the can) with the remaining ingredients. Stir well to dissolve skim milk powder.
2. Cook over low heat until potatoes are tender, about 20 minutes. Ladle into soup bowls.

Preparation time: 10 minutes
Cooking time: 20 minutes

Yield: 7 servings
Serving size: 1 cup

Nutrition per serving:
Calories: 90
Carbohydrate: . . . . .12 g
Protein: . . . . .8 g
Fat: . . . . .2 g

Exchanges: 1 carbohydrate
1 lean meat
Carbohydrate choices: 1

Saturated fat: . . . . .trace
Cholesterol: . . . . .9 mg
Dietary fiber: . . . .<1 g
Sodium: . . . . .359 mg
(omitting salt) . . . . . . .206 mg

Fish chowder

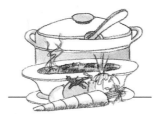

1 tablespoon margarine
1 cup chopped onion
½ cup diced celery
1½ cups diced raw potato
½ cup diced carrot
½ teaspoon dried leaf thyme
½ teaspoon salt (optional)
¼ teaspoon freshly ground black pepper
2 cups cold water
1 pound boned fish fillets, cut into bite-size pieces
2 cups skim milk

1. In a large, heavy saucepan, melt the margarine, add the onion and celery, and cook over medium-high heat, stirring, until onions are translucent, about 5 minutes.
2. Add the potatoes, carrot, thyme, salt (optional), pepper, and 2 cups of water. Cover and simmer until the vegetables are tender, about 20 minutes.
3. Add the fish and simmer 10 minutes. Add the milk and heat to a simmer; do not boil. Ladle into soup bowls.

Use any kind of fish you want in this soup, whether fresh, frozen, or smoked. Different fish will yield different flavors, so try this recipe with several varieties.

87

Preparation time: 15 minutes
Cooking time: 40 minutes

Yield: 8 servings
Serving size: 1 cup

Exchanges: 1 starch
      1 very lean meat
Carbohydrate choices: 1

Nutrition per serving:
Calories: 117
Carbohydrate: . . . . .12 g
Protein: . . . . .13 g
Fat: . . . . .2 g

Saturated fat: . . . . .trace
Cholesterol: . . . . .33 mg
Dietary fiber: . . . . .1 g
Sodium: . . . . .229 mg
(omitting salt) . . . . .95 mg

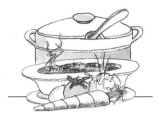

The salt pork is what gives this dish its distinctive taste. Try making this with a meaty ham bone instead of the salt pork for a milder flavor.

Hearty split pea soup

2 cups dried split peas
10 cups plus 2 cups cold water
1 cup diced lean salt pork, well rinsed
2 cups diced turnip
1 cup diced carrot
½ cup diced potato
½ cup chopped onion
⅓ cup chopped celery tops, including leaves
1 teaspoon salt (optional)
¼ teaspoon freshly ground black pepper

1. In a heavy, large saucepan, combine the split peas and 10 cups of water. Bring to a boil. Boil 2 minutes, turn off the heat, and allow to stand 1 hour.
2. Meanwhile, place the salt pork in another saucepan, cover with the remaining 2 cups of water, bring to a boil, reduce heat, and simmer 30 minutes. Strain liquid into a bowl and chill until the fat congeals on top. Discard the fat and add the remaining liquid to the peas. Trim lean meat from salt pork and add to peas. Discard fat.
3. Add remaining ingredients to saucepan and cook over low heat until vegetables are tender, about 1–1½ hours. Puree soup in a blender or food processor if a smoother texture is desired.

Preparation time: 10 minutes
Cooking time: 2–2½ hours

Exchanges: 2 starch
Carbohydrate choices: 2

Yield: 10 servings
Serving size: 1 cup

Nutrition per serving:
Calories: 158
Carbohydrate: . . . . .27 g
Protein: . . . . .10 g
Fat: . . . . .1 g

Saturated fat: . . . . .trace
Cholesterol: . . . . .4 mg
Dietary fiber: . . . . .7 g
Sodium: . . . . .351 mg
(omitting salt) . . . . . . .138 mg

Chapter 4

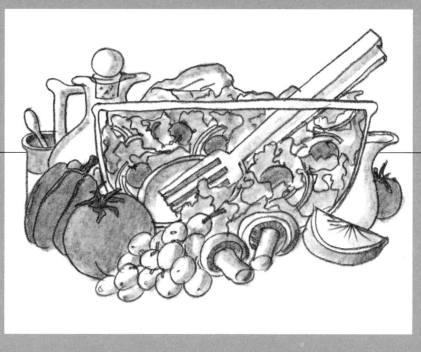

SALADS AND DRESSINGS

Though you might be tempted to think of a salad as a side dish to the main course, this chapter contains a number of recipes that will surprise you. Traditional recipes such as Potato Salad, Fancy Coleslaw, and Caesar Salad are presented here in low-fat versions. But the Tuna Salad can be a healthy meal in itself. And if you're looking for a light, refreshing dessert, our Festival Fruit Salad or Cucumber Lime Mold will more than satisfy. Salads can be an easy way of adding vegetables and fruits to your meal plan.

Of course, the key to any salad is a great dressing, and we have plenty of recipes for you to choose from. Try the low-calorie versions of favorites like Thousand Island, Slim-and-trim Italian, and Herb Buttermilk dressings. For fancier tastes, we have a tangy Raspberry Vinaigrette or a rich Wine and Mustard dressing. Try them all for yourself!

Orange and sprout salad

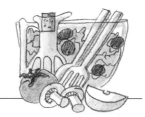

For the salad:

2 cups torn lettuce leaves

1 cup fresh bean sprouts, washed and patted dry

2 oranges, peeled and sectioned, or ½ cup canned mandarin oranges, drained and rinsed

2 stalks celery, sliced

2 tablespoons toasted slivered almonds

For the dressing:

2 tablespoons orange juice

1 tablespoon cider vinegar

1 tablespoon vegetable oil

½ teaspoon celery seed

¼ teaspoon salt (optional)

¼ teaspoon freshly ground black pepper

Liquid artificial sweetener equivalent to 1 tablespoon sugar (optional)

The sweetness of the orange juice combines with the tartness of the cider vinegar to make this dressing something special. You might wants to use the dressing on other salads as well.

91

Combine the lettuce, bean sprouts, orange segments, celery, and almonds in a salad bowl. In a small mixing bowl or covered jar, combine all of the dressing ingredients. Whisk or shake until well mixed. Pour over salad and toss well. Serve immediately.

Preparation time: 10 minutes

Yield: 4 servings
Serving size: 1 cup

Exchanges: ½ fruit
      1 vegetable
      1 fat
Carbohydrate choices: 1

Nutrition per serving:
Calories: 107
Carbohydrate: . . . . .11 g
Protein: . . . . .2 g
Fat: . . . . .5 g

Saturated fat: . . . . .1 g
Cholesterol: . . . . .0 mg
Dietary fiber: . . . . .4 g
Sodium: . . . . .156 mg
(omitting salt) . . . . .23 mg

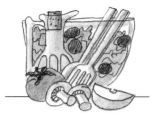

Molded cranberry salad

Cranberry salad is a favorite at holiday dinners. Make sure to let the gelatin slightly set before adding the celery and apple. Otherwise, all the fruit and vegetable pieces will sink right to the bottom.

1 envelope unflavored gelatin
1¾ cups plus ¼ cup sugar-free ginger ale
2 cups coarsely chopped fresh or frozen cranberries
1 tablespoon freshly squeezed lemon juice
2 teaspoons grated orange zest
Artificial sweetener equivalent to 5 teaspoons sugar
½ cup diced celery
½ cup diced apple

1. In a small bowl, sprinkle the gelatin over ¼ cup of the ginger ale and allow it to soften, about 5 minutes.
2. Meanwhile, in a medium saucepan, combine the remaining 1¾ cups of ginger ale, the cranberries, lemon juice, and grated orange zest. Bring to a boil, then immediately remove from the heat.
3. Add the softened gelatin and sweetener to the cranberry mixture and stir until the gelatin dissolves. Chill until partially set.
4. Stir in the celery and apple. Spoon into a 6-cup mold that has been rinsed first with cold water. Refrigerate at least 4 hours or overnight.

92

Preparation time: 20 minutes
Cooking time: 5 minutes
Chilling time: 4 hours

Exchanges: ½ fruit
Carbohydrate choices: ½

Yield: 6 servings
Serving size: ½ cup

Nutrition per serving:
Calories: 32
Carbohydrate: . . . . .6 g
Protein: . . . . .2 g
Fat: . . . . .0 g

Saturated fat: . . . . .0 g
Cholesterol: . . . . .0 mg
Dietary fiber: . . . . .2 g
Sodium: . . . . .29 mg

Jellied beet mold

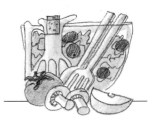

1 can (about 16 ounces) diced beets, drained, liquid reserved
¾ cup unsweetened orange juice
2 teaspoons cider vinegar
1 envelope unflavored gelatin
1 cup shredded zucchini
½ cup diced celery

Beets may not be your favorite vegetable, but this crunchy, colorful gelatin mold will definitely change your mind.

1. In a small saucepan, combine the beet liquid, orange juice, and vinegar. Sprinkle the gelatin over the top and allow it to soften, about 5 minutes.
2. Stir the mixture over low heat until the gelatin is dissolved, then pour it into a bowl and refrigerate until partially set.
3. Spread the shredded zucchini and celery out on paper towels to blot up excess moisture. Fold the reserved beets, zucchini, and celery into the cooled gelatin mixture.
4. Rinse a 1-quart mold with cold water. Spoon the gelatin mixture into the mold. Refrigerate at least 4 hours or overnight.

93

Preparation time: 20 minutes
Cooking time: 5 minutes
Chilling time: 4 hours

Exchanges: 2 vegetable
Carbohydrate choices: ½

Yield: 6 servings
Serving size: ½ cup

Nutrition per serving:
Calories: 46
Carbohydrate: . . . . .9 g
Protein: . . . . .2 g
Fat: . . . . .0 g
Saturated fat: . . . . .0 g
Cholesterol: . . . . .0 mg
Dietary fiber: . . . . .2 g
Sodium: . . . . .209 mg

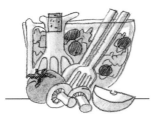

Salad Royale

With both horseradish and pineapple, this beet salad carries a welcome surprise kick.

1 can (about 16 ounces) diced beets, drained, liquid reserved
¾ cup unsweetened grape juice
2 teaspoons freshly squeezed lemon juice
1 envelope unflavored gelatin
1 can (about 15 ounces) unsweetened, crushed pineapple, drained
1 teaspoon bottled horseradish
⅛ teaspoon ground cinnamon

1. In a small saucepan, combine the beet liquid, grape juice, and lemon juice. Sprinkle the gelatin over the top and allow it to soften, about 5 minutes.
2. Stir the mixture over low heat until the gelatin is dissolved. Refrigerate until partially set.
3. Fold the reserved beets, crushed pineapple, horseradish, and cinnamon into the cooled gelatin mixture.
4. Rinse a 1-quart mold with cold water. Spoon the gelatin mixture into the mold. Refrigerate at least 4 hours or overnight.

94

Preparation time: 20 minutes
Cooking time: 5 minutes
Chilling time: 4 hours

Yield: 5 servings
Serving size: ½ cup

Exchanges: 1 fruit
          1 vegetable
Carbohydrate choices: 1½

Nutrition per serving:
Calories: 97
Carbohydrate: . . . . .21 g
Protein: . . . . .2 g
Fat: . . . . .trace

Saturated fat: . . . . .0 g
Cholesterol: . . . . .0 mg
Dietary fiber: . . . . .3 g
Sodium: . . . . .241 mg

Festival fruit salad

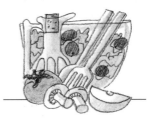

2 envelopes unflavored gelatin
2¼ cups plus ¼ cup sugar-free orange soda
2 tablespoons freshly squeezed lemon juice
½ teaspoon almond extract
½ cup plain nonfat yogurt
1 orange, peeled and sectioned
1 small banana, peeled and sliced
½ cup halved red grapes, seeded
½ cup halved seedless green grapes
⅓ cup drained, unsweetened pineapple chunks

Here's a great salad that can be used either as a side dish to your main course or a dessert.

1. In a small bowl, sprinkle the gelatin over ¼ cup of the orange soda and let it stand about 5 minutes to soften.
2. In a saucepan, combine the remaining 2¼ cups orange soda with the lemon juice. Bring to a boil, remove from heat, and add the gelatin mixture and almond extract. Chill until partially set.
3. Stir in the yogurt, then fold in the fruit. Rinse an 8" × 4" loaf pan with cold water. Spoon the gelatin mixture into the pan. Refrigerate at least 4 hours or overnight. Unmold and slice into 6 equal portions.

95

Preparation time: 20 minutes
Cooking time: 5 minutes
Chilling time: 4 hours

Exchanges: 1 fruit
Carbohydrate choices: 1

Yield: 6 servings
Serving size: 1 cup

Nutrition per serving:
Calories: 85
Carbohydrate: . . . . .17 g
Protein: . . . . .4 g
Fat: . . . . .trace

Saturated fat: . . . . .trace
Cholesterol: . . . . .trace
Dietary fiber: . . . . .1 g
Sodium: . . . . .15 mg

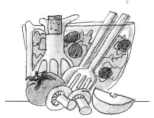

The ground ginger gives this dish a particularly interesting taste.

96

Sunburst salad

1 envelope unflavored gelatin
¼ cup cold water
½ cup boiling water
1 cup sugar-free ginger ale
¼ cup unsweetened orange juice
¼ teaspoon ground ginger
2 oranges, peeled and sectioned
1 cup finely shredded white cabbage
½ cup grated carrot
¼ cup chopped pecans or walnuts

1. In a mixing bowl, sprinkle the gelatin over ¼ cup of cold water and allow it to soften, about 5 minutes. Add ½ cup boiling water and stir to dissolve.
2. Stir in the ginger ale, orange juice, and ginger. Chill until partially set.
3. Stir in the orange sections, cabbage, carrot, and nuts. Rinse a 1-quart mold with cold water and spoon the gelatin mixture into the mold. Refrigerate at least 4 hours or overnight.

Preparation time: 20 minutes
Cooking time: 5 minutes
Chilling time: 4 hours

Yield: 4 servings
Serving size: 1 cup

Exchanges: 1 fruit
         1 fat
Carbohydrate choices: 1

Nutrition per serving:
Calories: 102
Carbohydrate: . . . . .13 g
Protein: . . . . .3 g
Fat: . . . . .4 g
Saturated fat: . . . . .trace
Cholesterol: . . . . .0 mg
Dietary fiber: . . . . .4 g
Sodium: . . . . .25 mg

Mixed melon salad

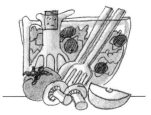

1 cup fresh or canned pineapple chunks,
   packed in juice
3 cups cantaloupe balls
2 cups watermelon balls
2 cups honeydew melon balls
3 tablespoons honey
3 tablespoons cider vinegar or other fruit vinegar
1 tablespoon vegetable oil
1 small shallot, minced
1 teaspoon Dijon mustard
1½ teaspoons poppy seeds

This salad is so versatile that it can be used for breakfast, lunch, dinner, or dessert. Make it ahead of time and enjoy it all through the day.

1. Combine fruits in a large bowl. Combine remaining ingredients in a small jar, cover tightly, and shake to blend.
2. Pour dressing over fruit and toss to coat. Cover and chill for 30 minutes before serving.

97

Preparation time: 15 minutes
Chilling time: 30 minutes

Exchanges: 1½ fruit
Carbohydrate choices: 1½

Yield: 8 cups
Serving size: 1 cup

Nutrition per serving:
Calories: 102
Carbohydrate: . . . . .21 g
Protein: . . . . .1 g
Fat: . . . . .2 g

Saturated fat: . . . .<1 g
Cholesterol: . . . . .0 mg
Dietary fiber: . . . . .1 g
Sodium: . . . . .9 mg

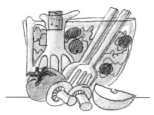

Cucumber lime mold

This cool, tart cucumber salad is a great accompaniment to hot and spicy foods.

1 tablespoon freshly squeezed lime juice

1 tablespoon white vinegar

1 cup cold water

1 envelope unflavored gelatin

1 cup low-fat cottage cheese

½ teaspoon salt (optional)

½ teaspoon Worcestershire sauce

3 drops hot pepper (or Tabasco) sauce

1½ cups shredded, peeled, seeded cucumber

1 tablespoon minced onion, rinsed in a sieve and drained

1. In a small saucepan, combine the lime juice and vinegar with 1 cup of water. Sprinkle the gelatin over the top and allow to soften, about 5 minutes.

2. Stir over low heat until the gelatin is dissolved. Pour into a medium bowl and refrigerate.

3. In a blender or food processor, blend the cottage cheese, salt (optional), Worcestershire sauce, and hot pepper (or Tabasco) sauce until smooth. Add to the gelatin mixture and stir to combine. Refrigerate until partially set.

4. Blot cucumber and onion between paper towels to remove excess moisture. Fold into gelatin mixture. Rinse a 1-quart mold with cold water and spoon the gelatin mixture into it. Refrigerate at least 4 hours or overnight.

98

Preparation time: 20 minutes
Cooking time: 5 minutes
Chilling time: 4 hours

Yield: 4 servings
Serving size: ½ cup

Exchanges: 1 lean meat
Carbohydrate choices: 0

Nutrition per serving:
Calories: 57
Carbohydrate: . . . . .3 g
Protein: . . . . .9 g
Fat: . . . . .1 g
Saturated fat: . . . . .trace
Cholesterol: . . . . .3 mg
Dietary fiber: . . . .<1 g
Sodium: . . . . .484 mg
(omitting salt) . . . . . . .217 mg

Cucumber and fruit salad

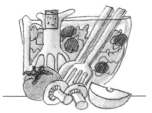

1 large seedless cucumber, peeled and sliced

2 medium red apples, cored and sliced

1 small cantaloupe or honeydew melon, peeled, seeded and sliced

¼ cup plain nonfat yogurt

2 tablespoons freshly squeezed lemon or lime juice

1 teaspoon minced fresh mint
or ½ teaspoon dried mint

Lettuce or spinach leaves, washed and dried

1 tablespoon sunflower seeds

Cantaloupe, cucumber, and apple combine to create the perfect summer salad. Serve this at your next picnic or backyard barbecue.

1. In a mixing bowl, combine the cucumber, apples, and cantaloupe (or honeydew) slices.

2. In a separate bowl, whisk together the yogurt, juice, and mint.

3. Pour dressing over cucumber mixture and toss well. Arrange decoratively on individual salad plates lined with lettuce or spinach leaves. Sprinkle with sunflower seeds.

99

Preparation time: 15 minutes

Yield: 8 servings

Serving size: ½ cup

Exchanges: 1 fruit
Carbohydrate choices: 1

Nutrition per serving:

Calories: 61	Saturated fat: . . . . .trace
Carbohydrate: . . . . .12 g	Cholesterol: . . . . .trace
Protein: . . . . .1 g	Dietary fiber: . . . . .2 g
Fat: . . . . .1 g	Sodium: . . . . .13 mg

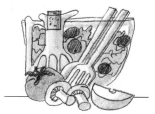

Marinated cucumbers

Here's an interesting take on the classic vinegar-marinated cucumbers. Not only is it tasty, but it's low-sodium, low-fat, and free for your meal plan.

2 medium cucumbers, peeled, halved, seeded, and sliced
½ cup Herb Buttermilk Dressing (recipe, p. 120)

Combine the cucumbers and dressing in a small bowl. Refrigerate overnight to blend flavors. Drain before serving.

Preparation time: 10 minutes
Chilling time: 8 hours

Exchanges: free
Carbohydrate choices: 0

Yield: 8 servings
Serving size: ¼ cup

Nutrition per serving:

Calories: 12	Saturated fat: . . . . .trace
Carbohydrate: . . . . .2 g	Cholesterol: . . . . .trace
Protein: . . . . .1 g	Dietary fiber: . . . . .1 g
Fat: . . . . .trace	Sodium: . . . . .11 mg

100

Mushroom salad

Try different types of mushrooms, either separately or at the same time, to give this salad a variety of flavors.

1 medium head romaine lettuce, washed and dried
1 cup sliced fresh mushrooms
½ cucumber, peeled, seeded, and diced
¼ cup Thousand Island Dressing (recipe, p. 114)
or commercial fat-free salad dressing
¼ cup sunflower or pumpkin seeds

1. Tear the lettuce into bite-size pieces and place them in a salad bowl. Add the sliced mushrooms, cucumber, and dressing.
2. Toss well and serve immediately. Garnish each serving with sunflower or pumpkin seeds.

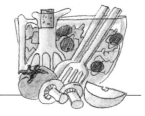

Preparation time: 10 minutes

Yield: 6 servings
Serving size: 1 cup

Exchanges: 1 vegetable
½ fat
Carbohydrate choices: ½

Nutrition per serving:
Calories: 59
Carbohydrate: . . . . .6 g
Protein: . . . . .2 g
Fat: . . . . .3 g

Saturated fat: . . . . .trace
Cholesterol: . . . . .trace
Dietary fiber: . . . . .2 g
Sodium: . . . . .50 mg

Tuna or salmon salad

**1 can (about 6 ounces) chunk, water-packed tuna,
  drained, or 1 can (about 7 ounces) salmon, drained**

⅓ cup low-fat cottage cheese

½ cup finely chopped celery

**¼ cup finely chopped onion, rinsed in a sieve
  and drained**

**2 tablespoons Cider Vinegar Dressing (recipe, p. 115)
  or fat-free mayonnaise**

2 tablespoons minced fresh parsley

½ tablespoon grated lemon zest

**1 teaspoon minced fresh tarragon
  or ¼ teaspoon dried tarragon**

In a mixing bowl, mash the tuna (or salmon) and cottage cheese together with a fork. Add the remaining ingredients and mix until well blended. Cover and refrigerate until ready to serve.

*Tuna or salmon salad
can be served as a first
course or be a meal
in itself. If you use this
in a sandwich, don't
forget to count the
bread slices in your
meal plan.*

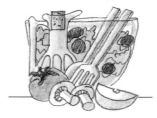

Crunchy tuna salad in pepper cups

Each serving of this main-course salad sits in its own cup—a neat presentation on a luncheon plate.

1 envelope unflavored gelatin

½ cup cold water

1 can (about 10 ounces) condensed consommé, undiluted

2 large, nicely shaped green peppers, halved crosswise, cored, and seeded

½ cup coarsely chopped onion

1 can (about 6 ounces) flaked, water-packed tuna, drained

2 medium tomatoes, peeled, seeded, and chopped

1 cup coarsely chopped iceberg lettuce

½ teaspoon grated lemon zest

1 tablespoon freshly squeezed lemon juice

½ teaspoon salt (optional)

¼ teaspoon freshly ground black pepper

4 whole, crisp lettuce leaves

¼ cup low-fat sour cream (or plain nonfat yogurt)

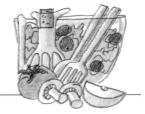

1. Sprinkle the gelatin over ½ cup water and allow it to soften, about 5 minutes.

2. Pour the consommé into a medium saucepan. Bring the consommé to a boil and add the pepper shells, cut side up. Cover and cook 3 minutes. Remove the shells, turn upside down to drain, then refrigerate.

3. Bring the consommé back to a boil, add the onion, and cook 30 seconds. Stir in the gelatin until it dissolves. Pour the mixture into a bowl and refrigerate until partially set.

4. Fold in the tuna, tomatoes, chopped lettuce, lemon zest, lemon juice, salt (optional), and pepper. Spoon into pepper shells, piling the mixture high. Refrigerate at least 4 hours, until set.

5. At serving time, place each pepper on a lettuce leaf; garnish with a dollop of sour cream (or yogurt).

Preparation time: 15 minutes
Cooking time: 10 minutes
Chilling time: 4 hours

Yield: 4 servings
Serving size: ½ filled green pepper

Exchanges: 2 vegetable
                  2 very lean meat
Carbohydrate choices: ½

Nutrition per serving:

With low-fat sour cream

Calories: 121
Carbohydrate: . . . . .8 g
Protein: . . . . .15 g
Fat: . . . . .3 g
Saturated fat: . . . . .3 g
Cholesterol: . . . . .5 mg
Dietary fiber: . . . . .2 g
Sodium: . . . . .790 mg
(omitting salt) . . . . . . .523 mg

With plain nonfat yogurt

Calories: 99
Carbohydrate: . . . . .8 g
Protein: . . . . .16 g
Fat: . . . . .trace
Saturated fat: . . . . .trace
Cholesterol: . . . . .5 mg
Dietary fiber: . . . . .2 g
Sodium: . . . . .786 mg
(omitting salt) . . . . . . .519 mg

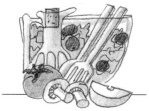

Four bean salad

Can you eat this salad right away, without chilling it overnight? Definitely, but allowing the beans to marinate in the dressing for a day or two will really bring out the flavors.

104

For the salad:

1 can (about 15 ounces) cut green beans, drained, or 1 package frozen cut green beans, cooked and cooled

1 can (about 15 ounces) cut wax beans, drained, or 1 package frozen cut wax beans, cooked and cooled

1 can (about 15 ounces) lima beans, drained, or 1 package frozen lima beans, cooked and cooled

1 can (about 15 ounces) red kidney beans, drained, or 1 package frozen red kidney beans, cooked and cooled

1 red onion, thinly sliced into half-circles

1 cup chopped celery

⅓ cup diced green pepper

For the dressing:

1 tablespoon Dijon mustard

¼ cup red wine vinegar

½ teaspoon sugar

1 teaspoon dried leaf thyme

½ teaspoon salt (optional)

¼ teaspoon freshly ground black pepper

1 clove garlic, finely minced

½ cup good-quality olive oil

1. In a large mixing bowl, combine all of the beans, the onion, celery, and green pepper.
2. In a smaller mixing bowl, whisk together the mustard, vinegar, sugar, thyme, salt (optional), pepper, and minced garlic. Whisking continuously, add the oil in a slow, thin stream. Whisk until well blended.
3. Pour the dressing over the bean mixture and toss to coat well. Cover and refrigerate 1–2 days before serving.

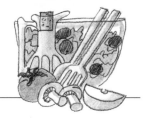

Preparation time: 10 minutes
Chilling time: 1–2 days

Yield: 8 servings
Serving size: ½ cup

Nutrition per serving:
Calories: 113
Carbohydrate: . . . . .16 g
Protein: . . . . .5 g
Fat: . . . . .3 g

Exchanges: 1 starch
    ½ fat
Carbohydrate choices: 1

Saturated fat: . . . . .trace
Cholesterol: . . . . .0 mg
Dietary fiber: . . . . .5 g
Sodium: . . . . .71 mg
(omitting salt) . . . . . . .44 mg

Fancy coleslaw

2 cups shredded cabbage
1 medium carrot, finely chopped
¼ cup diced green pepper
¼ cup Cider Vinegar Dressing (recipe, p. 115)
**   or fat-free mayonnaise**
2 tablespoons plain nonfat yogurt

Choice of one:
½ chopped red apple
⅓ cup drained unsweetened pineapple chunks
2 tablespoons raisins

In a large mixing bowl, combine the cabbage, carrot, and green pepper. In a small bowl, whisk together the salad dressing or mayonnaise and yogurt, and add this to the cabbage mixture. Add the apple, or pineapple, or raisins, and toss.

Cabbage is an easy and economical vegetable for creating crisp salads like this one. Adding apple, pineapple chunks, or raisins turns a basic coleslaw into a special-occasion dish.

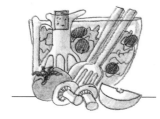

Preparation time: 10 minutes	Exchanges: 2 vegetable
Yield: 4 servings	Carbohydrate choices: ½

Serving size: ½ cup

Nutrition per serving:

Calories: 43	Saturated fat: . . . . .0 g
Carbohydrate: . . . . .9 g	Cholesterol: . . . . .trace
Protein: . . . . .2 g	Dietary fiber: . . . . .3 g
Fat: . . . . .0 g	Sodium: . . . . .161 mg

Caesar salad

Traditional Caesar salad dressing calls for a raw egg yolk, but we recommend a soft-boiled yolk to decrease the risk of salmonella. Better yet, substitute a tablespoon of fat-free mayonnaise in the yolk's place and eliminate the risk completely.

1 large head romaine lettuce, washed and dried

1 large clove garlic, minced

½ teaspoon salt (optional)

½ teaspoon dry mustard

2 tablespoons olive or vegetable oil

2 tablespoons freshly squeezed lemon juice

1 teaspoon Worcestershire sauce

1 soft-cooked egg yolk

3 anchovy fillets, soaked in warm water, drained and chopped (optional)

1 cup toasted bread cubes or croutons

4 slices crisp cooked bacon (or turkey bacon), crumbled

1 tablespoon grated Parmesan cheese

1. Tear lettuce into bite-size pieces, place in a salad bowl, and refrigerate.

2. Blend together garlic, salt (optional), mustard, oil, lemon juice, Worcestershire sauce, egg yolk, and anchovies (optional) until smooth (add water to thin, if necessary).

3. Add the croutons, bacon, and Parmesan to the salad bowl with the lettuce. Pour dressing over and toss well. Serve immediately.

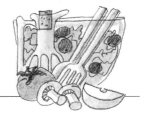

Preparation time: 10 minutes

Yield: 6 servings

Serving size: 1 cup

Exchanges: 1 vegetable
         1 lean meat
         1½ fat

Carbohydrate choices: ½

Nutrition per serving:

With anchovy		**Without anchovy**	
Calories:	.159	Calories:	.140
Carbohydrate:	.8 g	Carbohydrate:	.8 g
Protein:	.7 g	Protein:	.4 g
Fat:	.11 g	Fat:	.10 g
Saturated fat:	.3 g	Saturated fat:	.2 g
Cholesterol:	.57 mg	Cholesterol:	.50 mg
Dietary fiber:	.<1 g	Dietary fiber:	.<1 g
Sodium:	.436 mg	Sodium:	.422 mg
(omitting salt)	.258 mg	(omitting salt)	.244 mg

Celery Victor

**24 four-inch celery stalks or 6 celery hearts,
washed and halved lengthwise**

½ cup white wine vinegar

1 tablespoon freshly squeezed lemon juice

2 tablespoons minced fresh parsley

**1 tablespoon minced fresh oregano
or 1 teaspoon dried oregano**

½ teaspoon dried leaf thyme

1 whole bay leaf

½ teaspoon salt (optional)

¼ teaspoon freshly ground black pepper

Pinch cayenne pepper

6 whole lettuce leaves, washed and dried

2 tablespoons capers, rinsed and drained

2 tablespoons chopped pimento

The lemon-herb broth in this recipe lends a delicious flavor to this dish. For a slightly different texture and flavor, chill the celery for an hour or two before serving.

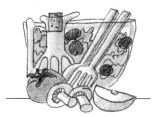

1. In a large, nonreactive saucepan with a lid, cook the celery in enough lightly salted water to cover until slightly tender but still crisp, about 7–10 minutes.

2. Drain off all but ½ cup of the water, leaving the celery in the pan. Add the vinegar, lemon juice, herbs, and seasonings. Bring to a boil, lower the heat to a simmer, cover, and cook about 5 minutes. Turn off heat and allow to cool.

3. When ready to serve, drain the celery and place decoratively on lettuce leaves. Garnish with capers and pimento.

108

Preparation time: 10 minutes
Cooking time: 15 minutes

Yield: 6 servings
Serving size: 4 celery stalks or
            ½ celery heart

Exchanges: free
Carbohydrate choices: 0

Nutrition per serving:
Calories: 15
Carbohydrate: . . . . .3 g
Protein: . . . . .1 g
Fat: . . . . .trace

Saturated fat: . . . . .trace
Cholesterol: . . . . .0 mg
Dietary fiber: . . . . .2 g
Sodium: . . . . .183 mg
(omitting salt) . . . . .76 mg

Marinated vegetable medley

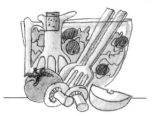

1/4 **cup cider vinegar**
1 **tablespoon vegetable oil**
1/4 **teaspoon onion powder**
1/2 **teaspoon freshly ground black pepper**
1 **cup cauliflower florets**
1 **cup broccoli florets**
1 **cup sliced celery**
1 **medium carrot, peeled and sliced**
1/2 **cucumber, peeled, seeded, and sliced**
1 **large tomato, cut into 8 wedges**

1. In a small mixing bowl, whisk together the vinegar, oil, onion powder, and pepper until well blended.
2. In a large bowl, combine the cauliflower, broccoli, celery, carrot, and cucumber.
3. Pour the dressing over the vegetables and toss until well coated. Cover and refrigerate at least 3 hours or up to 3 days. Add the tomato wedges just before serving.

Looking for a good vegetable dish but out of ideas? This one offers a crisp texture with a light pickled flavor.

109

Preparation time: 15 minutes
Chilling time: at least 3 hours

Exchanges: 1 vegetable
Carbohydrate choices: 1/2

Yield: 8 servings
Serving size: 1/2 cup

Nutrition per serving:
Calories: 38
Carbohydrate: . . . . .5 g
Protein: . . . . .1 g
Fat: . . . . .2 g
Saturated fat: . . . . .trace
Cholesterol: . . . . .0 mg
Dietary fiber: . . . . .2 g
Sodium: . . . . .24 mg

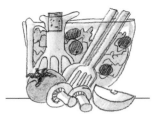

Spinach is a good source of potassium and vitamin A. And it tastes great—especially when it's prepared this way!

Spinach salad

1 small bunch fresh spinach, washed, stemmed, and dried
1 large red onion, thinly sliced into rings
1 large orange, peeled and sectioned
¼ cup orange juice
1 tablespoon olive or vegetable oil
1 clove garlic, minced
½ teaspoon salt (optional)
¼ teaspoon freshly ground black pepper

1. Tear spinach leaves into bite-size pieces and place in a salad bowl. Add the onion rings and orange segments.
2. In a small bowl, whisk together the orange juice, oil, garlic, salt (optional), and pepper. Pour over spinach mixture and toss well to coat.

110

Preparation time: 10 minutes

Yield: 4 servings
Serving size: 1½ cups

Exchanges: ½ fruit
 1 vegetable
 ½ fat
Carbohydrate choices: ½

Nutrition per serving:
Calories: 72
Carbohydrate: . . . . .9 g
Protein: . . . . .1 g
Fat: . . . . .3 g

Saturated fat: . . . . .trace
Cholesterol: . . . . .0 mg
Dietary fiber: . . . . .2 g
Sodium: . . . . .285 mg
(omitting salt) . . . . .18 mg

Crunchy layered salad

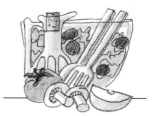

6 cups coarsely shredded lettuce
1 medium red onion, chopped
1 cup chopped green or red sweet pepper
1 cup chopped celery
1 cup frozen peas, uncooked
1 cup Cider Vinegar Dressing (recipe, p. 115)
** or fat-free mayonnaise**
3 slices bacon (or turkey bacon), crisply cooked
** and crumbled**
1 cup shredded low-fat Cheddar cheese

1. Place the lettuce in an even layer in a 9-inch square glass dish or salad bowl. Add alternating layers of onion, green pepper, celery, and peas.
2. Spoon the dressing or mayonnaise over the top layer, spreading to the edges of the dish. Sprinkle with crumbled bacon and cheese.
3. Cover tightly with plastic wrap and refrigerate at least 6 hours. (Will keep 1–2 days in the refrigerator if not mixed.) To serve, cut into squares.

A thin coating of dressing spread over this salad keeps the air out, so the lettuce and vegetables remain crisp and fresh while it chills.

111

Preparation time: 15 minutes
Chilling time: 6 hours

Yield: 9 servings
Serving size: 1 three-inch
                        square

Exchanges: 2 vegetable
                   ½ fat
Carbohydrate choices: ½

Nutrition per serving:

With bacon		**With turkey bacon**	
Calories:	77	Calories:	68
Carbohydrate:	. . . . .9 g	Carbohydrate:	. . . . .9 g
Protein:	. . . . .4 g	Protein:	. . . . .4 g
Fat:	. . . . .3 g	Fat:	. . . . .2 g
Saturated fat:	. . . . .2 g	Saturated fat:	. . . . .1 g
Cholesterol:	. . . . .15 mg	Cholesterol:	. . . . .13 mg
Dietary fiber:	. . . . .2 g	Dietary fiber:	. . . . .2 g
Sodium:	. . . . .516 mg	Sodium:	. . . . .496 mg
(omitting salt)	. . . . . . .258 mg	(omitting salt)	. . . . . . .244 mg

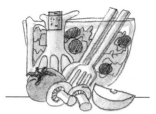

Potato salad

Baking potatoes (sometimes called Russets) tend to fall apart when blended together, so avoid using these. Idaho, Baby Red, and Yellow potatoes are ideal for this salad.

2 medium potatoes, washed and peeled
1 whole bay leaf
¼ cup minced onion, rinsed in a sieve and squeezed dry
¼ cup chopped celery
¼ cup Cider Vinegar Dressing (recipe, p. 115) or fat-free mayonnaise
1 teaspoon Dijon mustard
¼ teaspoon celery seed
½ teaspoon salt (optional)
½ teaspoon freshly ground black pepper

1. In a medium saucepan, place potatoes and bay leaf. Cover with cold water, bring to a boil, lower heat to a simmer and cook until tender, about 15–20 minutes. Drain, cover with cold water, and allow to sit about 5 minutes.
2. Drain and slice the potatoes into bite-size chunks. In a mixing bowl, combine the potatoes, onion, and celery.
3. In a small bowl, whisk together the dressing or mayonnaise, mustard, and celery seed; pour this over the potato mixture and toss well to coat. Season to taste with salt (optional) and pepper. Refrigerate 2–3 hours before serving.

112

Preparation time: 20 minutes
Cooking time: 25 minutes
Chilling time: 2–3 hours

Yield: 4 servings
Serving size: ½ cup

Exchanges: 1 starch
Carbohydrate choices: 1

Nutrition per serving:
Calories: 78
Carbohydrate: . . . . .18 g
Protein: . . . . .2 g
Fat: . . . . .0 g

Saturated fat: . . . . .0 g
Cholesterol: . . . . .trace
Dietary fiber: . . . . .2 g
Sodium: . . . . .417 mg
(omitting salt) . . . . . . .150 mg

Garbanzo garden green salad

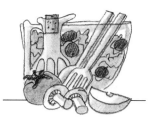

2 cups shredded lettuce
1¼ cups drained canned or home-cooked garbanzo beans
½ cup sliced celery
¼ cup diced green pepper
¼ cup chopped red onion
2 tablespoons minced fresh parsley
2 tablespoons freshly squeezed lemon juice
1 tablespoon olive or vegetable oil
1 clove garlic, minced
½ teaspoon salt (optional)
¼ teaspoon freshly ground black pepper

Garbanzo beans, also known as chickpeas, are not only tasty but rich in protein. They make a great addition to any tossed salad.

In a salad bowl, combine the lettuce, garbanzos, celery, green pepper, and onion. In a small mixing bowl, whisk together the parsley, lemon juice, oil, and minced garlic; pour over salad and toss well to coat. Season to taste with salt (optional) and pepper. Serve immediately.

113

Preparation time: 15 minutes
Yield: 6 servings
Serving size: ½ cup

Nutrition per serving:
Calories: 85
Carbohydrate: . . . . .11 g
Protein: . . . . .3 g
Fat: . . . . .3 g

Exchanges: ½ starch
     1 vegetable
     ½ fat
Carbohydrate choices: ½

Saturated fat: . . . . .trace
Cholesterol: . . . . .0 mg
Dietary fiber: . . . . .3 g
Sodium: . . . . .191 mg
(omitting salt) . . . . .13 mg

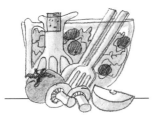

Thousand Island dressing

This dressing isn't just
for salads. Try it as
a dip for hot or cold
vegetables, a topping for
fish, or a sauce for beef.
Or use it as a sandwich
spread, instead of may-
onnaise or mustard.

1 cup Tomato French Dressing (recipe, below)
2 tablespoons chopped pickle relish
2 tablespoons capers, rinsed
2 tablespoons plain nonfat yogurt

Combine all the ingredients in a bowl and whisk to
blend. Store covered in the refrigerator for up to 1 month.

Preparation time: 5 minutes
Yield: 20 servings
Serving size: 1 tablespoon

Exchanges: free
Carbohydrate choices: 0

Nutrition per serving:
Calories: 13
Carbohydrate: . . . . .3 g
Protein: . . . . .1 g
Fat: . . . . .trace

Saturated fat: . . . . .0 g
Cholesterol: . . . . .0 mg
Dietary fiber: . . . . .0 g
Sodium: . . . . .11 mg

114

Tomato French dressing

*Tomato soup makes
a quick, convenient
base for this dressing.
Feel free to play with
different spices in
this recipe.*

1 can (about 10 ounces) low-sodium tomato soup,
    undiluted
2 tablespoons red wine vinegar
1 tablespoon minced fresh parsley
1 tablespoon minced fresh basil
    or 1 teaspoon dried basil
½ teaspoon dried leaf thyme
1 teaspoon dry mustard
½ teaspoon garlic powder
½ teaspoon Worcestershire sauce
¼ teaspoon freshly ground black pepper

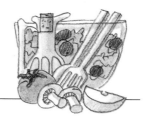

Combine all of the ingredients in a bowl and whisk until
well blended. Refrigerate at least 2 hours before using.
Store covered in the refrigerator for up to 1 month.

Preparation time: 5 minutes
Chilling time: at least 2 hours

Exchanges: free
Carbohydrate choices: 0

Yield: 16 servings
Serving size: 1 tablespoon

Nutrition per serving:
Calories: 15
Carbohydrate: . . . . .3 g
Protein: . . . . .1 g
Fat: . . . . .trace

Saturated fat: . . . . .trace
Cholesterol: . . . . .0 mg
Dietary fiber: . . . . .0 g
Sodium: . . . . .7 mg

Cider vinegar dressing

1 cup cider vinegar

3 eggs

¼ cup all-purpose flour

1 tablespoon dry mustard

1 teaspoon salt (optional)

¼ teaspoon freshly ground black pepper

2 cups cold water

2 tablespoons margarine

**Artificial sweetener equivalent to ½ cup sugar
(optional)**

*This dressing is so versa-
tile that we've used it in
several recipes through-
out this book. It will
soon become a favorite
of yours as well.*

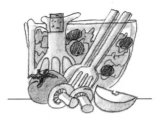

1. In a heavy saucepan, whisk together the vinegar, eggs, flour, mustard, salt (optional), pepper, and 2 cups of water. Cook over medium heat, stirring constantly, until smooth and thickened, about 6 minutes.

2. Remove from heat, stir in margarine and artificial sweetener (optional). Whisk until smooth. Store covered in refrigerator for up to 3 months.

Preparation time: 5 minutes
Cooking time: 10 minutes

Exchanges: free
Carbohydrate choices: 0

Yield: 35 servings
Serving size: 2 tablespoons

Nutrition per serving:
Calories: 14
Carbohydrate: . . . . .1 g
Protein: . . . . .1 g
Fat: . . . . .1 g

Saturated fat: . . . . .trace
Cholesterol: . . . . .0 mg
Dietary fiber: . . . . .0 g
Sodium: . . . . .88 mg
(omitting salt) . . . . .12 mg

116

Wine and mustard dressing

This dressing is perfect for an elegant dinner. Serve it over a mix of chopped Romaine lettuce, spinach, and chopped red cabbage.

⅓ cup vegetable oil

2 tablespoons lemon juice

2 teaspoons Worcestershire sauce

⅛ teaspoon salt

¼ teaspoon onion powder

⅛ teaspoon white pepper

¼ teaspoon dry mustard

1 teaspoon honey

¼ cup white wine

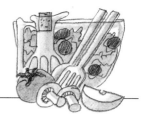

Combine all ingredients in a food processor or blender and mix for 1 minute. Store in refrigerator and mix well before using.

Preparation time: 5 minutes

Yield: ¾ cup
Serving size: 1 tablespoon

Exchanges: 1 fat
Carbohydrate choices: 0

Nutrition per serving:
Calories: 59
Carbohydrate: . . . . .trace
Protein: . . . . .trace
Fat: . . . . .6 g

Saturated fat: . . . . .trace
Cholesterol: . . . . .0 mg
Dietary fiber: . . . . .0 g
Sodium: . . . . .30 mg

Slim-and-trim Italian dressing

⅓ **cup canned low-sodium chicken broth**

1 tablespoon vegetable oil

1 tablespoon freshly squeezed lemon juice

1 tablespoon red wine vinegar

1 clove garlic, peeled and halved

1 teaspoon minced Italian parsley

**1 teaspoon minced fresh basil
  or ½ teaspoon dried basil**

¼ **teaspoon dried oregano**

¼ **teaspoon dried leaf thyme**

¼ **teaspoon salt (optional)**

¼ **teaspoon freshly ground black pepper**

Store-bought Italian dressing is one of the most popular kinds of dressings—and also one of the most fattening. Try this slimmed-down version of the original.

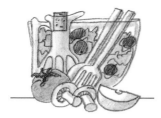

Combine all of the ingredients in a bowl, and whisk until well blended. Refrigerate at least 30 minutes before serving. Remove garlic before using.

Preparation time: 10 minutes
Chilling time: 30 minutes

Yield: 8 servings
Serving size: 1 tablespoon

Exchanges: free
Carbohydrate choices: 0

Nutrition per serving:
Calories: 17
Carbohydrate: . . . . .trace
Protein: . . . . .trace
Fat: . . . . .2 g

Saturated fat: . . . . .trace
Cholesterol: . . . . .0 mg
Dietary fiber: . . . . .0 g
Sodium: . . . . .69 mg
(omitting salt) . . . . .2 mg

Raspberry vinaigrette

Keeping raspberry seeds out of this dressing can be tricky, but here's a secret: If you wind up with seeds in your vinegar, strain them out using cheesecloth instead of a sieve.

For the raspberry vinegar:
1½ cups fresh raspberries or thawed, unsweetened frozen raspberries
¾ cup white vinegar

For the dressing:
¼ cup raspberry vinegar
1 clove garlic, minced
1 green onion (white portion only), minced
1 tablespoon fresh rosemary, finely chopped, or 1½ teaspoons dried rosemary, crushed
⅛ teaspoon salt (optional)
⅛ teaspoon black pepper
¾ cup olive oil

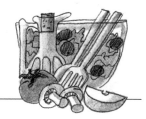

1. Combine raspberries and vinegar in a bowl and let soak for 30 minutes. Place a fine wire-mesh strainer over a second bowl, and pour raspberries and vinegar through strainer. Use a large spoon to force raspberry juice through the strainer, being careful not to let raspberry seeds pass through. Yield is one cup. One-quarter cup will be used in the next step. Remainder should be tightly covered and refrigerated for future use.

2. In a small bowl, whisk together 1/4 cup of raspberry vinegar, garlic, onion, rosemary, salt, and pepper. Slowly whisk in olive oil. Refrigerate at least 1 hour to allow flavors to blend.

Preparation time: 15 minutes Exchanges: 2 fat
Standing time: 30 minutes Carbohydrate choices: 0
Chilling time: 1 hour

Yield: 1 cup
Serving size: 1 tablespoon

Nutrition per serving:
Calories: . . . . .96 Saturated fat: . . . . .1 g
Carbohydrate: . . . . .1 g Cholesterol: . . . . .0 mg
Protein: . . . .<1 g Dietary fiber: . . . .<1 g
Fat: . . . . .10 g Sodium: . . . . .19 mg
             (omitting salt) . . . . .2 mg

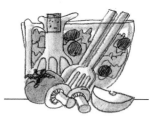

Herb buttermilk dressing

If you like creamy salad dressings, this one is for you. The buttermilk gives a wonderful flavor without the fat.

1½ cups buttermilk
1 tablespoon minced fresh parsley
1 tablespoon minced onion, rinsed in a sieve
   and drained
½ teaspoon garlic powder or 1 clove garlic, minced
½ teaspoon dried leaf thyme
½ teaspoon dried tarragon
   or 1 teaspoon minced fresh tarragon
½ teaspoon salt (optional)
¼ teaspoon freshly ground black pepper
1 teaspoon cider vinegar
½ teaspoon Worcestershire sauce

Combine all of the ingredients in a mixing bowl, and whisk until well blended. Refrigerate about 2 hours to allow flavors to blend. Store covered in the refrigerator for up to 1 month.

120

Preparation time: 10 minutes
Chilling time: 2 hours

Yield: 12 servings
Serving size: 2 tablespoons

Nutrition per serving:
Calories: 13
Carbohydrate: . . . . .1 g
Protein: . . . . .1 g
Fat: . . . . .trace

Exchanges: free
Carbohydrate choices: 0

Saturated fat: . . . . .trace
Cholesterol: . . . . .1 mg
Dietary fiber: . . . . .0 g
Sodium: . . . . .123 mg
(omitting salt) . . . . . . .34 mg

Chapter 5

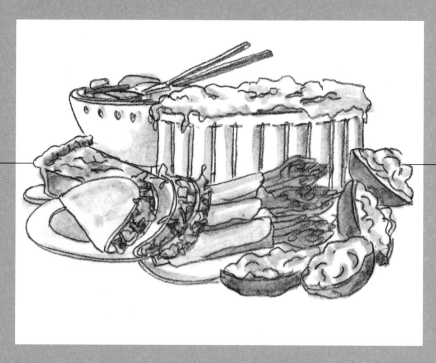

ONE-DISH MEALS

*W*ho isn't pressed for time these days? If we aren't running around worried about work, then we are worried about things that need to be done around the house, errands that need to be run, bills that have to be paid—sometimes it seems as if life is rushing past us.

One thing you won't have to worry about is dinner. The recipes in this chapter are designed for those days when you are pressed for time and can't deal with the hassle of making a big meal. One-dish meals can be real time-savers both before and after dinner—just think, no sink full of dishes when you are done.

The recipes here are as delicious as they are easy to make. Traditional fare like Country Cabbage Rolls and Shepherd's Pie will satisfy those who hunger for home cooking. Have a taste for something more exotic? Try Chinese tonight, with Pineapple Pork Stir-Fry or Chinese Chicken and Snow Peas. If Mexican is more to your liking, recipes for Enchiladas or Tacos await you. And there's no longer a reason for you to avoid Italian, not with our Low-Cal Lasagna recipe.

Chicken crepes

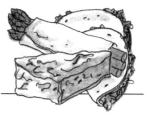

1¼ cups low-sodium chicken broth
1 teaspoon cornstarch
2 tablespoons raisins
8 dried apricot halves, coarsely chopped
½ teaspoon cinnamon
½ teaspoon chili powder
1½ cups cooked chicken, cut in chunks
4 Crepes (recipe, p. 362)
2 tablespoons slivered almonds, toasted

The combination of raisins, apricots, and cinnamon gives this chicken recipe a distinctive and delectable flavor.

1. In a medium saucepan, combine the broth and cornstarch; whisk to dissolve. Add the raisins, apricots, cinnamon, and chili powder; bring to a boil. Reduce heat and simmer uncovered, stirring occasionally, until thickened and reduced, about 10 minutes.
2. Add the chicken chunks to the sauce and simmer, stirring occasionally, about 5 minutes.
3. Place warmed crepes on warm serving plates. Divide the filling between the crepes, reserving a small amount for the top. Roll or fold the crepes. Spoon reserved filling on top. Garnish with toasted almonds. Serve immediately.

123

Preparation time: 15 minutes
Cooking time: 15 minutes

Yield: 4 servings
Serving size: ½ cup filling with 1 crepe

Exchanges: 1½ carbohydrate
3 lean meat
Carbohydrate choices: 1½

Nutrition per serving:
Calories: 253
Carbohydrate: . . . . .21 g
Protein: . . . . .26 g
Fat: . . . . .7 g

Saturated fat: . . . . .2 g
Cholesterol: . . . . .58 mg
Dietary fiber: . . . . .3 g
Sodium: . . . . .106 mg

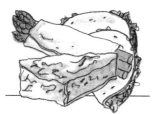

Chinese chicken and snow peas

*Everyone likes stir-fry—
especially the cook who
knows how easy it is!
Fresh snow peas might
be difficult to find, so
feel free to substitute
with thawed, frozen
peas or green beans.*

124

**1 pound boneless chicken breasts,
skinned and sliced diagonally into ½-inch strips**
2 teaspoons cornstarch
2 tablespoons vegetable oil
2 stalks celery, sliced diagonally
1 green onion, thinly sliced diagonally
1 clove garlic, minced
1 tablespoon fresh minced ginger
½ cup low-sodium chicken broth
4 ounces fresh snow peas, stems and strings removed
1 tablespoon low-sodium soy sauce (or more to taste)
¼ cup sliced water chestnuts
2 cups hot, cooked long-grain rice

1. In a mixing bowl, toss the chicken strips with the cornstarch. Heat 1 tablespoon of the oil in a wok or frying pan until hot. Stir-fry the chicken pieces in the wok until golden, about 5 minutes. Remove the chicken to a warm plate.
2. Heat the remaining oil in the wok and add the celery, onion, garlic, and ginger; stir-fry until fragrant, about 4 minutes. Add the chicken broth and simmer 4 minutes.
3. Add the snow peas, soy sauce, water chestnuts, and chicken strips. Cover and cook about 2 more minutes, or until the chicken is reheated and the snow peas are crisp-tender. Serve immediately over hot rice.

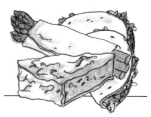

Preparation time: 10 minutes
Cooking time: 15 minutes

Yield: 4 servings
Serving size: 2 cups
over ½ cup rice

Exchanges: 2 starch
3 lean meat
Carbohydrate choices: 2

Nutrition per serving:
Calories: 334
Carbohydrate: . . . . .28 g
Protein: . . . . .33 g
Fat: . . . . .10 g
Saturated fat: . . . . .2 g
Cholesterol: . . . . .71 mg
Dietary fiber: . . . . .4 g
Sodium: . . . . .735 mg

125

Quick crustless quiche

Nonfat cooking spray
1 cup chopped broccoli, blanched and refreshed
1½ cups shredded low-fat Swiss cheese
¼ cup chopped onion
3 slices lean luncheon meat, chopped
2 cups skim milk
2 eggs (or ½ cup egg substitute)
2 egg whites
½ cup all-purpose flour
1 teaspoon baking powder
½ teaspoon salt (optional)
¼ teaspoon freshly ground black pepper
⅛ teaspoon freshly grated nutmeg

Without the traditional pastry crust, this quiche is not only much lower in fat and calories, but also much easier to make.

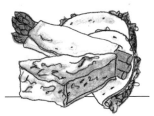

1. Coat a 9-inch pie plate with cooking spray. Combine the broccoli, cheese, onion, and meat; spread in the prepared pie plate. Preheat the oven to 325°F.

2. In a blender, food processor, or large mixing bowl, combine the milk, eggs (or egg substitute), egg whites, flour, baking powder, salt (optional), pepper, and nutmeg. Blend or whisk vigorously until smooth.

3. Pour egg mixture over vegetables in the pie plate. Bake until set, or until a knife inserted in the center comes out clean, about 45 minutes. Let stand 5 minutes before serving.

Preparation time: 10 minutes
Baking time: 45 minutes

Yield: 6 servings
Serving size: ⅙ pie

Exchanges: 1 starch
          2 lean meat
Carbohydrate choices: 1

Nutrition per serving:

	With eggs	*With egg substitute*
Calories:	204	199
Carbohydrate:	14 g	15 g
Protein:	18 g	18 g
Fat:	8 g	7 g
Saturated fat:	4 g	4 g
Cholesterol:	69 mg	24 mg
Dietary fiber:	1 g	1 g
Sodium:	1,013 mg	1,028 mg
(omitting salt)	835 mg	850 mg

Low-cal lasagna

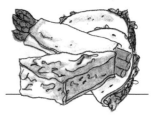

½ cup freshly grated Parmesan cheese
1 cup Basic White Sauce (recipe, p. 354)
1 pound lean ground beef, cooked and drained of fat
1 package frozen chopped spinach, thawed
3 cups Spaghetti Sauce (recipe p. 357)
9 lasagna noodles, cooked and drained
8 ounces shredded low-fat mozzarella cheese

1. Preheat oven to 350°F. Stir all but 1–2 tablespoons of the Parmesan cheese into the White Sauce. Set aside.
2. Spoon about ¾ cup of the Spaghetti Sauce into the bottom of a greased 13" × 9" baking pan. Top with 2 cooked lasagna noodles, half the spinach, half the beef, a third of the Parmesan–White Sauce, and another ¾ cup of spaghetti sauce. Repeat this layering, ending with the last 3 noodles, the remainder of the Parmesan–White Sauce, mozzarella, spaghetti sauce, and Parmesan cheese.
3. Cover pan with foil and bake 30–35 minutes. Remove foil and bake uncovered 10–15 minutes longer, or until lightly browned. Let stand 5 minutes before serving.

No need to avoid your favorite dish again—not with this delicious, low-calorie version! Serve it with a green salad for a complete, healthy meal.

127

Preparation time: 15 minutes
Cooking time: 50 minutes

Yield: 9 servings
Serving size: one 3" × 4" piece

Exchanges: 1 starch
1 vegetable
3 medium-fat meat
Carbohydrate choices: 1½

Nutrition per serving:
Calories: 323
Carbohydrate: . . . . .26 g
Protein: . . . . .25 g
Fat: . . . . .13 g

Saturated fat: . . . . .7 g
Cholesterol: . . . . .58 mg
Dietary fiber: . . . . .3 g
Sodium: . . . . .703 mg

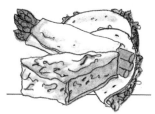

Pizza lover's pizza

Nothing will ever make pizza fat-free, but this recipe is as close as you can get. Try this instead of take-out!

For the crust:

1 teaspoon sugar

½ cup warm water (about 110°F)

1½ teaspoons (½ package) active dry yeast

1 cup plus 2 tablespoons all-purpose flour

1½ teaspoons baking powder

½ teaspoon salt

1 tablespoon olive oil

For the topping:

1 cup Spaghetti Sauce (recipe, p. 357)

1 onion, chopped

1 green pepper, chopped

2 cups sliced mushrooms

3 ounces pepperoni (or Canadian bacon), sliced

8 ounces shredded low-fat mozzarella cheese

2 tablespoons grated Parmesan cheese

128

1. In a small bowl, dissolve the sugar in the warm water. Sprinkle the yeast over the water, stir, and allow to proof, about 5 minutes. Preheat the oven to 375°F.

2. In a mixing bowl, combine ½ cup flour, baking powder, and salt. Add the yeast mixture and the olive oil, and beat vigorously, about 100 strokes. Gradually stir in the remaining ½ cup flour. Turn out onto a floured board and knead the dough until soft and smooth, about 5 minutes, adding 1 or 2 more tablespoons flour if necessary. Cover the dough with a damp dish towel and allow to sit at room temperature at least 10 minutes.

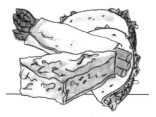

3. Stretch and pat the dough into a 12-inch round onto an oiled baking sheet or pizza pan, forming a lip around the rim of the dough. Bake 10 minutes.

4. Remove the crust from the oven and top with sauce, onions, peppers, mushrooms, pepperoni (or Canadian bacon), and cheeses. Return to oven and bake until crust is crisp and cheeses are bubbly, about 20–25 minutes. Cut into 8 wedges.

129

Preparation time: 30 minutes
Baking time: 35 minutes

Yield: 4 servings
Serving size: 2 slices

Exchanges: 2 starch
  1 vegetable
  1 medium-fat meat
  1½ fat
Carbohydrate choices: 2

Nutrition per serving:

With pepperoni

Calories: 347
Carbohydrate: . . . . .36 g
Protein: . . . . .16 g
Fat: . . . . .15 g
Saturated fat: . . . . .6 g
Cholesterol: . . . . .27 mg
Dietary fiber: . . . . .4 g
Sodium: . . . . .884 mg

With Canadian bacon

Calories: 327
Carbohydrate: . . . . .35 g
Protein: . . . . .17 g
Fat: . . . . .13 g
Saturated fat: . . . . .5 g
Cholesterol: . . . . .27 mg
Dietary fiber: . . . . .4 g
Sodium: . . . . .983 mg

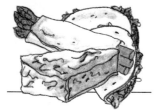

Beef and spinach bake

1 package frozen chopped spinach (10 ounces)
Nonfat cooking spray
1 pound ground chuck beef
½ cup chopped celery
½ cup chopped green pepper
½ cup chopped onion
¾ cup cooked rice
1 egg, beaten
¼ teaspoon salt (optional)
½ teaspoon dried thyme
¼ teaspoon black pepper
½ cup shredded reduced-fat Cheddar cheese

1. Preheat oven to 350°F. Cook spinach according to package directions. Drain well and set aside. Coat a large nonstick skillet with cooking spray. Add ground chuck, celery, green pepper, and onion. Cook over medium heat until browned and crumbled. Drain off fat.
2. Combine spinach, meat mixture, rice, egg, salt (optional), thyme, and pepper in a medium bowl and mix well. Place mixture in a 2-quart baking dish coated with cooking spray. Cover and bake 20 minutes. Top with cheese and bake uncovered 5 minutes longer, until cheese melts.

Preparation time: 20 minutes
Baking time: 25 minutes

Yield: 6 servings
Serving size: 1 cup

Exchanges: 1 starch
           2 medium-fat meat
           1 fat
Carbohydrate choices: 1

Nutrition per serving:
Calories: 267
Carbohydrate: . . . . .12 g
Protein: . . . . .20 g
Fat: . . . . .15 g

Saturated fat: . . . . .6 g
Cholesterol: . . . . .90 mg
Dietary fiber: . . . . .2 g
Sodium: . . . . .236 mg
(omitting salt) . . . . . . .147 mg

Curried lamb

2 teaspoons vegetable oil
1 cup chopped onion
1–2 tablespoons curry powder (or to taste)
2 tablespoons all-purpose flour
2 cups low-sodium beef or chicken broth
½ teaspoon salt (optional)
¼ teaspoon freshly ground black pepper
¾ pound cooked lean lamb, cut into cubes
¼ teaspoon cinnamon
1 Granny Smith apple, peeled, cored, and chopped

1. In a heavy saucepan, sauté the onion in the oil until translucent. Add the curry powder and flour, and cook, stirring, over medium heat 2–3 minutes.
2. Add the broth and cook until thickened, 3–5 minutes. Add the meat and seasonings to the sauce, cover, and cook over low heat 15–20 minutes. Add the chopped apple in the last 5 minutes of cooking.

This curry takes very little effort and is a great way to use up leftover lamb roast. Serve this over steamed rice.

131

Preparation time: 10 minutes
Cooking time: 40 minutes

Yield: 4 servings
Serving size: 1 cup

Exchanges: ½ carbohydrate
3 lean meat
½ fat
Carbohydrate choices: ½

Nutrition per serving:
Calories: 237
Carbohydrate: . . . . .10 g
Protein: . . . . .23 g
Fat: . . . . .12 g

Saturated fat: . . . . .4 g
Cholesterol: . . . . .73 mg
Dietary fiber: . . . . .2 g
Sodium: . . . . .364 mg
(omitting salt) . . . . .97 mg

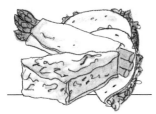

Ham-stuffed potatoes

A baked potato for lunch? Absolutely. With this ham and potato combination, you'll be looking forward to it.

4 small baking potatoes, scrubbed and pierced with a fork

¼ cup dry white wine

4 tablespoons cold water

2 teaspoons margarine

1 teaspoon minced fresh tarragon or ½ teaspoon dried tarragon

3 cups sliced fresh mushrooms

2 tablespoons tomato paste

2 green onions, finely chopped

8 ounces (about 2 cups) coarsely chopped cooked ham

⅓ cup evaporated skim milk

1. Bake the potatoes in a 400°F oven for 45 minutes (or MICROWAVE on High, wrapped individually in microwavable paper toweling, 5–10 minutes, depending on size), until tender. Wrap in foil to keep warm.
2. In a medium saucepan, combine the wine, 2 tablespoons water, margarine, and tarragon and bring to a boil. Add the mushrooms, cover, and cook 2 minutes. Add the tomato paste, green onions, and the remaining 2 tablespoons of water, and cook, stirring, 2 more minutes. Remove from heat and fold in the chopped ham.
3. Slice the baked potatoes in half lengthwise and scoop out most of the interior, reserving the shells. Mash the potato pulp and add it to the mushroom–ham mixture, along with the evaporated milk. Cook, stirring, over low heat just until heated through.
4. Spoon the filling into the reserved potato shells. Serve immediately, or place in an oiled baking dish for later reheating.

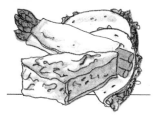

Preparation time: 10 minutes
Cooking time: 1 hour

Yield: 4 servings
Serving size: 1 stuffed potato

Nutrition per serving:
Calories: 242
Carbohydrate: . . . . .30 g
Protein: . . . . .16 g
Fat: . . . . .6 g

Exchanges: 2 starch
            2 lean meat
Carbohydrate choices: 2

Saturated fat: . . . . .2 g
Cholesterol: . . . . .23 mg
Dietary fiber: . . . . .4 g
Sodium: . . . . .777 mg

133

Ham and asparagus roll-ups

12 slices (about 1 ounce each) cooked ham
¾ cup shredded low-fat Cheddar cheese
24 fresh asparagus spears, ends trimmed, blanched
1 cup plus 2 tablespoons Cheese Sauce
** (recipe, p. 355)**
¼ teaspoon sweet paprika

1. Preheat oven to 350°F. Sprinkle each slice of ham with cheese (about ½ ounce) and roll up two asparagus spears inside each. Arrange in a shallow glass baking dish.
2. Pour the Cheese Sauce over the roll-ups and sprinkle with paprika. Bake 15–20 minutes (or MICROWAVE on High, covered, about 5–7 minutes, depending on size) or until sauce bubbles.

Not only does this make a good meal on its own, but these roll-ups are great appetizers for the next time you entertain.

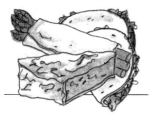

Preparation time: 10 minutes
Cooking time: 20 minutes

Yield: 6 servings
Serving size: 2 roll-ups with
              sauce

Exchanges: 3 lean meat
           1 vegetable
Carbohydrate choices: ½

Nutrition per serving:
Calories: 192
Carbohydrate: . . . . .5 g
Protein: . . . . .22 g
Fat: . . . . .9 g

Saturated fat: . . . . .3 g
Cholesterol: . . . . .36 mg
Dietary fiber: . . . . .1 g
Sodium: . . . . .1,212 mg

Chili con carne

Chili is probably the original one-dish meal. Notice how substituting ground turkey for beef dramatically lowers the overall calories, fat, and cholesterol.

1 teaspoon vegetable oil

1½ pounds lean ground beef (or ground turkey)

1 cup chopped onion

1 clove garlic, minced

2 cans (about 16 ounces each) whole tomatoes, chopped

1 can (about 14 ounces) tomato sauce

1–2 teaspoons chili powder (or to taste)

1 teaspoon salt (optional)

½ teaspoon dried oregano

½ teaspoon ground cumin

½ teaspoon freshly ground black pepper

1 whole bay leaf

1 can (about 15 ounces) kidney beans, rinsed and drained

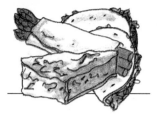

1. Film a large, heavy pot with the oil. Add the meat, onion, and green pepper and cook over medium-high heat, stirring, until the meat is thoroughly cooked. Drain off excess fat.

2. Add the garlic, tomatoes, tomato sauce, chili powder, salt (optional), oregano, cumin, black pepper, and bay leaf. Cover loosely and simmer about 1 hour, stirring occasionally. Taste for seasoning and add more if desired.

3. Add kidney beans and cook 20–30 minutes. Remove bay leaf and serve.

Preparation time: 10 minutes
Cooking time: 1¾ hours

Yield: 7–8 servings
Serving size: 1 cup

Nutrition per serving:

With ground beef	**With ground turkey**
Exchanges: 1 starch	Exchanges: 1 starch
1 vegetable	1 vegetable
3 medium-fat meat	3 lean meat
Carbohydrate choices: 1½	Carbohydrate choices: 1½
Calories: 330	Calories: 250
Carbohydrate: . . . . .23 g	Carbohydrate: . . . . .23 g
Protein: . . . . .28 g	Protein: . . . . .29 g
Fat: . . . . .14 g	Fat: . . . . .4 g
Saturated fat: . . . . .6 g	Saturated fat: . . . . .1 g
Cholesterol: . . . . .74 mg	Cholesterol: . . . . .56 mg
Dietary fiber: . . . . .7 g	Dietary fiber: . . . . .7 g
Sodium: . . . . .847 mg	Sodium: . . . . .834 mg
(omitting salt) . . . . . .542 mg	(omitting salt) . . . . . .529 mg

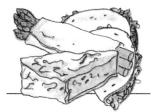

Enchiladas

Here's a mild version of a South-of-the-Border favorite. If you like your meals a little hotter, feel free to add cayenne pepper or Tabasco sauce to the meat mixture.

136

12 six-inch Whole Wheat Flour Tortillas (recipe, p. 365) or commercial whole wheat tortillas
1 pound lean ground beef (or ground turkey)
1 clove garlic, minced
2 green bell peppers, seeded and diced
1 onion, chopped
¼ cup minced fresh cilantro or parsley
2 tablespoons freshly squeezed lime juice or lemon juice
1 teaspoon salt (optional)
½ teaspoon ground cumin
¼ teaspoon chili powder (or more to taste)
¼ teaspoon freshly ground black pepper
2 cups cold water
1½ cups low-fat cottage cheese
2 tablespoons freshly grated Parmesan cheese
½ cup shredded low-fat mozzarella cheese

Fresh tomato sauce:
4 firm Italian tomatoes, peeled, seeded, and chopped
1 green bell pepper, seeded and chopped
¼ cup chopped onion
1 tablespoon chopped fresh cilantro or parsley
¼ cup cold water

1. Cook the tortillas until lightly browned but still pliable. In a sauté pan, over medium heat, brown the meat with the garlic until the meat is no longer pink. Drain off the fat.
2. Add the green pepper, onion, cilantro or parsley, lime or lemon juice, spices and seasonings, plus 2 cups of water, and simmer, uncovered, until the liquid is reduced by half, about 15–20 minutes. Preheat oven to 350°F.

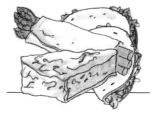

3. Add the cottage cheese and Parmesan to the meat mixture and cook, stirring, an additional 5 minutes. Spoon about 2–3 tablespoons of the mixture into each tortilla and roll up. Place the rolls in a lightly oiled shallow baking dish. Pour the remaining meat mixture over the filled enchiladas and bake 15 minutes.

4. Meanwhile, make the tomato sauce: In a small saucepan, combine the tomatoes, pepper, onion, cilantro or parsley, and ¼ cup water. Cook over medium heat, stirring, until the vegetables are tender, about 7–8 minutes.

5. Remove the enchiladas from the oven, top with the tomato sauce, and sprinkle with mozzarella cheese. Return to the oven for 5 minutes, or until the cheese is melted. Serve immediately.

Preparation time: 20 minutes
Cooking time: 50 minutes

Yield: 12 servings
Serving size: 1 enchilada
with sauce

Nutrition per serving:

With ground beef
Exchanges: 1 starch
2 medium-fat meat
Carbohydrate choices: 1

Calories:	.214
Carbohydrate:	.19 g
Protein:	.16 g
Fat:	.8 g
Saturated fat:	.3 g
Cholesterol:	.33 mg
Dietary fiber:	.2 g
Sodium:	.471 mg
(omitting salt)	.293 mg

With ground turkey
Exchanges: 1 starch
2 lean meat
Carbohydrate choices: 1

Calories:	.183
Carbohydrate:	.19 g
Protein:	.17 g
Fat:	.4 g
Saturated fat:	.2 g
Cholesterol:	.26 mg
Dietary fiber:	.2 g
Sodium:	.466 mg
(omitting salt)	.288 mg

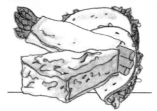

Tacos

Tacos are great on a busy night. Let everyone make his own buffet-style. Kids especially will love it.

1 teaspoon vegetable oil

¼ cup minced onion

¼ cup chopped green bell pepper

1 pound lean ground beef

1 teaspoon chili powder (or to taste)

½ teaspoon salt (optional)

¼ teaspoon freshly ground black pepper

1 teaspoon Worcestershire sauce (optional)

3–4 drops hot pepper (or Tabasco) sauce (or to taste)

1 can (about 6 ounces) tomato paste

¼ cup cold water

1 can (about 15 ounces) red kidney beans, rinsed and drained

12 six-inch Whole Wheat Flour Tortillas (recipe, p. 365) or commercial whole wheat tortillas

Topping:

3 cups assorted fresh vegetables (lettuce, tomatoes, cucumber, celery)

½ cup low-fat Cheddar cheese

1. Heat the oil in a saucepan. Sauté the onion and green pepper over medium heat about 2–3 minutes. Add the meat and cook, stirring, until brown; drain excess fat. Season with chili powder, salt (optional), pepper, Worcestershire (optional), and hot pepper (or Tabasco) sauce.

2. In a small bowl, whisk the tomato paste with ¼ cup water until smooth and pour into meat mixture. Add kidney beans and simmer, stirring occasionally, for 20 minutes. (Mixture should be thick.)

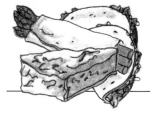

3. Meanwhile, prepare the tortillas according to the recipe on page 365*. Fold each in half after removing from the frying pan. Fill each shell with ¹⁄₁₂ of the sauce (about ¼ cup); top with ¼ cup chopped fresh vegetables and sprinkle with 2 teaspoons shredded cheese. Serve immediately.

If you use packaged whole wheat tortillas instead, heat them on a dry griddle or frying pan, flipping them until they are toasty and pliable.

Preparation time: 10 minutes
Cooking time: 30 minutes

Yield: 12 servings
Serving size: 1 taco

Exchanges: 1 starch
          2 vegetable
          2 medium-fat meat
Carbohydrate choices: 2

Nutrition per serving:
Calories: 259
Carbohydrate: . . . . .30 g
Protein: . . . . .15 g
Fat: . . . . .9 g

Saturated fat: . . . . .3 g
Cholesterol: . . . . .29 mg
Dietary fiber: . . . . .4 g
Sodium: . . . . .483 mg
(omitting salt) . . . . . .394 mg

Reuben casserole

4 cups mashed potatoes (without butter, milk, or salt)
¹⁄₃ cup fat-free sour cream
¼ cup skim milk
¼ teaspoon salt (optional)
¼ teaspoon black pepper
Nonfat cooking spray
4 cups cabbage, thinly sliced
¼ pound deli corned beef, finely chopped
½ teaspoon caraway seeds
¼ cup fat-free Thousand Island dressing
¾ cup plus ¼ cup shredded Swiss cheese
Paprika

You've never tasted anything quite like this casserole version of the famous sandwich.

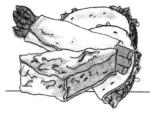

1. Preheat oven to 350°F. Combine potatoes, sour cream, milk, salt (optional), and pepper. Blend well and set aside.

2. Coat a large nonstick skillet with cooking spray and place over medium-high heat until hot. Add cabbage, corned beef, and caraway seeds; sauté for 4 minutes or until cabbage wilts. Remove from heat and stir in Thousand Island dressing. Set aside.

3. Spread half of the potato mixture in the bottom of an 11" × 17" baking dish coated with cooking spray. Top with cabbage mixture and sprinkle with ¾ cup cheese. Spread remaining potatoes over cheese and top with the remaining ¼ cup cheese. Sprinkle with paprika. Bake 40 minutes or until golden brown.

140

Preparation time: 30 minutes
Baking time: 40 minutes

Yield: 6 servings
Serving size: 1 cup

Exchanges: 2 starch
    1 high-fat meat
Carbohydrate choices: 2

Nutrition per serving:
Calories: 258
Carbohydrate: . . . . .30 g
Protein: . . . . .14 g
Fat: . . . . .10 g

Saturated fat: . . . . .5 g
Cholesterol: . . . . .34 mg
Dietary fiber: . . . . .2 g
Sodium: . . . . .470 mg
(omitting salt) . . . . . . .381 mg

Pineapple pork stir-fry

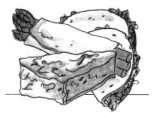

1 tablespoon vegetable oil

1½ pounds lean pork shoulder, leg, or loin, cut into bite-size cubes

1 can (about 15 ounces) unsweetened pineapple chunks, drained, juice reserved

1 tablespoon low-sodium soy sauce

1 teaspoon ground ginger

¼ teaspoon freshly ground black pepper

2 teaspoons cornstarch

1 green pepper, cored, seeded, and cut in chunks

1 tablespoon unsweetened shredded coconut

Pork is one of the most versatile meats. Here it goes well with pineapple and green pepper in a quick stir-fry dish that is both delicious and colorful.

1. Heat the oil in a wok or frying pan and stir-fry the pork until lightly browned. Drain off fat.

2. Combine pineapple liquid, soy sauce, ginger, and black pepper and pour over pork. Cover and simmer 20 minutes.

3. Whisk cornstarch into 1 tablespoon of water and stir into pork mixture. Cook about 3 minutes, until sauce thickens.

4. Stir in the pineapple chunks and green pepper. Cook 2–3 minutes longer, stirring, until the sauce coats and glazes the pork cubes. Garnish each serving with shredded coconut.

Preparation time: 10 minutes
Cooking time: 35 minutes

Yield: 9 servings
Serving size: ½ cup

Exchanges: 2 medium-fat meat
½ fruit
Carbohydrate choices: ½

Nutrition per serving:
Calories: 194
Carbohydrate: . . . . .8 g
Protein: . . . . .18 g
Fat: . . . . .9 g

Saturated fat: . . . . .4 g
Cholesterol: . . . . .52 mg
Dietary fiber: . . . .<1 g
Sodium: . . . . .108 mg

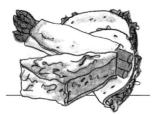

Shepherd's pie

This pie is tasty enough with ground beef, but try substituting other kinds of beef, pork, lamb, or turkey. If you're looking for a way to use leftover steak or roast, this recipe is it.

142

2 cups potatoes, peeled, cut into chunks
2 tablespoons freshly grated Parmesan cheese
1 pound lean ground meat
2 cups low-sodium beef broth
1 tablespoon all-purpose flour
2 teaspoons Worcestershire sauce
¼ teaspoon celery powder
¼ cup chopped onion
1½ cups frozen mixed vegetables
1 cup sliced fresh mushrooms

1. In a medium saucepan, cover the potatoes with cold water, salt lightly, and bring to a boil. Lower heat to a simmer and cook until tender, about 15–20 minutes.
2. Drain the potatoes, reserving about 3 tablespoons of cooking liquid. Mash the potatoes with the reserved liquid until fluffy; fold in Parmesan cheese, and set aside.
3. Brown the meat in a frying pan. Then, using a slotted spoon, transfer the cooked meat to a bowl; set aside. Drain fat from the pan. Preheat oven to 375°F.
4. In a mixing bowl, whisk together the broth, flour, Worcestershire, and celery powder until smooth. Add this mixture, along with the onions and vegetables, to the frying pan and cook, stirring occasionally, until thickened, about 5 minutes. Stir in the mushrooms and browned meat.
5. Spoon the mixture into a lightly oiled casserole dish. Top with mashed potatoes, spreading evenly over the top, and bake 30 minutes. Serve immediately.

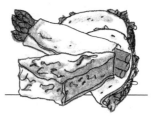

Preparation time: 20 minutes
Cooking time: 1 hour

Yield: 5 servings
Serving size: 1 cup

Exchanges: 1 starch
           3 medium-fat meat
           1 vegetable
Carbohydrate choices: 1½

Nutrition per serving:
Calories: 318
Carbohydrate: . . . . .25 g
Protein: . . . . .25 g
Fat: . . . . .13 g

Saturated fat: . . . . .6 g
Cholesterol: . . . . .70 mg
Dietary fiber: . . . . .3 g
Sodium: . . . . .213 mg

Turkey tetrazzini

2 tablespoons margarine

½ pound fresh mushrooms, cleaned and sliced

1 tablespoon freshly squeezed lemon juice

6 tablespoons all-purpose flour

2½ cups low-sodium chicken broth

1 cup skim milk

¼ dry sherry

2 tablespoons minced fresh parsley

1 teaspoon salt (optional)

½ teaspoon freshly grated nutmeg

½ teaspoon onion powder

¼ teaspoon paprika

¼ teaspoon white pepper

½ pound spaghetti or thin noodles

4 cups cooked turkey, cut into bite-size pieces

¼ cup freshly grated Parmesan cheese

*Wondering what to do
with that leftover turkey?
Here's a wonderful
after-Thanksgiving idea.*

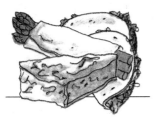

1. In a heavy frying pan, sauté the mushrooms in 1 table-spoon of the margarine until soft. Add the lemon juice and remaining tablespoon of margarine. Blend in the flour until smooth and cook over low heat 1–2 minutes.
2. Add the broth and milk, bring to a boil, lower heat and cook, stirring, until thickened, 2–3 minutes. Add the sherry, parsley, and seasonings and cook 2–3 more minutes. Preheat oven to 350°F.
3. Cook the spaghetti according to package directions. Drain well. Coat the bottom of a lightly oiled 10-cup casserole with sauce. Layer the mushrooms, spaghetti, and turkey over the sauce. Top with remaining sauce. Sprinkle with Parmesan cheese. Bake 30–40 minutes, or until bubbly.

144

Preparation time: 10 minutes
Cooking time: 50 minutes

Yield: 8 servings
Serving size: 1 cup

Exchanges: 2½ starch
          3 lean meat
Carbohydrate choices: 2½

Nutrition per serving:
Calories: 339
Carbohydrate: . . . . .39 g
Protein: . . . . .31 g
Fat: . . . . .6 g

Saturated fat: . . . . .2 g
Cholesterol: . . . . .59 mg
Dietary fiber: . . . . .2 g
Sodium: . . . . .422 mg
(omitting salt) . . . . . . .155 mg

Country cabbage rolls

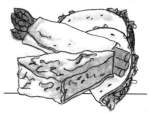

24 medium cabbage leaves (1 medium-sized head)
1 pound lean ground pork
½ pound lean ground beef
½ cup uncooked rice
2 cups tomato juice
⅓ cup chopped onion
1 clove garlic, minced
1 teaspoon salt (optional)
½ teaspoon freshly ground black pepper

These cabbage rolls may spend some time in the oven, but they are worth the wait. These will remind you of the ones your grandmother used to make.

1. Core the cabbage, wrap in plastic wrap, and freeze overnight to wilt the leaves. To separate leaves, run the frozen head under warm water at the core. Trim the center rib on each of the 24 leaves to give them a uniform thickness, but do not remove the ribs.
2. In a mixing bowl, combine the pork, beef, rice, ½ cup tomato juice, onion, garlic, and seasonings. Work together with your hands until well blended. Preheat the oven to 300°F.
3. Place one heaping tablespoon of the meat mixture on the rib end of a cabbage leaf. Roll up and tuck in the sides. Repeat with all of the leaves. Pack the cabbage rolls tightly into a lightly oiled 2-quart casserole.
4. Pour the remaining 1½ cups of tomato juice over the rolls. Cover tightly and bake 2 hours. Reduce heat to 250°F and bake an additional hour.

145

Preparation time: 30 minutes
Baking time: 2 hours

Yield: 24 cabbage rolls
Serving size: 3 cabbage rolls

Exchanges: ½ starch
　　　　　　 3 medium-fat meat
Carbohydrate choices: ½

Nutrition per serving:
Calories: 237
Carbohydrate: . . . . .11 g
Protein: . . . . .22 g
Fat: . . . . .11 g

Saturated fat: . . . . .5 g
Cholesterol: . . . . .65 mg
Dietary fiber: . . . . .2 g
Sodium: . . . . .545 mg
(omitting salt) . . . . . .278 mg

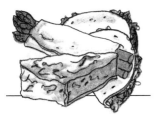

Savory luncheon buns

Though these buns hide a savory surprise, they are surprisingly low in calories. Serve them with soup or a salad.

For the buns:
2 teaspoons sugar
1 cup warm water
2 packages active dry yeast
½ cup margarine
⅓ cup sugar
1 teaspoon salt
1 cup cold water
2 eggs
6 cups all-purpose flour

For the filling:
1 pound finely chopped ham, about 3 cups
1 can (about 4 ounces) shrimp, rinsed, drained, and chopped
¼ cup minced fresh parsley
¼ cup chopped green onion or minced fresh chives
Sesame or poppy seeds (optional)

1. Dissolve the sugar in 1 cup of warm (110°F) water. Add the yeast, stir, and allow to proof 5–10 minutes.
2. In a medium saucepan, combine the margarine, ⅓ cup sugar, salt, and 1 cup water. Heat just until the margarine is melted. Cool to lukewarm.
3. In a mixing bowl, beat the eggs with the yeast mixture. Beat in 3 cups of the flour and the lukewarm margarine mixture. Gradually stir in enough of the remaining flour to make a soft dough.
4. Turn the dough out onto a lightly floured board and knead 8–10 minutes, until smooth and elastic. Place in a lightly oiled bowl, turning to oil all sides. Cover and place in a warm spot until doubled in size, about 1 hour.
5. Meanwhile, prepare the filling: In a mixing bowl, combine the ham, shrimp, parsley, and green onion or chives until well mixed. Set aside.

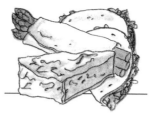

6. Punch the dough down and roll out on a floured board to an 18-inch square, about ¼-inch thick. Using a 3½-inch cutter, cut out 36 rounds from the dough. Place about 2 tablespoons of the filling in the center of each dough round. Pinch edges together tightly and roll between palms to form a bun.

7. Place the buns seam-side down, at least 2 inches apart, on a lightly greased baking sheet. If desired, brush the tops with water or milk, sprinkle with sesame or poppy seeds, and press the seeds lightly into the dough.

8. Cover the filled buns loosely with plastic wrap and set aside in a warm spot to rise until double, about 30 minutes. Bake in a 400°F oven for 12–15 minutes, or until golden brown.

147

Preparation time: 45 minutes
Rising time: 1½ hours
Baking time: 15 minutes

Yield: 36 filled buns
Serving size: 1 bun

Exchanges: 1 starch
       ½ medium-fat meat
Carbohydrate choices: 1

Nutrition per serving:
Calories: 121
Carbohydrate: . . . . .17 g
Protein: . . . . .5 g
Fat: . . . . .3 g

Saturated fat: . . . . .1 g
Cholesterol: . . . . .29 mg
Dietary fiber: . . . .<1 g
Sodium: . . . . .225 mg

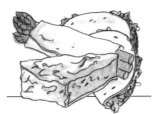

Easy oven stew

The name of this dish says it all. What could be easier than leaving this stew in the oven while you're running errands, then coming back to a finished meal?

148

1 pound lean stewing beef, cut into bite-size cubes
1 can (about 10 ounces) low-sodium tomato soup, undiluted
1 cup low-sodium beef broth
2 medium onions, chopped
2 large carrots, peeled and thickly sliced
1 bay leaf
½ teaspoon salt (optional)
¼ teaspoon freshly ground black pepper
¾ cup frozen peas

1. Preheat oven to 250°F.
2. In a medium-size casserole with a lid, combine the beef, soup, broth, onions, carrots, bay leaf, and seasonings. Stir well. Bring to a boil on the top of the stove. Cover, transfer to oven, and bake until the meat is very tender, about 3–4 hours. Stir once during cooking period.
3. Add the peas to the slow-baked stew during the last 15 minutes of cooking time.

Preparation time: 10 minutes
Cooking time: 3–4 hours

Yield: 4 servings
Serving size: 1 cup

Nutrition per serving:
Calories: 292
Carbohydrate: . . . . .27 g
Protein: . . . . .29 g
Fat: . . . . .7 g

Exchanges: 1 starch
3 lean meat
2 vegetable
Carbohydrate choices: 2

Saturated fat: . . . . .3 g
Cholesterol: . . . . .71 mg
Dietary fiber: . . . . .3 g
Sodium: . . . . .399 mg
(omitting salt) . . . . . . .132 mg

Chapter 6

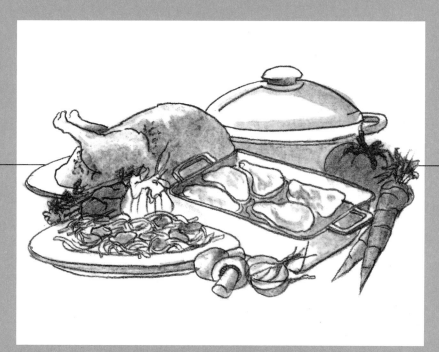

POULTRY

*C*ooks and health-conscious eaters all agree that chicken is a favorite. It is a versatile ingredient that lends itself to almost any method of preparation while being one of the leanest sources of protein in the diet. Removing the skin helps to keep fat and cholesterol levels very low.

Individually packaged, boneless, skinless chicken breasts can be expensive to purchase, but you can keep your grocery costs low by buying chickens whole and cutting them up yourself. Store breasts, legs, thighs, and wings in the freezer for up to two months by packaging them in airtight, zip-top storage bags.

You'll be pleased with the variety of recipes included here. Many are slimmed-down versions of your favorites. Instead of fattening fried chicken, try our delicious Oven "Fried" Chicken. Or try the "Creamed" Chicken, which uses skim milk and cornstarch in place of heavy cream. The Spicy Broiled Chicken makes a great summertime treat on the grill, and Pita Chicken Salad Sandwiches can be prepared ahead of time for a brown-bag lunch. Several of the recipes here can be made in the microwave for ease and speed.

Chicken, broccoli, and rice bake

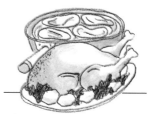

Nonfat cooking spray

1 package (10 ounces) frozen chopped broccoli, thawed

1 cup cooked white rice

2 cups diced cooked chicken breast

1 can (10¾ ounces) Campbell's Healthy Request cream of chicken soup

¼ cup reduced-fat mayonnaise

¼ cup skim milk

⅛ teaspoon curry powder

1 teaspoon dill

½ teaspoon lemon juice

1 tablespoon Seasoned Bread Crumbs (recipe, p. 363) or commercial bread crumbs

Paprika

This is a great way to use up leftover chicken. It works well with turkey also.

1. Preheat oven to 350°F. Coat an 8" × 8" pan with cooking spray. Layer broccoli in bottom of pan. Top evenly with rice and then chicken.

2. In a large bowl, whisk together soup, mayonnaise, milk, curry powder, dill, and lemon juice. Pour evenly over chicken.

3. Sprinkle top of casserole with bread crumbs and paprika. Spray cooking spray over bread crumbs to help them crisp during baking. Bake uncovered for 25–30 minutes, or until bubbly.

151

Preparation time: 15 minutes
Cooking time: 30 minutes

Yield: 4 servings
Serving size: ¼ recipe

Exchanges: 1 starch
           1 vegetable
           2 lean meat
           ½ fat
Carbohydrate choices: 1

Nutrition per serving:

Calories: 244	Saturated fat: . . . . 2 g
Carbohydrate: . . . . 20 g	Cholesterol: . . . . 60 mg
Protein: . . . . 23 g	Dietary fiber: . . . . 2 g
Fat: . . . . 8 g	Sodium: . . . . 382 mg

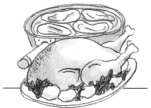

Quick chicken casserole

152

Cannellini beans, sometimes called white kidney beans, aren't the only kind of beans that work in this casserole. Try green beans or black-eyed peas for variety.

2 cans (14½ ounces each) no-salt-added chopped tomatoes, undrained

1 teaspoon olive oil

½ cup shallots, thinly sliced

2 cloves garlic, minced

1 pound boneless, skinless chicken breast halves, cut into bite-size pieces

1 teaspoon ground coriander

¼ teaspoon salt (optional)

¼ teaspoon ground pepper

1½ teaspoons dried thyme

2 cans (19 ounces each) cannellini beans, drained and rinsed

1. Preheat oven to 350°F. Drain tomatoes, reserving 1 cup liquid, and set both aside.

2. Heat oil in large skillet. Add shallots and garlic and sauté until tender. Add chicken, coriander, salt (optional), and pepper; stir well. Cook until chicken pieces are lightly browned.

3. Stir in tomatoes, reserved tomato liquid, thyme, and beans. Bring to a boil. Pour mixture into a 3-quart casserole, cover, and bake 20–25 minutes, until chicken is cooked thoroughly.

Preparation time: 15 minutes
Cooking time: 25 minutes

Yield: 7 servings
Serving size: about 1 cup

Exchanges: 2 starch
　　　　　 3 very lean meat
Carbohydrate choices: 2

Nutrition per serving:
Calories: 249
Carbohydrate:. . . . . 28 g
Protein: . . . . 24 g
Fat:. . . . . 5 g

Saturated fat: . . . . 1 g
Cholesterol:. . . . . 37 mg
Dietary fiber: . . . . 3 g
Sodium:. . . . . 596 mg
(omitting salt) . . . . 520 mg

Lime chicken

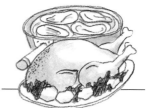

6 chicken breast halves, boneless and skinless
1 fresh lime
⅓ cup flour
1 teaspoon salt
2 teaspoons paprika
1 tablespoon vegetable oil
2 tablespoons brown sugar
½ cup chicken broth
½ cup white wine
2 tablespoons chopped fresh mint

Here's a simple but fla-vorful method that can be adapted for use with any kind of herb or spice. Eliminate the lime and brown sugar, use cayenne pepper and fresh minced oregano instead of paprika in the chicken coating, and you'll be surprised how different the dish turns out.

1. Preheat oven to 375°F. Wash chicken and pat dry. Grate zest from lime and set aside. Squeeze juice from lime over chicken. Then place chicken in a plastic bag containing the flour, salt, and paprika, and shake until chicken pieces are coated.
2. Heat oil in a nonstick oven-proof skillet and brown chicken on both sides. Combine lime zest and brown sugar. Sprinkle over chicken. Add broth and wine to pan. Sprinkle mint over top. Cover pan and bake 45 minutes. Garnish with extra lime slices or mint leaves if desired.

153

Preparation time: 15 minutes
Cooking time: 55 minutes

Yield: 6 servings
Serving size: 1 chicken breast
　　　　　　　with sauce

Exchanges: ½ carbohydrate
　　　　　　3 lean meat
Carbohydrate choices: ½

Nutrition per serving:
Calories: 200
Carbohydrate: . . . . 10 g
Protein: . . . . 20 g
Fat: . . . . 7 g

Saturated fat: . . . . 2 g
Cholesterol: . . . . 64 mg
Dietary fiber: . . . . trace
Sodium: . . . . 443 mg

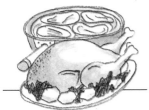

Caribbean stewed chicken

The lime juice, ginger, and cinnamon give this dish its Caribbean flavor, but the rosemary and thyme bring out the hearty taste of chicken. If there is cooking liquid left when you're finished, save it (refrigerated and covered) for use in another stew.

3 pounds chicken pieces
1 large onion, chopped
1 large tomato, peeled, seeded, and chopped
2 tablespoons freshly squeezed lime or lemon juice
1 tablespoon chopped fresh parsley
½ teaspoon dried thyme leaves
½ teaspoon dried rosemary, crumbled
¼ teaspoon ground ginger
¼ teaspoon ground cinnamon
3 cups low-sodium chicken broth
½ teaspoon salt (optional)
¼ teaspoon freshly ground black pepper
1 tablespoon margarine
2 tablespoons all-purpose flour
¼ teaspoon grated nutmeg

1. Remove the skin and all visible fat from the chicken pieces. Place the chicken, onion, tomato, lime juice, parsley, thyme, rosemary, ginger, and cinnamon in a mixing bowl; cover and refrigerate 2 hours, turning the chicken pieces after 1 hour.

2. Transfer the chicken mixture to a Dutch oven or covered casserole dish. Add the chicken broth, salt (optional), and pepper and simmer until the chicken is tender, about 1½ hours. (Or MICROWAVE on High, covered, in a microwave-safe dish, for 12–15 minutes.)

3. In a small saucepan, melt the margarine over medium-low heat. Add the flour and nutmeg and stir with a wooden spoon until well blended. Strain 1½ cups of the cooking liquid from the chicken into the flour mixture. Cook the sauce, stirring continuously, until thickened and smooth, about 3–4 minutes.

4. Place the chicken pieces on a warm platter and serve with the sauce hot.

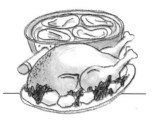

Preparation time: 10 minutes
Chilling time: 2 hours
Cooking time: 1½ hours

Yield: 6 servings
Serving size: ⅙ recipe

Nutrition per serving:

Exchanges: 3 lean meat
Carbohydrate choices: 0

Calories: 170	Saturated fat: . . . . 2 g
Carbohydrate: . . . . 4 g	Cholesterol: . . . . 67 mg
Protein: . . . . 23 g	Dietary fiber: . . . . <1 g
Fat: . . . . 7 g	Sodium: . . . . 309 mg
	(omitting salt) . . . . 131 mg

Chicken linguine stir-fry

155

1 box (8 ounces) linguine

1 tablespoon olive oil

1 pound boneless, skinless chicken breast, cut into bite-size pieces

1 medium onion, coarsely chopped

1 small zucchini, quartered and sliced into bite-size pieces

8 ounces fresh mushrooms, quartered

3 cloves garlic, crushed

¼ teaspoon crushed dried oregano

½ teaspoon dried basil

¼ teaspoon dried thyme

¾ teaspoon salt (optional)

½ teaspoon freshly ground black pepper

⅓ cup grated Parmesan cheese

2 Roma (plum) tomatoes, seeded and finely chopped

The secret to a great stir-fry is high heat and constant motion. Keep all the ingredients in the wok moving and they will cook, not burn.

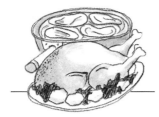

1. Bring a large pot of water to a rolling boil and add linguine. Cook for 7–9 minutes, until pasta is tender but firm. Drain and set aside.

2. While the pasta is cooking, heat the oil in the wok. Add the chicken and cook, stirring constantly, for 4–5 minutes. Remove chicken from wok and set aside.

3. Add onion to the wok and cook, stirring constantly, 1–2 minutes. Add zucchini, mushrooms, garlic, oregano, basil, thyme, salt (optional), and pepper. Continue cooking, stirring constantly, 3–4 minutes.

4. Add the drained linguine and cooked chicken to the mixture in the wok; toss well. Turn down the heat and cook 3–4 minutes, stirring frequently, to allow the linguine to absorb the flavors. Toss well again, then sprinkle with Parmesan cheese and chopped tomato. Serve immediately.

Preparation time: 20 minutes
Cooking time: 20 minutes

Yield: 4 servings
Serving size: 2 cups

Exchanges: 3 starch
    2 vegetable
    4 very lean meat
    ½ fat
Carbohydrate choices: 3

Nutrition per serving:

Calories: 449	Saturated fat: . . . . 1 g
Carbohydrate:. . . . . 52 g	Cholesterol:. . . . . 79 mg
Protein: . . . . 40 g	Dietary fiber: . . . . 2 g
Fat:. . . . . 9 g	Sodium:. . . . . 653 mg
	(omitting salt) . . . . 253 mg

Chicken divan

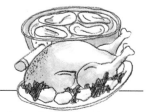

2 packages (10 ounces each) frozen broccoli spears, thawed
1 tablespoon lemon juice
6 chicken breast halves, boneless and skinless
2 tablespoons margarine
3 tablespoons flour
2 cups skim milk
⅛ teaspoon white pepper
½ teaspoon curry powder
¼ cup white wine
½ cup reduced-fat shredded Cheddar cheese
½ cup bread crumbs

If you have never eaten this divine chicken dish before—and even if you have—you must try this healthy version of the original. Serve this over hot white rice.

1. Preheat oven to 350°F. Place broccoli spears in a single layer on the bottom of a shallow, oiled baking dish. Sprinkle with lemon juice. Lay chicken breasts on top of broccoli.
2. Melt margarine over medium-low heat in a skillet. Blend in flour and stir until smooth. Cook mixture for 5 minutes, stirring constantly. Add milk and stir until thickened. Add pepper, curry, wine, and cheese, stirring to combine. Pour sauce over chicken. Sprinkle with bread crumbs.
3. Cover and bake for 1 hour. Remove cover and broil until golden brown on top.

157

Preparation time: 20 minutes
Cooking time: 60 minutes

Yield: 6 servings
Serving size: 1 chicken breast and ⅙ sauce and broccoli

Exchanges: 1 carbohydrate
5 lean meat
½ fat
Carbohydrate choices: 1

Nutrition per serving:
Calories: 380
Carbohydrate: . . . . 17 g
Protein: . . . . 42 g
Fat: . . . . 15 g
Saturated fat: . . . . 4 g
Cholesterol: . . . . 88 mg
Dietary fiber: . . . . 0 g
Sodium: . . . . 286 mg

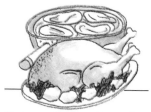

Chicken ratatouille stew

Ratatouille is a French word for recipes that combine onions, tomatoes, eggplant, zucchini, and green peppers. You can see what a great source of vegetables this dish can be.

1 teaspoon vegetable oil
2 tablespoons chopped shallot
2 cloves garlic, minced
1 can (14 ounces) chopped tomatoes
1 small eggplant, cut into 1-inch cubes
1 small zucchini, cut into 1/2-inch slices
1 small yellow squash, cut into 1/2-inch slices
1 red bell pepper, diced
1 green bell pepper, diced
1/2 teaspoon dried oregano
1/2 teaspoon dried rosemary
1/2 teaspoon dried basil
1/4 teaspoon ground black pepper
12 ounces boneless, skinless chicken breast meat,
    cut into 1-inch cubes, cooked

1. In a large, nonstick sauté pan, heat the oil and add shallot and garlic. Cook for 3–5 minutes over medium heat, until shallot is wilted and clear.
2. Add the tomato, eggplant, zucchini, squash, red and green pepper, oregano, rosemary, basil, and black pepper. Stir to combine ingredients and cook for 5–7 minutes, until vegetables are tender.
3. Add the cooked chicken and cook for an additional 3–5 minutes, until the chicken is reheated. Serve immediately.

Preparation time: 15 minutes
Cooking time: 20 minutes

Yield: 6 servings
Serving size: 1 cup

Exchanges: 2 vegetable
             2 lean meat
Carbohydrate choices: 1/2

Nutrition per serving:
Calories: 143
Carbohydrate: . . . . 9 g
Protein: . . . . 16 g
Fat: . . . . 5 g
Saturated fat: . . . . 1 g
Cholesterol: . . . . 32 mg
Dietary fiber: . . . . 2 g
Sodium: . . . . 145 mg

Oven "fried" chicken

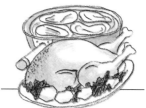

⅓ cup dry unseasoned bread crumbs
2 teaspoons sesame seeds
1½ tablespoons grated Parmesan cheese
¼ cup fat-free mayonnaise
¼ teaspoon salt (optional)
⅛ teaspoon garlic powder
2 dashes cayenne pepper
¼ teaspoon poultry seasoning
4 boneless, skinless chicken breast halves
Nonfat cooking spray

This healthy version of an old-time favorite might even be tastier than the original. For some extra crunch, add crushed, unsweetened corn or bran flakes to the bread crumb mixture before coating the chicken.

1. Preheat oven to 425°F. Place bread crumbs, sesame seeds, and Parmesan cheese in a large zip-top bag and shake gently to combine.
2. In a small bowl, whisk together mayonnaise, salt (optional), garlic powder, cayenne pepper, and poultry seasoning. Using a pastry brush, coat both sides of each piece of chicken with the mayonnaise mixture. Place chicken, one piece at a time, into the zip-top bag and shake to coat chicken well.
3. Transfer chicken to a foil-lined baking sheet coated with cooking spray. Spray chicken evenly with cooking spray. Bake for 20–25 minutes.

159

Preparation time: 10 minutes
Baking time: 25 minutes

Yield: 4 servings
Serving size: ½ breast

Exchanges: ½ starch
           5 very lean meat
           1 fat
Carbohydrate choices: ½

Nutrition per serving:
Calories: 238
Carbohydrate: . . . . 9 g
Protein: . . . . 37 g
Fat: . . . . 6 g

Saturated fat: . . . . 2 g
Cholesterol: . . . . 76 mg
Dietary fiber: . . . . 1 g
Sodium: . . . . 446 mg
(omitting salt): . . . . 313 mg

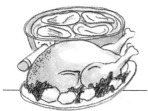

"Creamed" chicken

This chicken can be prepared ahead of time and reheated just before serving. It can be served in a variety of ways— over rice and noodles, inside soft tortilla shells, or inside dough pockets.

160

2 chicken breasts, skin on and bone in
2 cups low-sodium chicken broth
1 teaspoon marjoram
½ teaspoon salt (optional)
1 stalk celery, chopped
1 small onion, chopped
1 tablespoon skim milk powder
1 teaspoon cornstarch
¼ teaspoon white pepper
1 tablespoon fresh minced parsley (optional)

1. Place chicken, broth, marjoram, and salt (optional) in a saucepan. Bring to a boil, reduce heat, cover, and simmer until the chicken is tender, about 20 minutes. Allow chicken to cool in broth.
2. When cool enough to handle, remove chicken from broth and reserve broth. Remove and discard the skin and bones, then cut chicken into bite-size pieces. Set aside.
3. Degrease the chicken broth. Bring the broth to a boil in a small saucepan, add the chopped celery and onion, and cook until the liquid is reduced by about half and the vegetables are soft, about 10 minutes.
4. In a small bowl, mix the milk powder, cornstarch, pepper, and 1–2 tablespoons of water until it is a smooth paste. Add the cornstarch mixture to the reduced broth and cook until thickened, about 3 minutes. Add chicken pieces and cook until heated through. Serve garnished with minced parsley.

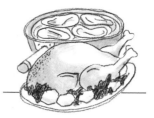

Preparation time: 10 minutes
Cooking time: 40 minutes

Yield: 3 servings
Serving size: ½ cup

Nutrition per serving:
Calories: 167
Carbohydrate:. . . . . 6 g
Protein: . . . . 25 g
Fat:. . . . . 4 g

Exchanges: 3 lean meat
1 vegetable
Carbohydrate choices: ½

Saturated fat: . . . . 1 g
Cholesterol: . . . . 63 mg
Dietary fiber: . . . . 1 g
Sodium:. . . . . 723 mg
(omitting salt) . . . . . . 190 mg

Pita chicken salad sandwiches

2 cups diced cooked chicken breast
¼ cup sliced green onions
½ cup chopped celery
½ cup red grapes, halved
½ cup nonfat sour cream
¼ cup light mayonnaise
½ teaspoon chili powder
3 pita breads, 6 inches across, cut in half
   to make pockets
¾ cup shredded lettuce

1. Combine chicken, onion, celery, and grapes. In a separate bowl, combine sour cream, mayonnaise, and chili powder. Combine the sour cream mixture and chicken mixture.
2. Place ½ cup of the mixture inside each pita pocket. Garnish with lettuce.

Want a meal in no time flat? These pita sandwiches are just the thing. Try plain nonfat yogurt in place of the sour cream and mayonnaise, add 2 teaspoons of minced fresh mint, and enjoy these with a slightly Middle Eastern flavor.

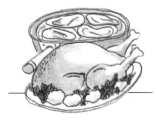

Preparation time: 10 minutes

Yield: 6 servings
Serving size: 1 sandwich

Exchanges: 1 starch
           2 lean meat
Carbohydrate choices: 1½

Nutrition per serving:
Calories: 203
Carbohydrate: . . . . 20 g
Protein: . . . . 18 g
Fat: . . . . 5 g

Saturated fat: . . . . 1 g
Cholesterol: . . . . 44 mg
Dietary fiber: . . . . 1 g
Sodium: . . . . 271 mg

Chicken parmigiana

Here's a healthier version of a traditional Chicken parmigiana, with low-fat mozzarella standing in for the Parmesan and bread crumbs.

1 can (about 14 ounces) whole tomatoes

**1 tablespoon minced fresh basil leaves
   or 1 teaspoon dried basil**

**1 tablespoon minced fresh tarragon
   or 1 teaspoon dried tarragon**

½ teaspoon salt (optional)

¼ teaspoon freshly ground black pepper

2 teaspoons olive oil

1 clove garlic, minced

4 chicken breasts (about 2 pounds total), skinned

2 tablespoons chopped fresh parsley, or to taste

½ cup shredded low-fat mozzarella cheese

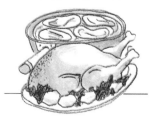

1. Puree the tomatoes with the basil, tarragon, salt (optional), and pepper in a blender or food processor until smooth. Set aside.

2. In a sauté pan large enough to hold the chicken in a single layer, heat the oil and sauté the garlic for about 30 seconds. Add the chicken breasts and brown on both sides.

3. Pour the tomato mixture over the chicken, bring to a boil, reduce heat, cover, and simmer until tender, about 15–20 minutes.

4. Remove the chicken and place in a warm oven-proof dish. Stir the parsley into the sauce and spoon it over the chicken breasts. Sprinkle the chicken breasts with mozzarella cheese and place under a heated broiler 1 minute, just until the cheese melts.

163

Preparation time: 10 minutes
Cooking time: 30 minutes

Yield: 4 servings
Serving size: 1 chicken breast
            with sauce

Exchanges: 4 lean meat
          1 vegetable
Carbohydrate choices: 0

Nutrition per serving:
Calories: 220
Carbohydrate: . . . . 5 g
Protein: . . . . 33 g
Fat: . . . . 7 g

Saturated fat: . . . . 2 g
Cholesterol: . . . . 81 mg
Dietary fiber: . . . . 2 g
Sodium: . . . . 587 mg
(omitting salt) . . . . 320 mg

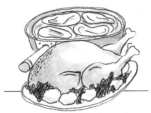

Spicy broiled chicken

This chicken dish is low in sodium but high in flavor. You'll love the combination of spices here.

1 cup plain nonfat yogurt
1 tablespoon minced or grated ginger root
2 large cloves garlic, peeled and minced
1 tablespoon paprika
1 teaspoon coriander
1 teaspoon cumin
1 teaspoon ground black pepper
½ teaspoon cayenne pepper
2 pounds boneless, skinless chicken breasts
  (4 split breasts)
Nonfat cooking spray

1. In a small bowl, combine all ingredients except the chicken. Place the chicken pieces in a flat dish and cover evenly with yogurt mixture. Refrigerate the chicken for at least 6 hours.
2. Spray a broiler rack with nonfat cooking spray. Place coated chicken pieces on the broiler rack, broiling 10–15 minutes per side. Serve immediately.

Preparation time: 10 minutes
Chilling time: 6 hours
Broiling time: 30 minutes

Exchanges: 4 very lean meat
Carbohydrate choices: 0

Yield: 8 servings
Serving size: ½ breast

Nutrition per serving:
Calories: 159
Carbohydrate:. . . . . 3 g
Protein: . . . . 26 g
Fat:. . . . . 4 g

Saturated fat: . . . . 1 g
Cholesterol:. . . . . 73 mg
Dietary fiber: . . . . <1 g
Sodium:. . . . . 79 mg

Baked chicken with wine sauce

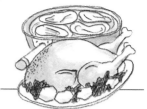

**2 pounds chicken breasts or thighs,
    skinned and boned**
**¼ cup Seasoned Bread Crumbs (recipe, p. 363)
    or commercial bread crumbs**
2 tablespoons vegetable oil
1 tablespoon cornstarch
1½ cups low-sodium chicken broth
½ cup dry white wine (not "cooking wine")

1. Preheat oven to 425°F. Rinse the chicken pieces under cold water and shake off excess water. Coat with bread crumbs.
2. Spread the oil in a shallow baking pan and arrange chicken pieces flat in the pan. Bake until tender, about 30 minutes, turning halfway.
3. After turning the chicken halfway through baking, combine the cornstarch with ½ cup of the broth and set aside. In a small saucepan, combine the remaining 1 cup of broth and the wine; bring to a boil and simmer until reduced by half, about 10 minutes. Stir in the cornstarch mixture and cook, stirring, until the sauce is clear and thickened. Serve the sauce hot over the chicken.

This dish is great for entertaining—it tastes like you put hours of work into it, but it is so easy to make. For variety, try adding sautéed mushrooms to the white wine sauce in the last 2–3 minutes of cooking.

165

Preparation time: 10 minutes
Cooking time: 30 minutes

Yield: 4 servings
Serving size: ¼ recipe

Exchanges: 3 lean meat
Carbohydrate choices: 0

Nutrition per serving:
Calories: 187
Carbohydrate:. . . . . 4 g
Protein: . . . . 27 g
Fat:. . . . . 5 g
Saturated fat: . . . . 1 g
Cholesterol:. . . . . 67 mg
Dietary fiber: . . . . 0 g
Sodium:. . . . . 109 mg

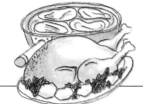

Chicken paprika

Did you know that paprika comes in a wide range of flavors? The paprika you generally buy in the grocery store is very mild in flavor and is used primarily for coloring or beautifying a dish. Try a Hungarian paprika (available in sweet, half-sweet, and hot) or a Spanish paprika (mild) to give this dish a different taste.

166

2 teaspoons vegetable oil
1 cup chopped onion
2 teaspoons paprika (sweet or hot, to taste)
½ teaspoon salt (optional)
¼ teaspoon freshly ground black pepper
2 pounds chicken breasts or legs, skinned
¾ cup low-sodium chicken broth
1 small green bell pepper, seeded and diced
1 tablespoon all-purpose flour
½ cup skim milk
⅓ cup low-fat sour cream (or plain nonfat yogurt)

1. In a heavy frying pan, heat the oil and sauté the onion until wilted, 3–5 minutes. Stir in paprika, salt (optional), and pepper. Add the chicken pieces and brown on both sides.

2. Add the chicken broth to the pan, cover, and simmer until the chicken is tender (about 30 minutes for breasts, 45 minutes for legs). (Or MICROWAVE on High, covered, in a microwave-safe dish, for 12–15 minutes.)

3. Add the green pepper and cook 5 minutes longer. (Or about 1 minute longer in the MICROWAVE.) In a small bowl, whisk the flour and milk together until smooth, then add it to the pan with the chicken. Cook, stirring, until thickened, about 3–5 minutes. Off the heat, stir in the sour cream or yogurt. Serve immediately.

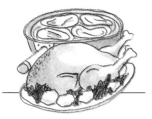

Preparation time: 10 minutes
Cooking time: 45–55 minutes

Yield: 4 servings
Serving size: ¼ recipe

Exchanges: 3 lean meat
       1 vegetable
Carbohydrate choices: ½

Nutrition per serving:

With low-fat sour cream	**With plain nonfat yogurt**
Calories: 215	Calories: 198
Carbohydrate:. . . . . 7 g	Carbohydrate:. . . . . 8 g
Protein: . . . . 29 g	Protein: . . . . 29 g
Fat:. . . . . 7 g	Fat:. . . . . 5 g
Saturated fat: . . . . 3 g	Saturated fat: . . . . 1 g
Cholesterol:. . . . . 67 mg	Cholesterol:. . . . . 66 mg
Dietary fiber: . . . . <1 g	Dietary fiber: . . . . <1 g
Sodium:. . . . . 364 mg	Sodium:. . . . . 370 mg
(omitting salt) . . . . 97 mg	(omitting salt) . . . . . . 103 mg

Chicken and vegetable skewers

2 small yellow squash, cut crosswise into 4 slices each

2 small zucchini, cut crosswise into 4 slices each

½ cup olive oil

⅓ cup lemon juice

8 cloves of garlic, peeled

1 tablespoon chopped fresh rosemary

¼ teaspoon salt (optional)

¼ teaspoon pepper

2 whole boneless, skinless chicken breasts,
    cut into 1½-inch strips

1 medium onion, cut into 8 wedges

8 cherry tomatoes

8 long sprigs of fresh rosemary

Marinate this delectable dish the day before your cookout so you can let the ingredients enrich the flavor. The taste of the fresh rosemary will make you glad you planned these skewers in advance.

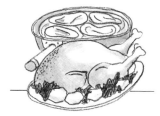

1. Place yellow squash and zucchini in a medium saucepan of boiling water. Cook for 3 minutes, drain, and rinse under cold water. Set aside.

2. Combine olive oil, lemon juice, garlic, chopped rosemary, salt (optional), and pepper in a large mixing bowl. Add squash, zucchini, chicken, and onion, mixing gently. Cover and marinate in the refrigerator for 8 hours.

3. On each of the skewers, arrange the ingredients in this order: chicken, yellow squash, zucchini, onion, chicken, tomato, garlic clove. Wrap each skewer with a long sprig of rosemary. Place skewers on grill rack and cook, turning once, for 8–10 minutes.

Preparation time: 15 minutes
Marinating time: 8 hours
Cooking time: 10 minutes

Yield: 4 servings
Serving size: 2 skewers

Nutrition per serving:
Calories: 245
Carbohydrate: . . . . 11 g
Protein: . . . . 28 g
Fat: . . . . 10 g

Exchanges: 2 vegetable
        3 lean meat
        ½ fat
Carbohydrate choices: 1

Saturated fat: . . . . 2 g
Cholesterol: . . . . 72 mg
Dietary fiber: . . . . 2 g
Sodium: . . . . 143 mg
(omitting salt) . . . . 10 mg

Curried chicken salad

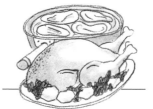

This curried chicken salad works great in sandwiches or with crackers at a party.

3 cups diced cooked chicken breast
1 carrot, grated
1 onion, finely chopped
2 stalks celery, chopped
½ cup raisins
3 tablespoons lemon juice
2 teaspoons curry powder
1 tablespoon honey
¼ cup light mayonnaise
1 small head romaine lettuce, washed and dried
2 tomatoes, cored and sliced into wedges
1 cup julienned radish

1. In a large bowl, combine chicken, carrot, onion, celery, and raisins. In a separate bowl, combine lemon juice, curry, honey, and mayonnaise. Stir curry mixture into chicken mixture; blend well. Chill for 1 hour.
2. Line plates with lettuce leaves, mound chicken salad on the lettuce, and garnish the sides with tomato wedges and julienned radish. Serve immediately.

169

Preparation time: 15 minutes
Chilling time: 1 hour

Yield: 6 servings
Serving size: 1 cup

Exchanges: 1½ carbohydrate
2 lean meat
Carbohydrate choices: 1½

Nutrition per serving:
Calories: 229
Carbohydrate: . . . . 21 g
Protein: . . . . 23 g
Fat: . . . . 6 g

Saturated fat: . . . . 1 g
Cholesterol: . . . . 63 mg
Dietary fiber: . . . . 3 g
Sodium: . . . . 156 mg

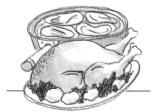

Turkey roll-ups

This is a great lunch or dinner idea when you are pressed for time—especially if you're near a microwave.

12 slices (1 ounce each) oven-roasted turkey breast
6 slices (¾ ounce each) fat-free processed mozzarella cheese
16 ounces frozen broccoli spears (12 spears), thawed and well drained
Nonfat cooking spray
1 jar (12 ounces) fat-free turkey gravy

1. Preheat oven to 350°F. On a clean countertop, lay out two turkey slices, overlapping somewhat and oriented so that you will be able to roll them into a cylinder shape. Lay one slice of cheese on the turkey slice closest to you. Place two broccoli spears on the cheese, and roll the turkey and cheese around the broccoli. Secure with a toothpick. Repeat to make six roll-ups in all.
2. Place roll-ups in a baking dish coated with cooking spray. Cover roll-ups with gravy and cover baking pan with foil. Bake 25–30 minutes or until heated through. (Or MICROWAVE, in a microwave-safe dish covered with plastic wrap (instead of foil), on High for 5–6 minutes, or until heated through.)

170

Preparation time: 10 minutes
Baking time: 25 minutes

Yield: 6 servings
Serving size: 1 roll-up

Exchanges: 2 vegetable
        2 very lean meat
Carbohydrate choices: ½

Nutrition per serving:
Calories: 125
Carbohydrate:. . . . . 10 g
Protein: . . . . 19 g
Fat:. . . . . 1 g

Saturated fat: . . . . <1 g
Cholesterol:. . . . . 29 mg
Dietary fiber: . . . . 1 g
Sodium: . . . . 1,176 mg

Chapter 7

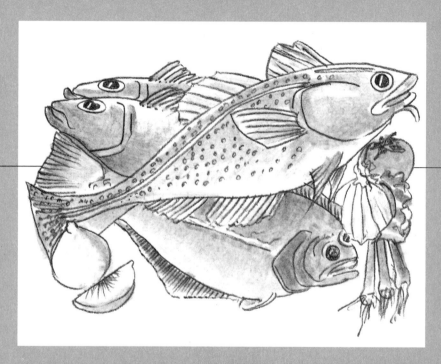

FISH

*A*ll the nutrition experts agree that fish is good for you. Not only are fish high in protein, but most varieties of fish also are very low in saturated fat and cholesterol. In fact, many varieties contain omega-3 fatty acids, which have been shown to help prevent heart disease and improve your cholesterol. Plus fish tastes great!

The key to cooking fish is to purchase fresh fish and prepare it the same day—or better yet, the same day it was caught. Be sure to buy fish that is shiny, with good color (do not buy fish that seems dull in color or appearance). The fish should smell mild and fresh, and the meat should be firm to the touch and not separated from the bones. Never purchase fish with cloudy or milky eyes—this is a sure sign it has not been kept fresh on ice.

With these delicious recipes, you will want to enjoy fish every day!

Tuna, broccoli, and pasta casserole

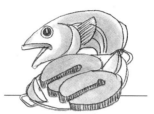

8 ounces penne pasta, dry
1 cup chopped broccoli
½ cup finely chopped onion
3 ounces Brie cheese, rind removed
1½ cups skim milk
1 teaspoon Dijon mustard
4 green onions, sliced
½ cup chopped celery
½ cup diced red bell pepper
1 can (6½ ounces) water-packed tuna,
    drained and flaked
¼ teaspoon pepper
¼ teaspoon salt (optional)

Tuna casserole is as American as mom and apple pie. You'll love this lighter version with Brie cheese and Dijon mustard.

1. Preheat oven to 350°F. In a medium saucepan, cook pasta according to package directions, adding the broccoli to the boiling water for the last 5 minutes. Drain well and place pasta and broccoli in casserole dish.
2. While the mixture is still hot, add the onion and Brie cheese, stirring until the cheese is melted. Add the milk, mustard, green onions, celery, and bell peppers. Stir well. Mix in the tuna, pepper, and salt (optional). Bake about 30 minutes, or until the mixture is bubbly, stirring halfway through. Let stand 5 minutes before serving.

173

Preparation time: 25 minutes
Baking time: 30 minutes

Yield: 6 servings
Serving size: 1 cup

Exchanges: 2 starch
    1 vegetable
    2 very lean meat,
Carbohydrate choices: 2

Nutrition per serving:
Calories: 263
Carbohydrate:. . . . . 34 g
Protein: . . . . 20 g
Fat:. . . . . 5 g

Saturated fat: . . . . 3 g
Cholesterol: . . . . 23 mg
Dietary fiber: . . . . 1 g
Sodium:. . . . . 358 mg
(omitting salt) . . . . 269 mg

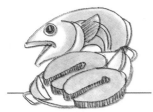

Spanish fish

This spicy fish dish needs very little attention. While it simmers, prepare a side dish that would go well with this, such as Asparagus with Mustard Vinaigrette (recipe, p. 241).

1 medium onion, chopped
1 green pepper, chopped
1 tablespoon vegetable oil
½ cup white wine
1 can (15 ounces) no-salt-added tomato sauce
1 can (15 ounces) chopped tomatoes
1 bay leaf
½ teaspoon garlic powder
¼ teaspoon oregano
½ teaspoon hot pepper (or Tabasco) sauce
1 pound fresh fish fillets,
    divided into 4 equal portions

1. Sauté onion and green pepper in oil for 2 minutes in a large nonstick skillet. Add wine, tomato sauce, tomatoes, bay leaf, garlic powder, oregano, and hot pepper sauce. Simmer for 10 minutes, stirring frequently.
2. Add fish to sauce. Cover and simmer 20 minutes longer, or until fish flakes easily with fork. Remove bay leaf. Serve immediately.

174

Preparation time: 10 minutes
Cooking time: 35 minutes

Yield: 4 servings
Serving size: 1 portion fish
    and sauce

Exchanges: 1 carbohydrate
    3 very lean meat
    1 fat
Carbohydrate choices: 1

Nutrition per serving:
Calories: 222
Carbohydrate: . . . . 13 g
Protein: . . . . 26 g
Fat: . . . . 6 g

Saturated fat: . . . . 0 g
Cholesterol: . . . . 36 mg
Dietary fiber: . . . . 2 g
Sodium: . . . . 291 mg

Poached fish

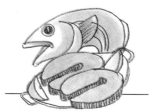

1½ cups clam juice or water
1 medium onion, sliced
4 slices of lemon
3 sprigs of parsley
6 whole black peppercorns
1 whole bay leaf
1 pound fresh fillets

What could be easier and faster than this poached fish recipe? You can also try a low-sodium vegetable or chicken broth in place of the clam juice or water.

1. Combine the clam juice (or water), onion, lemon, parsley, peppercorns, and bay leaf in a medium, nonreactive sauté pan. Bring to a boil. (Or MICROWAVE on High, covered, in a microwave-safe dish, until boiling.)
2. Arrange the fish fillets in a single layer on top of the poaching liquid. Lower heat, cover the pan, and simmer until the fish is just cooked, 8–10 minutes. (Or MICROWAVE on High, about 2 minutes.)
3. Carefully lift fish from the pan with a slotted spoon. Lift cooked onions and lemon slices to serve with fish, if desired.

175

Preparation time: 5 minutes
Cooking time: 15 minutes

Yield: 4 servings
Serving size: 3½ ounces

Exchanges: 3 very lean meat
Carbohydrate choices: 0

Nutrition per serving:
Calories: 115
Carbohydrate:. . . . . 1 g
Protein: . . . . 25 g
Fat:. . . . . 1 g
Saturated fat: . . . . trace
Cholesterol:. . . . . 55 mg
Dietary fiber: . . . . 0 g
Sodium:. . . . . 188 mg

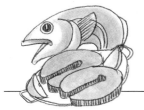

Here's another great recipe that takes no time at all to make. For an extra crispy texture, spray the crumb-coated fish lightly with a vegetable oil cooking spray before baking.

Crispy baked fish

1 pound fresh fish fillets
2 tablespoons Cider Vinegar Dressing (recipe, p. 115) or fat-free mayonnaise
½ cup Seasoned Bread Crumbs (recipe, p. 363) or commercial bread crumbs

1. Preheat oven to 425°F. Pat fillets with paper towels. Brush with dressing. Coat with bread crumbs, pressing crumbs into fish.
2. Place fish on a lightly-greased baking sheet and bake until the fish is just done and the bread crumbs are golden, 10–12 minutes.

176

Preparation time: 5 minutes
Cooking time: 10 minutes

Yield: 4 servings
Serving size: 3½ ounces

Nutrition per serving:
Calories: 125
Carbohydrate:. . . . . 4 g
Protein: . . . . 25 g
Fat:. . . . . 1 g

Exchanges: 3 very lean meat
Carbohydrate choices: 0

Saturated fat:. . . . . trace
Cholesterol:. . . . . 55 mg
Dietary fiber: . . . . 0 g
Sodium:. . . . . 175 mg

Creole fish bake

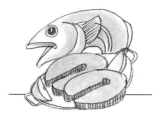

1 can (about 14 ounces) crushed tomatoes
1 cup frozen mixed vegetables
1 green bell pepper, seeded and diced
½ cup clam juice or chicken broth
1 small onion, minced
1 clove garlic, minced
⅓ cup minced fresh parsley
1 teaspoon dried thyme leaf
½ teaspoon salt (optional)
½ teaspoon freshly ground black pepper
2–3 drops hot pepper (or Tabasco) sauce (optional)
1 pound fresh fish fillets
1 lemon, cut into 6 wedges

Use any kind of fish you like in this fish stew from the oven. If you like your foods spicy, feel free to add more hot sauce.

1. Preheat oven to 400°F. In a medium saucepan, combine the tomatoes, mixed vegetables, diced green pepper, clam juice or chicken broth, onion, garlic, parsley, thyme, and seasonings. Cook over medium heat until the peppers are soft and the flavors have melded, about 10–15 minutes. (Or MICROWAVE on High, covered, for about 5 minutes.) Pour the sauce into an 8-cup casserole.
2. Cut the fish into 1-inch chunks and add them to the casserole. Bake until the fish is opaque, about 10 minutes. (Or MICROWAVE on High about 2 more minutes.) Serve with lemon wedge as garnish.

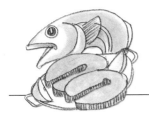

Preparation time: 10 minutes
Cooking time: 25 minutes

Yield: 6 servings
Serving size: 1 cup

Nutrition per serving:
Calories: 106
Carbohydrate: . . . . 7 g
Protein: . . . . 18 g
Fat: . . . . 1 g

Exchanges: 1 vegetable
          2 very lean meat
Carbohydrate choices: ½

Saturated fat: . . . . trace
Cholesterol: . . . . 39 mg
Dietary fiber: . . . . 3 g
Sodium: . . . . 431 mg
(omitting salt) . . . . 253 mg

Louisiana stir-fry

Looking for a low-fat meal that's high in taste? Try this quick dish from New Orleans.

Nonfat cooking spray
2 teaspoons corn oil
1 pound shrimp, peeled and deveined (or frozen, cooked shrimp that have been thawed)
1 bag (14 ounces) frozen broccoli florets
1 can (11 ounces) corn with red and green pepper, drained
½ cup coarsely chopped onion
⅛–¼ teaspoon hot pepper (or Tabasco) sauce
1 tablespoon Cajun seasoning
1 can (14½ ounces) diced tomatoes
Hot rice (optional)
8 lemon wedges (optional)

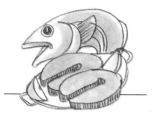

1. Coat a cool, nonstick wok with cooking spray. Heat wok and add oil. Add shrimp and cook until they turn pink. (If using precooked shrimp, add shrimp during last minute of cooking.) Remove shrimp and set aside.

2. Place frozen broccoli in wok and cook for 3 minutes, stirring constantly. Add corn, onion, hot pepper sauce, and Cajun seasoning. Cook 2 minutes more, stirring frequently. Add tomatoes and cook until hot and bubbly, about 3 minutes.

3. Add cooked shrimp and heat 1 more minute, stirring frequently. Serve immediately (over hot rice with a squeeze of lemon, if desired).

NOTE: *If you need to watch your sodium intake, look for a low-salt or no-salt Cajun seasoning.*

179

Preparation time: 5 minutes
  (when using frozen, cooked
  shrimp)
Cooking time: 15 minutes

Yield: 4 servings
Serving size: 2 cups

Exchanges: ½ starch
          3 vegetable
          4 very lean meat
Carbohydrate choices: 1½

Nutrition per serving:
Calories: 239
Carbohydrate: . . . . 23 g
Protein: . . . . 30 g
Fat: . . . . 3 g

Saturated fat: . . . . <1 g
Cholesterol: . . . . 165 mg
Dietary fiber: . . . . 1 g
Sodium: . . . . 1,864 mg

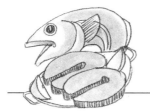

Stuffed baked fillets

Serve these stuffed fillets with a Mushroom or Velouté Sauce (recipes, p. 353 and p. 359). For a different approach, spread the filling on four long, thin fillets; roll up, secure with a toothpick, cover, and bake as directed.

180

½ **cup finely chopped celery**
⅓ **cup finely chopped sweet red or green bell pepper**
3 green onions, finely chopped
⅔ **cup low-sodium chicken broth**
3 tablespoons dry bread crumbs
2 tablespoons chopped fresh parsley
2 tablespoons chopped walnuts or almonds
1 tablespoon freshly squeezed lemon juice
½ **teaspoon grated lemon zest**
½ **teaspoon salt (optional)**
1 pound fresh fish fillets
Paprika (optional)

1. In a small sauté pan, combine the celery, bell pepper, onions, and broth. Cover and cook over medium heat until the vegetables are tender, about 6–8 minutes. Preheat oven to 425°F.
2. Stir in the bread crumbs, parsley, nuts, lemon juice, lemon zest, and salt (optional). Place half of the fillets in an oiled, shallow baking dish. Top with the vegetable mixture. Cover with remaining fillets. Pour remaining mixture over fish. Sprinkle with paprika, if desired. Cover loosely.
3. Bake until fish is just cooked, about 10–15 minutes. (Or MICROWAVE on High, covered, in a microwave-safe dish for 3–5 minutes.)

Preparation time: 10 minutes
Cooking time: 25 minutes

Yield: 4 servings
Serving size: ¼ recipe

Exchanges: 1 vegetable
            3 very lean meat
Carbohydrate choices: ½

Nutrition per serving:
Calories: 155
Carbohydrate:. . . . . 5 g
Protein: . . . . 26 g
Fat:. . . . . 3 g

Saturated fat:. . . . . trace
Cholesterol:. . . . . 56 mg
Dietary fiber: . . . . 1 g
Sodium:. . . . . 497 mg
(omitting salt) . . . . 230 mg

Tuna salad with couscous

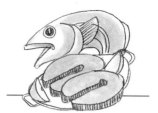

1/2 cup water
1/3 cup uncooked couscous
1/4 cup red wine vinegar
2 tablespoons olive oil
1 tablespoon Dijon mustard
1 teaspoon dried parsley flakes
1/4 teaspoon salt (optional)
1/4 teaspoon black pepper
1 teaspoon sugar
1 clove garlic, minced
1 cup chopped green pepper
1/2 cup chopped red pepper
1 cup peeled, chopped cucumber
1 cup chopped onion
1 can (11 ounces) whole-kernel corn, drained
1 can (6 ounces) water-packed tuna, drained and
   flaked

If you've never tried couscous before, you don't know what you're missing. This tuna salad dish will soon have you serving couscous with every dinner.

1. Bring water to a boil in a medium saucepan; stir in couscous. Remove from heat, cover, and allow to stand 5 minutes. Fluff with a fork. Transfer couscous to a bowl, cover, and chill.
2. Combine vinegar, oil, mustard, parsley, salt (optional), pepper, sugar, and garlic in a large bowl. Blend ingredients using a whisk or fork. Add prepared couscous, peppers, cucumber, onion, corn, and tuna, tossing well. Serve chilled.

181

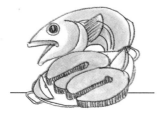

Preparation time: 15 minutes
Cooking time: 5 minutes
Chilling time: 1 hour

Yield: 7 servings
Serving size: 1 cup

Exchanges: 1½ starch
1 fat
Carbohydrate choices: 1½

Nutrition per serving:
Calories: 150
Carbohydrate:. . . . . 20 g
Protein: . . . . 8 g
Fat:. . . . . 5 g

Saturated fat: . . . . <1 g
Cholesterol: . . . . 340 mg
Dietary fiber: . . . . 3 g
Sodium:. . . . . 340 mg
(omitting salt) . . . . 264 mg

Pacific salmon pie

Salmon and Swiss cheese are baked together in this rice-crusted pie that can be served hot soon after it emerges from the oven or at room temperature.

2 cups cold water

½ cup long-grain white rice

1 teaspoon salt (optional)

3 teaspoons margarine

1 cup finely chopped celery

½ cup finely chopped onion

2 eggs (or ½ cup egg substitute)

½ teaspoon freshly ground black pepper

½ cup shredded low-fat Swiss cheese

1 can (about 7 ounces) salmon, undrained and flaked

½ cup skim milk

¼ teaspoon ground nutmeg

¼ teaspoon ground cinnamon

¼ teaspoon curry powder (optional)

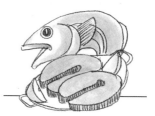

1. In a medium saucepan, bring 2 cups of water to a boil. Add the rice and salt (optional) and bring back to a boil; reduce heat, cover, and simmer until all the water is absorbed and the rice is tender, 15–20 minutes.

2. Lightly grease a 9-inch pie plate with 1 teaspoon of the margarine. Melt the remaining 2 teaspoons margarine in a frying pan and sauté the celery and onion until tender, about 5 minutes. Preheat the oven to 375°F.

3. In a small bowl, beat 1 egg (or ¼ cup of the egg substitute) with the pepper and mix into the cooked rice. Press the rice mixture into the bottom and up the sides of the pie plate to form a crust. Sprinkle half the cheese over the rice, spread with half the celery-onion mixture, and all of the salmon. Top with the remaining celery-onion mixture and cheese.

4. Beat together the remaining egg (or ¼ cup egg substitute), milk, and spices, and pour this mixture over the ingredients in the pie plate. Bake until set, about 30–35 minutes (a tester inserted in the center should come out clean). Cool 5 minutes before serving.

Preparation time: 15 minutes
Cooking time: 1 hour

Yield: 6 servings
Serving size: ⅙ pie

Exchanges: 1 starch
2 lean meat
Carbohydrate choices: 1

Nutrition per serving:

With eggs
Calories: 211
Carbohydrate:. . . . . 17 g
Protein: . . . . 16 g
Fat:. . . . . 8 g
Saturated fat: . . . . 2 g
Cholesterol: . . . . 110 mg
Dietary fiber: . . . . 1 g
Sodium: . . . . 1,105 mg
(omitting salt) . . . . 750 mg

With egg substitute
Calories: 193
Carbohydrate:. . . . . 17 g
Protein: . . . . 16 g
Fat:. . . . . 7 g
Saturated fat: . . . . 2 g
Cholesterol: . . . . 19 mg
Dietary fiber: . . . . 1 g
Sodium: . . . . 1,109 mg
(omitting salt) . . . . 754 mg

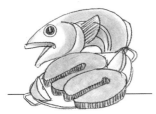

Smoked salmon gives this pasta dish a particularly hearty flavor.

Dilled salmon pasta with asparagus

2 tablespoons margarine
2 tablespoons olive oil
½ medium red onion, sliced
1 pound fresh asparagus, trimmed and cut diagonally into 1-inch lengths
4 ounces smoked salmon, sliced into thin strips
¼ teaspoon ground black pepper
16 ounces tubular pasta (such as penne or ziti)
2 tablespoons chopped fresh dill

1. Heat the margarine and oil in a large skillet. Add the onion and cook over low heat, stirring, until tender, about 5 minutes. Add the asparagus and sauté until crisp-tender, about 5 minutes. Add the salmon to the skillet. Sprinkle with pepper, and stir the mixture to blend for 2–3 minutes.

2. Bring a large pot of water to boil and cook the pasta until al dente, about 8–10 minutes. Drain pasta and return it to the cooking pot. Add the asparagus mixture. Stir in the dill and toss to blend.

184

Preparation time: 5 minutes
Cooking time: 25 minutes

Yield: 8 servings
Serving size: 2 cups

Exchanges: 2½ starch
1 vegetable
1½ fat
Carbohydrate choices: 3

Nutrition per serving:
Calories: 302
Carbohydrate: . . . . 46 g
Protein: . . . . 11 g
Fat: . . . . 8 g

Saturated fat: . . . . 1 g
Cholesterol: . . . . 3 mg
Dietary fiber: . . . . 3 g
Sodium: . . . . 148 mg

Confetti salmon cakes

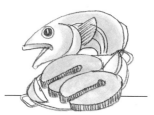

1 can (15 ounces) red salmon packed in oil
1 tablespoon vegetable oil
1 medium onion, finely chopped
¼ cup finely chopped green pepper
¼ cup finely chopped red pepper
20 saltines, crushed
1 tablespoon minced fresh dill
½ teaspoon ground black pepper
¼ cup skim milk
1 tablespoon lemon juice
1 egg white, beaten
Nonfat cooking spray

Here's a low-fat entrée that's high in calcium— and delicious, too!

1. Drain and flake salmon, discarding large bones and skin. Set aside.
2. Heat the oil in a medium saucepan. Add onion and chopped peppers and sauté over medium heat until they begin to soften, about 5 minutes. Remove pan from heat and lightly stir in the salmon, saltines, dill, pepper, milk, and lemon juice. Add the egg white and mix gently. Form the salmon mixture into 6 even-size patties.
3. Spray a nonstick skillet with cooking spray. Carefully sauté patties about 3 minutes on each side until evenly browned and crusty, taking care not to break them or let them burn. Serve immediately.

185

Preparation time: 20 minutes
Cooking time: 15 minutes

Yield: 6 servings
Serving size: 1 patty

Exchanges: 1 starch
        2 medium-fat meat
Carbohydrate choices: 1

Nutrition per serving:
Calories: 210
Carbohydrate:. . . . . 11 g
Protein: . . . . 17 g
Fat:. . . . . 11 g

Saturated fat: . . . . 2 g
Cholesterol: . . . . 42 mg
Dietary fiber: . . . . 2 g
Sodium:. . . . . 443 mg

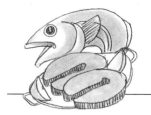

Broiled fish fillets almondine

Toasted almonds give this broiled fish a wonderful flavor. You can also use pecan slivers in place of almonds.

1 pound fresh fish fillets
2 tablespoons vegetable oil
¼ cup slivered almonds
2 tablespoons freshly squeezed lemon juice
½ teaspoon salt (optional)
¼ teaspoon white pepper

1. Place fish fillets on a broiler pan or ovenproof shallow baking dish. Brush lightly with 1 tablespoon of the oil. Broil about 4 inches from heat for about 3 minutes.
2. Remove pan from broiler and turn each piece of fish. Mix together the remaining tablespoon oil, almond slivers, lemon juice, and seasonings. Spoon almond mixture over fillets.
3. Return fish to broiler and broil until fish is just cooked and the almonds are toasted, about 3–4 more minutes.

186

Preparation time: 10 minutes
Broiling time: 10 minutes

Yield: 4 servings
Serving size: 3½ ounces

Exchanges: 3 lean meat
1 fat
Carbohydrate choices: 0

Nutrition per serving:
Calories: 205
Carbohydrate:. . . . . 2 g
Protein: . . . . 23 g
Fat:. . . . . 11 g

Saturated fat: . . . . 1 g
Cholesterol:. . . . . 49 mg
Dietary fiber: . . . . 1 g
Sodium:. . . . . 336 mg
(omitting salt) . . . . 69 mg

Chapter 8

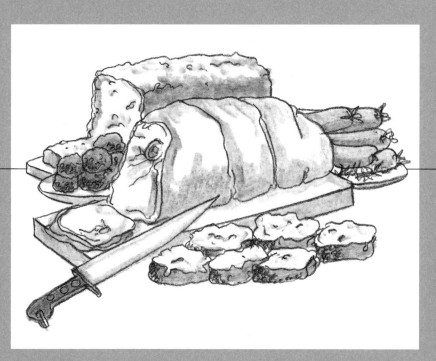

MEATS

There is no doubt that beef, pork, and lamb rank high as main-course favorites, yet many of us have avoided these meats for health reasons. The good news is that you do not have to avoid your favorite dishes any longer. Nutritionally, lean meats can be good for you. The first key is to select cuts of meat with less marbling and trim any excess fat from these cuts.

When looking for beef, choose ground round over higher-fat ground chuck. If you want steak, opt for the leaner sirloin. Choose beef tenderloin for roasting and trim away any fat you see. The same holds true for both pork and lamb— stick with the tenderloin for the leanest cut.

The second key to incorporating lean meats into a healthy diet is selecting a low-fat method of cooking. These recipes will help you in that area. The large amounts of oil, cream, butter, and cheese you might find in traditional recipes are replaced here in creative and delicious ways. You will probably never notice they are gone.

Braised steak and peppers

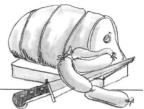

1½ pounds lean round steak, cut into ¼-inch strips
2 tablespoons all-purpose flour
½ teaspoon salt (optional)
¼ teaspoon freshly ground black pepper
1 tablespoon vegetable oil
1¾ cups low-sodium beef broth
1 cup canned tomatoes with juice
1 medium onion, sliced
1 clove garlic, minced
1 large or 2 small green bell peppers,
    seeded and cut into ¼-inch strips
1½ teaspoons Worcestershire sauce

Almost any vegetable can be substituted for the green peppers used here. Serve this over rice or cooked egg noodles.

1. Dust steak strips with flour and sprinkle with salt (optional) and pepper. Heat the oil in a large nonreactive frying pan and stir-fry until browned on all sides. Drain off any fat.
2. Add the broth, tomato juice (reserve the tomatoes for later), onion, and garlic to the meat. Cover and simmer until the meat is tender, about 1–1½ hours. (Or MICROWAVE on High, covered, in a microwave-safe dish, for 12–15 minutes.)
3. Chop the reserved tomatoes if whole, and add them, along with the green peppers and Worcestershire sauce, to the meat. Cook, stirring, 5–10 minutes, until peppers are tender.

189

Preparation time: 15 minutes
Cooking time: 1¾ hours

Yield: 6 servings
Serving size: ⅙ recipe

Exchanges: 1 vegetable
        3 medium-fat meat
Carbohydrate choices: 0

Nutrition per serving:
Calories: 233
Carbohydrate: . . . . 5 g
Protein: . . . . 23 g
Fat: . . . . 13 g

Saturated fat: . . . . 5 g
Cholesterol: . . . . 54 mg
Dietary fiber: . . . . 1 g
Sodium: . . . . 328 mg
(omitting salt) . . . . 150 mg

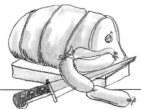

Steak fajitas

This is the ultimate in fast dinners. You can make it extra-special by whipping up your own homemade salsa—combine chopped tomatoes, onions, cilantro, minced garlic, and 1–2 seeded, chopped jalapeño peppers in a bowl and mix well.

190

¾ **pound lean flank steak, fat trimmed off and sliced across the grain into thin strips**
2 **teaspoons chili powder**
1 **teaspoon ground cumin**
⅛ **teaspoon garlic powder**
¼ **teaspoon black pepper**
6 **eight-inch flour tortillas**
1 **teaspoon vegetable oil**
1 **large onion, sliced**
1 **each green, red, and yellow bell peppers, cut into thin strips**
2 **cloves garlic, minced**
3 **tablespoons lime juice**
6 **tablespoons nonfat sour cream**
Salsa (optional)
Fresh cilantro sprigs (optional)

1. Combine steak, chili powder, cumin, garlic powder, and black pepper in a zip-top plastic bag; shake thoroughly to coat. Warm the tortillas according to the package directions.
2. Heat oil in a large nonstick skillet over medium-high heat. Add steak, onion, bell peppers, and garlic. Sauté 6–8 minutes, until the steak is thoroughly cooked. Remove from heat and stir in the lime juice.
3. Divide the mixture evenly among the warm tortillas, top each with 1 tablespoon sour cream, and roll up. Serve with salsa if desired and garnish with cilantro.

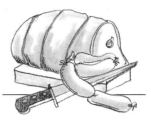

Preparation time: 10 minutes
Cooking time: 8 minutes

Yield: 6 servings
Serving size: 1 fajita

Exchanges: 2 starch
2 lean meat
Carbohydrate choices: 2

Nutrition per serving:
Calories: 266
Carbohydrate: . . . . 30 g
Protein: . . . . 18 g
Fat: . . . . 8 g
Saturated fat: . . . . 2 g
Cholesterol: . . . . 28 mg
Dietary fiber: . . . . 2 g
Sodium: . . . . 250 mg

Beef steak with herb garnish

2 tablespoons chopped green onion

2 tablespoons minced fresh parsley

**2 tablespoons freshly squeezed lemon juice
or red wine vinegar**

1 tablespoon olive oil

1–2 cloves garlic, minced

½ teaspoon salt (optional)

¼ teaspoon freshly ground black pepper

**1 pound boneless beef fillet, eye round,
or sirloin steak, cut into 4 portions**

1. In a small bowl, combine the onion, parsley, lemon juice or vinegar, olive oil, garlic, and seasonings. Cover and let stand at room temperature at least 2 hours for the flavors to meld.
2. Broil or sauté the steak to your desired doneness, a few minutes on each side, depending on thickness. Spoon herb garnish over each portion just before serving.

The blended herb garnish is what makes this steak so wonderful. Serve it the old-fashioned way, with a baked potato and green salad.

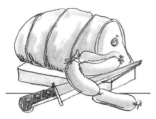

Preparation time: 10 minutes
Marinating time: 2 hours
Cooking time: 10 minutes

Yield: 4 servings
Serving size: 3 ounces

Exchanges: 3 medium-fat meat
Carbohydrate choices: 0

Nutrition per serving:
Calories: 207
Carbohydrate: . . . . 1 g
Protein: . . . . 26 g
Fat: . . . . 11 g

Saturated fat: . . . . 4 g
Cholesterol: . . . . 65 mg
Dietary fiber: . . . . 0 g
Sodium: . . . . 324 mg
(omitting salt) . . . . 57 mg

Salisbury steak with mushroom sauce

Salisbury steak takes ground beef to a new level. Topped with Mushroom Sauce, this is an elegant entrée.

1¼ pounds lean ground beef

¼ cup dry bread crumbs or cracker crumbs

½ cup finely chopped onion

1 clove garlic, minced

1 teaspoon Dijon mustard

½ teaspoon salt (optional)

¼ teaspoon freshly ground black pepper

1 egg, beaten (or ¼ cup liquid egg substitute)

Nonfat cooking spray

1½ cups (1½ batches) Mushroom Sauce (recipe, p. 353)

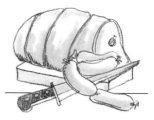

1. In a mixing bowl, combine the beef, crumbs, onion, garlic, mustard, and seasonings; add egg (or egg substitute) and mix thoroughly. Divide mixture into 6 portions and shape into patties.

2. Spray a frying pan with nonfat cooking spray. Cook the patties, turning often, over medium-high heat, to desired doneness, about 8–10 minutes total, depending on thickness.

3. Heat the Mushroom Sauce and spoon it over the patties.

193

Preparation time: 10 minutes
Cooking time: 10 minutes

Yield: 6 servings
Serving size: 1 patty with
⅙ sauce

Exchanges: ½ carbohydrate
3 medium-fat meat
Carbohydrate choices: ½

Nutrition per serving:

With egg
Calories: 252
Carbohydrate:. . . . . 7 g
Protein: . . . . 25 g
Fat:. . . . . 14 g
Saturated fat: . . . . 6 g
Cholesterol: . . . . 118 mg
Dietary fiber: . . . . 0 g
Sodium:. . . . . 284 mg
(omitting salt) . . . . 106 mg

With egg substitute
Calories: 243
Carbohydrate:. . . . . 7 g
Protein: . . . . 25 g
Fat:. . . . . 13 g
Saturated fat: . . . . 6 g
Cholesterol: . . . . 72 mg
Dietary fiber: . . . . 0 g
Sodium:. . . . . 286 mg
(omitting salt) . . . . 108 mg

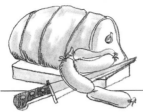

The sauce that covers these steaks is very flavorful and so simple to make. You also can substitute dry red wine for white in this recipe.

Minute steak deluxe

1 pound minute steaks
1 clove garlic, peeled and cut in half
½ teaspoon salt (optional)
¼ teaspoon freshly ground black pepper
1 tablespoon margarine
1 shallot, peeled and minced (optional)
1 tablespoon cognac or brandy
⅓ cup dry white wine
⅓ cup evaporated skim milk
¼ cup minced fresh parsley

1. Rub steaks on both sides with the cut surfaces of the garlic clove. Season to taste with salt (optional) and pepper.
2. Melt margarine in a heavy nonreactive skillet. Add steaks and cook over medium-high heat to desired doneness, about 1–2 minutes per side. Remove steaks to a platter and keep warm.
3. Add the shallot (optional) and cognac or brandy to the skillet and cook over medium heat about 1 minute, scraping up pan juices. Add the wine and cook, stirring, until reduced by half. Add the milk and parsley, reduce heat, and cook 2–3 more minutes, until heated through.
4. Return the steaks to the sauce to reheat briefly. Spoon sauce over steaks and serve.

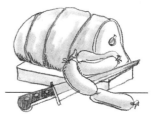

Preparation time: 5 minutes
Cooking time: 10 minutes

Yield: 4 servings
Serving size: 3 ounces meat
　　　　　with ¼ sauce

Exchanges: 3 medium-fat meat
Carbohydrate choices: 0

Nutrition per serving:
Calories: 241
Carbohydrate: . . . . 3 g
Protein: . . . . 23 g
Fat: . . . . 16 g

Saturated fat: . . . . 6 g
Cholesterol: . . . . 72 mg
Dietary fiber: . . . . 0 g
Sodium: . . . . 378 mg
(omitting salt) . . . . . . 111 mg

195

Scottish cheeseburgers

1 pound lean ground beef (or ground turkey)

1 egg, beaten (or ¼ cup liquid egg substitute)

¼ cup quick rolled oats

½ teaspoon salt (optional)

¼ teaspoon freshly ground black pepper

¼ cup minced onion

½ cup low-fat Swiss cheese or part-skim mozzarella

The Scots put oatmeal in just about everything—which may account for their robust good health. Don't forget to account for the hamburger bun when figuring this into your meal plan.

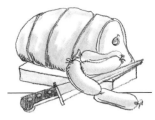

1. In a mixing bowl, combine the meat, egg (or egg substitute), oats, salt (optional), pepper, and onion; mix until well blended, but do not overmix.

2. Divide meat mixture into 8 portions; shape each into a flat patty. Top each of 4 patties with one-quarter of the cheese. Cover each with remaining patty. Pinch edges to form 4 firm burgers.

3. Broil or grill the burgers a few minutes on each side, to your desired doneness. Avoid overcooking or the cheese might leak out.

Preparation time: 15 minutes
Cooking time: 10 minutes

Yield: 4 servings
Serving size: 1 burger

Nutrition per serving:

With ground beef and egg

Exchanges: 3 medium-fat meat
½ fat
Carbohydrate choices: 0

Calories: 261
Carbohydrate:. . . . . 3 g
Protein: . . . . 24 g
Fat:. . . . . 16 g
Saturated fat: . . . . 6 g
Cholesterol: . . . . 134 mg
Dietary fiber: . . . . <1 g
Sodium:. . . . . 522 mg
(omitting salt) . . . . 255 mg

With ground turkey and egg substitute

Exchanges: 4 very lean meat
1 fat
Carbohydrate choices: 0

Calories: 204
Carbohydrate:. . . . . 4 g
Protein: . . . . 29 g
Fat:. . . . . 7 g
Saturated fat: . . . . 2 g
Cholesterol: . . . . 61 mg
Dietary fiber: . . . . <1 g
Sodium:. . . . . 523 mg
(omitting salt) . . . . 256 mg

Cilantro burgers

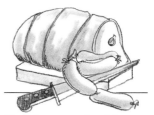

Try these veggie-rich burgers at your next barbecue.

1 pound ground round
½ cup chopped cilantro
¼ cup chopped red onion
¼ cup tiny capers, drained
¼ cup Dijon mustard
2 ripe plum tomatoes, seeded and diced
¼ cup chopped green bell pepper
2 tablespoons Seasoned Bread Crumbs
(recipe, p. 363) or commercial bread crumbs
1 egg white
1 teaspoon caraway seeds
1 teaspoon black pepper

1. Combine all the ingredients in a bowl and mix together with your hand. Divide the mixture into four equal portions, and shape them into ½-inch-thick patties.
2. Grill or broil the patties for about 5 minutes on each side, or until they reach the desired degree of doneness.

197

Preparation time: 10 minutes
Cooking time: 10 minutes

Yield: 4 servings
Serving size: 1 patty

Exchanges: 3 medium-fat meat
1 vegetable
Carbohydrate choices: ½

Nutrition per serving:
Calories: 268
Carbohydrate: . . . . 8 g
Protein: . . . . 24 g
Fat: . . . . 15 g

Saturated fat: . . . . 6 g
Cholesterol: . . . . 58 mg
Dietary fiber: . . . . 2 g
Sodium: . . . . 515 mg

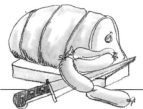

This is great as a stew, but add a can of red kidney beans and ½ teaspoon of cayenne pepper and you've got a fine Texas chili on your hands.

Tex-Mex beef stew

**1 pound lean round steak, trimmed
  and cut into 1-inch cubes**
1¼ cups water
1 large baking potato, cubed
2 carrots, sliced
½ cup light beer
1 red bell pepper, chopped
⅓ cup chopped fresh cilantro
1 can (16 ounces) chopped tomatoes
1 onion, chopped
1 clove garlic, chopped
1 jalapeño pepper, seeded and chopped (optional)
2 teaspoons dried oregano
1½ teaspoons chili powder
½ teaspoon beef-flavored bouillon granules
2 tablespoons flour
2 tablespoons water

1. Sauté round steak in a large Dutch oven until seared on all sides, about 3–4 minutes. Add remaining ingredients except for flour and water. Mix well and bring to a boil. Cover and reduce heat to simmer; cook 1 hour until meat is tender, stirring occasionally.
2. Combine flour and water, stirring to make a smooth paste. Gradually add paste to meat mixture and cook, stirring frequently, until thickened and bubbly.

Preparation time: 15 minutes
Cooking time: 1¼ hours

Yield: 6 servings
Serving size: 1 cup

Exchanges: 1 starch
　　　　　　 2 lean meat
Carbohydrate choices: 1

Nutrition per serving:
Calories: 184
Carbohydrate: . . . . 16 g
Protein: . . . . 20 g
Fat: . . . . 4 g

Saturated fat: . . . . 1 g
Cholesterol: . . . . 58 mg
Dietary fiber: . . . . 2 g
Sodium: . . . . 282 mg

Homestyle pot roast

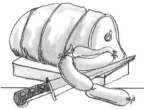

**3½ pounds boneless lean beef brisket,
  cross rib, chuck, or rump roast**
1 teaspoon dry mustard
½ teaspoon salt (optional)
½ cup chopped onion
1 can (about 8 ounces) tomato sauce
2 tablespoons red wine vinegar
1 teaspoon dried leaf thyme
¼ teaspoon freshly ground black pepper

1. Trim all fat from the roast. Rub the roast with the dry mustard and salt (optional). Place the meat in a lightly oiled ovenproof casserole. Preheat oven to 325°F.
2. In a small bowl, combine the remaining ingredients and mix together. Pour tomato mixture over the roast and cover tightly.
3. Bake until the meat is very tender, about 3 hours. (Or MICROWAVE on High, covered, for 65–70 minutes, turning meat over halfway through cooking time.)

To turn this into a simple one-dish meal, add sliced carrots, cubes of Russet potatoes, and 1–1½ cups of water to the tomato mixture in the last 45 minutes of cooking.

199

Preparation time: 10 minutes
Cooking time: 3 hours

Exchanges: 3 lean meat
Carbohydrate choices: 0

Yield: 10 servings
Serving size: 3 ounces

Nutrition per serving:
Calories: 191
Carbohydrate:. . . . . 2 g
Protein: . . . . 24 g
Fat:. . . . . 10 g

Saturated fat: . . . . 4 g
Cholesterol:. . . . . 70 mg
Dietary fiber: . . . . 1 g
Sodium:. . . . . 309 mg
(omitting salt) . . . . 202 mg

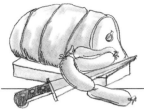

Savory stuffed peppers

4 medium green peppers
½ pound extra-lean ground beef
½ cup chopped onion
1 cup drained, canned whole tomatoes
1 cup cooked wild rice
1 tablespoon Worcestershire sauce
½ teaspoon Italian seasoning
½ cup soft bread crumbs
Nonfat cooking spray
1 cup canned tomato sauce

1. Slice off stem end of peppers and remove and discard seeds and membranes. Submerge the peppers in a pan of boiling water and cook 5–10 minutes; drain.

2. Preheat oven to 350°F. Brown ground beef and onion in a nonstick skillet over medium heat. Drain and pat dry with paper towels. Return meat mixture to skillet. Add tomatoes, breaking them into pieces with a cooking spoon, and cook until liquid evaporates. Remove meat mixture from heat; stir in wild rice, Worcestershire sauce, and Italian seasoning.

3. Spoon ½ cup of rice mixture into each pepper; sprinkle evenly with bread crumbs. Place peppers in a baking dish coated with cooking spray. Bake for 20 minutes, or until lightly browned. Spoon tomato sauce over peppers and return to oven until heated.

200

Preparation time: 10 minutes
Cooking time: 35 minutes

Yield: 4 servings
Serving size: 1 stuffed pepper

Nutrition per serving:
Calories: 243
Carbohydrate: . . . . 34 g
Protein: . . . . 19 g
Fat: . . . . 4 g

Exchanges: 2 starch
1 vegetable
1 lean meat
Carbohydrate choices: 2½

Saturated fat: . . . . <1 g
Cholesterol: . . . . 36 mg
Dietary fiber: . . . . 5 g
Sodium: . . . . 653 mg

Meatballs

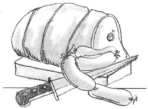

1 egg (or ¼ cup liquid egg substitute)
3 tablespoons ketchup
¼ cup dry bread crumbs
¼ cup minced fresh parsley
1 teaspoon dried oregano
½ teaspoon salt (optional)
¼ teaspoon freshly ground black pepper
½ cup cold water
1 pound lean ground beef or pork or turkey
Nonfat cooking spray

1. In a mixing bowl. combine the egg (or egg substitute), ketchup, herbs, seasonings, and ½ cup water; mix with a fork until well blended. Add the ground meat and mix thoroughly, but do not overmix. Preheat oven to 350°F.
2. Shape 2 tablespoons of the meat mixture into a round ball; repeat with the rest of the mixture. Place meatballs in equidistant rows on a baking sheet that has been sprayed with nonfat cooking spray and bake until meat is thoroughly cooked, about 15–20 minutes.

Add these savory meatballs to either Spaghetti Sauce (recipe, p. 357) or Stroganoff Sauce (recipe, p. 358) and serve over noodles. And here's a hint to keep the meat mixture from sticking to your hands: either run your hands under cold water for ten seconds or spray them with cooking spray.

201

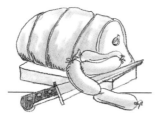

Preparation time: 10 minutes
Cooking time: 20 minutes

Yield: 6 servings
Serving size: 4 meatballs

Nutrition per serving:

With egg and ground beef

Exchanges: 2 medium-fat meat
Carbohydrate choices: 0

Calories: 161
Carbohydrate:. . . . . 5 g
Protein: . . . . 15 g
Fat:. . . . . 9 g
Saturated fat: . . . . 4 g
Cholesterol: . . . . 91 mg
Dietary fiber: . . . . 0 g
Sodium:. . . . . 337 mg
(omitting salt) . . . . . . 159 mg

**With egg substitute and
ground turkey**

Exchanges: 2 lean meat
Carbohydrate choices: 0

Calories: 127
Carbohydrate:. . . . . 5 g
Protein: . . . . 19 g
Fat:. . . . . 3 g
Saturated fat: . . . . 1 g
Cholesterol: . . . . 45 mg
Dietary fiber: . . . . 0 g
Sodium:. . . . . 341 mg
(omitting salt) . . . . . . 163 mg

Veggie meat loaf

The addition of vegetables to a traditional meat loaf cuts down on the amount of meat in each serving—and it's a great way to add fiber! Try this trick the next time you find yourself a little short on ground beef.

2 medium carrots, peeled and finely chopped

1 stalk celery, finely chopped

1 small onion, finely chopped

1 cup low-sodium beef broth (or water)

¼ cup Seasoned Bread Crumbs (recipe, p. 363) or commercial bread crumbs

¼ cup minced fresh parsley

1 egg, beaten (or ¼ cup liquid egg substitute)

1 teaspoon salt (optional)

½ teaspoon freshly ground black pepper

1 pound lean ground beef (or lean ground pork or lean ground turkey)

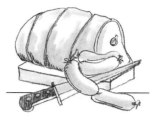

1. Preheat oven to 350°F. Combine the carrots, celery, and onion in a saucepan with ½ cup broth (or water). Cook, uncovered, over medium heat until softened, about 7 minutes, stirring occasionally. Remove from heat and set aside.

2. In a mixing bowl, combine the remaining ½ cup broth, bread crumbs, parsley, egg (or egg substitute), salt (optional), pepper, and meat. Mix thoroughly using your hands. Form the mixture into a loaf in a shallow baking pan large enough for the juices to drain away from the meat. Bake until the meat is no longer pink, about 50–60 minutes. (Or MICROWAVE on High, covered, in a microwave-safe dish, about 8 minutes.) Remove from oven to warm serving platter. Cut into 6 equal slices.

203

Preparation time: 15 minutes
Cooking time: 1¼ hours

Yield: 6 servings
Serving size: 1 slice

Exchanges: 1 vegetable
         2 medium-fat meat
Carbohydrate choices: ½

Nutrition per serving:

With egg
Calories: 184
Carbohydrate:. . . . . 7 g
Protein: . . . . 16 g
Fat:. . . . . 10 g
Saturated fat: . . . . 4 g
Cholesterol:. . . . . 95 mg
Dietary fiber: . . . . 1 g
Sodium:. . . . . 477 mg
(omitting salt) . . . . . . 122 mg

With egg substitute
Calories: 175
Carbohydrate:. . . . . 7 g
Protein: . . . . 16 g
Fat:. . . . . 9 g
Saturated fat: . . . . 4 g
Cholesterol:. . . . . 49 mg
Dietary fiber: . . . . 1 g
Sodium:. . . . . 478 mg
(omitting salt) . . . . . . 123 mg

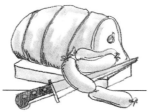

204

This classic beef stew is best made a day or two ahead of serving to allow the flavors to combine.

Beef Burgundy

2 slices bacon (or turkey bacon), chopped
2 cups chopped onion
2 pounds lean stewing beef, cut into 1-inch cubes
2 tablespoons all-purpose flour
1 teaspoon salt (optional)
1 teaspoon dried leaf thyme
½ teaspoon freshly ground black pepper
1 clove garlic, minced
1½ cups dry red wine (not "cooking wine")
1½ cups low-sodium beef broth
1 tablespoon tomato paste
½ pound fresh mushrooms, cleaned and sliced

1. In a nonstick skillet or lightly oiled frying pan, cook the bacon until crisp and drain on paper towels. (Or MICROWAVE on High, wrapped loosely in paper towel, 2–3 minutes.)
2. Remove all but a film of the bacon fat from the skillet. Cook the onions until tender, about 5 minutes. Remove the onions from the skillet with a slotted spoon and set aside.
3. Add the meat to the skillet and brown on all sides. Add the flour, salt (optional), thyme, pepper, and garlic, and cook, stirring, for 1 minute. Stir in bacon, wine, broth, and tomato paste. Stir well, reduce heat to low, and simmer, uncovered, until meat is very tender, about 2 hours. Add mushrooms and reserved onion and simmer 20 minutes longer.

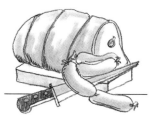

| Preparation time: 15 minutes | Exchanges: 2 lean meat |
| Cooking time: 2½ hours | Carbohydrate choices: 0 |

Yield: 12 servings
Serving size: ½ cup

Nutrition per serving:

Calories: 128	Saturated fat: . . . . 2 g
Carbohydrate:. . . . . 4 g	Cholesterol: . . . . 42 mg
Protein: . . . . 16 g	Dietary fiber: . . . . <1 g
Fat:. . . . . 5 g	Sodium:. . . . . 232 mg
	(omitting salt) . . . . 54 mg

Pork-stuffed lamb roast

7 pounds leg of lamb

1½ pounds pork tenderloin

1 teaspoon mixed herbs (dried basil, marjoram, oregano)

½ teaspoon freshly ground black pepper

¼ teaspoon garlic powder

1 cup Velouté Sauce (recipe, p. 359)

Holiday guests will love this stuffed lamb roast— and you will love how easy it is to prepare. Just pop it in the oven and let it cook.

1. Ask your butcher to bone a leg of lamb and replace the bone with a pork tenderloin. Have him roll and tie the roast securely. Preheat the oven to 350°F.

2. Crush the herbs in the palm of your hand and rub them into the surface of the roast. Sprinkle with pepper and garlic powder.

3. Place the roast on a rack in a roasting pan. Roast 2–2¼ hours, or until a meat thermometer registers an internal temperature of 140°F (for medium). Remove from oven, tent with foil, and allow to rest at least 10 minutes before carving. Serve with Velouté Sauce.

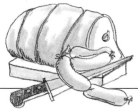

Preparation time: 5 minutes
Roasting time: 2–2¼ hours

Yield: 20 servings
Serving size: 3 ounces

Exchanges: 3 lean meat
Carbohydrate choices: 0

Nutrition per serving:
Calories: 148
Carbohydrate:. . . . . 0 g
Protein: . . . . 22 g
Fat:. . . . . 6 g

Saturated fat: . . . . 3 g
Cholesterol:. . . . . 69 mg
Dietary fiber: . . . . 0 g
Sodium:. . . . . 112 mg

Spicy baked pork chops

Why settle for plain old pork chops when this spicy casserole will have your family asking for more?

2 tablespoons plus 1 tablespoon chili seasoning mix
2 tablespoons all-purpose flour
4 boneless pork loin chops, ½-inch thick (about 4 ounces each)
Nonfat cooking spray
1½ teaspoons corn oil
1 cup uncooked instant white rice
1 cup water
1 can (about 8 ounces) tomato sauce
½ cup coarsely chopped onion
½ cup coarsely chopped yellow pepper
½ cup coarsely chopped green pepper

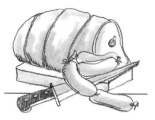

1. Preheat oven to 350°F. Combine 2 tablespoons chili seasoning mix with flour in a large zip-top bag. Add pork chops and shake to coat well.

2. Coat a large, nonstick skillet with cooking spray, add oil, and heat until oil is hot. Add chops and sprinkle with remaining coating. Brown pork chops quickly over medium-high heat, about 3–4 minutes each side. Remove from heat and set aside.

3. Coat a 2-quart casserole dish with cooking spray; set aside. In a large bowl, stir together the remaining 1 table-spoon chili seasoning mix, rice, water, and tomato sauce. Pour into casserole dish. Arrange pork chops over rice and sprinkle with onion, yellow pepper, and green pepper.

4. Bake, covered, for 35–40 minutes, or until rice is bubbly and pork chops are no longer pink in the center.

207

Preparation time: 25 minutes
Baking time: 35–40 minutes

Yield: 4 servings
Serving size: 1 pork chop with
¼ rice mixture

Exchanges: 2 starch
1 vegetable
4 very lean meat
1 fat
Carbohydrate choices: 2½

Nutrition per serving:
Calories: 373
Carbohydrate:. . . . . 34 g
Protein: . . . . 39 g
Fat:. . . . . 9 g

Saturated fat: . . . . 4 g
Cholesterol: . . . . 66 mg
Dietary fiber: . . . . 2 g
Sodium:. . . . . 965 mg

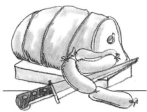

Stuffed butterfly pork chops

If you do not have a food processor to shred your vegetables, use the widest holes on a cheese grater and grate the vegetables sideways rather than lengthwise.

208

1–2 medium zucchini, shredded and drained (about 1 cup)

1 medium carrot, peeled and shredded (about ⅓ cup)

Nonfat cooking spray

2 tablespoons olive oil

1 tablespoon minced onion

¼ cup fresh whole wheat bread crumbs

¼ teaspoon crushed dried rosemary leaves

¼ teaspoon dried sage

2 pork chops, ½-inch thick, butterflied and trimmed of fat

¼ teaspoon dry mustard

1. In a mixing bowl, toss the zucchini and carrot together well. Lightly coat a shallow baking dish with cooking spray and sprinkle ⅓ cup of the zucchini-carrot mixture over the bottom of the dish. Preheat oven to 325°F.

2. In a medium frying pan, heat the olive oil and sauté the onion until wilted. Add the bread crumbs, herbs, and remaining cup of zucchini-carrot mixture, and cook, stirring, 2–3 minutes, until carrots are soft.

3. Spoon into the butterflied pork chops; fold over and secure with toothpicks. Rub chops with dry mustard and place them on the shredded vegetables in the baking dish. Cover and bake 20–25 minutes; turn the chops and bake 10 minutes longer, uncovered.

Preparation time: 20 minutes
Cooking time: 40 minutes

Yield: 2 servings
Serving size: 1 stuffed chop

Exchanges: ½ starch
     1 vegetable
     3 lean meat
     1 fat
Carbohydrate choices: 1

Nutrition per serving:
Calories: 288
Carbohydrate:. . . . . 15 g
Protein: . . . . 24 g
Fat:. . . . . 14 g

Saturated fat: . . . . 4 g
Cholesterol:. . . . . 69 mg
Dietary fiber: . . . . 2 g
Sodium:. . . . . 149 mg

Cherry-glazed pork roast

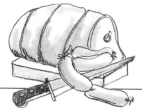

2 jars (12 ounces each) cherry preserves
2 tablespoons red wine vinegar
⅛ teaspoon cinnamon
⅛ teaspoon nutmeg
Dash ground cloves
2 tablespoons cornstarch
2 tablespoons water
1 rolled pork loin roast (about 4 pounds)

The fruit preserves are what make this roast recipe delicious. For a change of pace, substitute blackberry preserves for cherry. For a more Caribbean flavor, use mango preserves. The possibilities are endless.

1. Preheat oven to 325°F. Combine cherry preserves, vinegar, cinnamon, nutmeg, and cloves in a small saucepan. Heat to boiling.

2. Dissolve the cornstarch in the water and stir it into the cherry mixture. Cook the mixture, stirring constantly, until it is clear and slightly thickened, about 1 minute.

3. Place the pork loin on a rack in a shallow roasting pan. Do not add water and do not cover. Roast the pork loin until a meat thermometer registers 170°F, about 30–40 minutes per pound. Baste with a portion of the cherry glaze during the last half hour of roasting, and serve the remaining glaze with the meat at the table.

209

Preparation time: 10 minutes
Cooking time: 2–2½ hours

Yield: 12 servings
Serving size: 4 ounces

Exchanges: 2 carbohydrate
       4 very lean meat
Carbohydrate choices: 2

Nutrition per serving:
Calories: 294
Carbohydrate: . . . . 29 g
Protein: . . . . 32 g
Fat: . . . . 6 g

Saturated fat: . . . . 2 g
Cholesterol: . . . . 96 mg
Dietary fiber: . . . . 0 g
Sodium: . . . . 80 mg

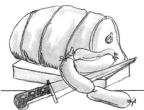

Brown 'n' serve sausage

This is an excellent alternative to store-bought sausage. Ask your butcher to trim and grind the pork for you. Choose pork shoulder or loin for the best taste. The two-step cooking method given here will remove most of the fat.

210

1 pound lean ground pork
¼ cup cracker crumbs
1 teaspoon salt (optional)
1 teaspoon dried sage
½ teaspoon dried leaf thyme
½ teaspoon dried oregano
¼ teaspoon freshly ground black pepper
¼ teaspoon ground cloves
¼ cup cold water

1. In a mixing bowl, combine all of the ingredients. Mix until thoroughly combined, but do not overmix.
2. Divide the meat mixture into 12 portions. With wet hands, form each portion into a sausage-shape roll or flat patty. Place in a nonstick or lightly oiled frying pan. Cook the sausages over medium heat, turning often, until browned on both sides. Drain well on paper towels.
3. If serving immediately, return sausages to a clean frying pan and cook over medium heat, turning once or twice, until sausages are crisp, about 4 minutes.
4. If not serving immediately, wrap once-cooked sausages well and refrigerate up to 5 days or freeze up to 2 months. When ready to serve, cook as described in Step 3.

Preparation time: 10 minutes
Cooking time: 15 minutes

Yield: 12 servings
Serving size: 1 sausage

Exchanges: 1 lean meat
Carbohydrate choices: 0

Nutrition per serving:
Calories: 57
Carbohydrate: . . . . 2 g
Protein: . . . . 8 g
Fat: . . . . 2 g
Saturated fat: . . . . 1 g
Cholesterol: . . . . 14 mg
Dietary fiber: . . . . 0 g
Sodium: . . . . 542 mg

Sweet 'n' sour no-cook ham kabobs

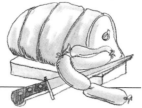

2 ten-inch skewers
6 cherry tomatoes
4 one-inch pineapple chunks (about ¼ cup)
⅓ green bell pepper, cut into 4 strips
4 one-inch ham chunks (½ ounce each)
2 tablespoons Wish-Bone Oriental dressing
   or similar sweet 'n' sour dressing

If you have baked ham left over from holiday dinner, this is a great way to use it. Try making these kabobs in the morning and letting them marinate until lunchtime.

On each skewer, place a tomato, a pineapple chunk, a pepper strip, and a ham cube. Repeat and end with a tomato. Lay kabobs in a shallow dish and drizzle with dressing. If desired, cover and refrigerate 1–2 hours to allow flavors to blend.

211

Preparation time: 10 minutes
Chilling time (optional):
   1–2 hours

Yield: 1 serving
Serving size: 2 kabobs

Nutrition per serving:
Calories: 233
Carbohydrate: . . . . 22 g
Protein: . . . . 16 g
Fat: . . . . 9 g

Exchanges: 1 fruit
          2 vegetable
          2 lean meat
          1 fat
Carbohydrate choices: 1½

Saturated fat: . . . . 2 g
Cholesterol: . . . . 16 mg
Dietary fiber: . . . . 3 g
Sodium: . . . . 1,205 mg

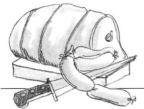

Liver, onions, and tomatoes

212

8 ounces beef, pork, or calf's liver, sliced thin
1 tablespoon all-purpose flour
¼ teaspoon salt (optional)
¼ teaspoon freshly ground black pepper
1 tablespoon olive oil
1 medium onion, sliced thin
1 medium tomato, peeled, seeded, and sliced
1 tablespoon freshly squeezed lemon juice

1. Combine the flour, salt (optional), and pepper; dredge the liver in the flour mixture.
2. In a heavy sauté pan, heat half the oil and cook the liver over medium-high heat until just cooked and tender, 1–2 minutes each side. (Do not overcook.) Remove liver to a serving dish and keep warm.
3. Add remaining oil to pan, along with onion slices. Cook, stirring, over medium heat until the onions are soft and golden, about 7–10 minutes. Add the tomato slices and cook 1–2 more minutes.
4. Return the cooked liver to the pan to reheat briefly. Sprinkle with lemon juice and serve.

Preparation time: 15 minutes
Cooking time: 20 minutes

Yield: 4 servings
Serving size: 2 ounces

Exchanges: 1 vegetable
            2 lean meat
Carbohydrate choices: 0

Nutrition per serving:
Calories: 131
Carbohydrate: . . . . 6 g
Protein: . . . . 13 g
Fat: . . . . 6 g

Saturated fat: . . . . 2 g
Cholesterol: . . . . 193 mg
Dietary fiber: . . . . <1 g
Sodium: . . . . 169 mg
(omitting salt) . . . . 36 mg

Chapter 9

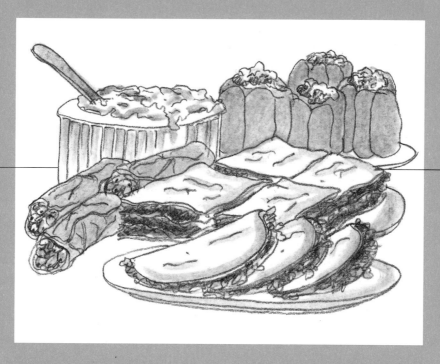

MEATLESS MAIN DISHES

*M*eatless meals aren't just for vegetarians anymore. Anyone who is looking to reduce saturated fat intake, lower cholesterol levels, or eat healthier should try to incorporate at least one meatless main dish into the meal plan each week. The recipes here call for lots of ingredients that are high in fiber and low in fat, such as beans, peas, lentils, cracked wheat, and vegetables.

The good news is that you don't have to skip great taste just because you're skipping meat. There are flavorful and healthy recipes here that you are sure to love. The Creamy Macaroni and Cheese is as tasty as your old favorite—but with half the fat. The Spinach Lasagna and Hearty Vegetable Chili might just make you forget the ground beef is missing. Whatever your taste, there is sure to be a recipe for you.

Tofu chop suey

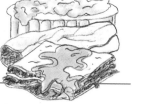

8 ounces tofu
2 teaspoons vegetable oil
1 tablespoon minced fresh ginger
1 clove garlic, minced
1–2 green onions, sliced thin
1 cup sliced celery
¼ red bell pepper, seeded and sliced thin
1½ cups bean sprouts, rinsed and well drained
¼ cup low-sodium chicken broth or vegetable broth
1 tablespoon low-sodium soy sauce
Freshly ground black pepper and salt (optional)

Tofu, a staple in many vegetarian diets, is an excellent source of protein. To get a crispy texture similar to fried chicken, sauté the tofu over medium-high heat in the oil and remove when browned on all sides before proceeding with Step 2.

1. Drain the tofu. Dice it into ¾-inch cubes, place between layers of paper towels, and weight down with a dinner plate; let stand 10 minutes to compress and remove excess water.
2. Heat oil in a wok or frying pan. Add the ginger, garlic, onions, celery, and red pepper, and stir-fry over medium-high heat 1–2 minutes.
3. Add the bean sprouts, broth, soy sauce, and diced tofu and stir-fry until the vegetables are crisp-tender and the liquid is evaporated. Season to taste with salt (optional) and pepper.

215

Preparation time: 20 minutes
Cooking time: 10 minutes

Yield: 4 servings
Serving size: 1 cup

Nutrition per serving:
Calories: 135
Carbohydrate:. . . . . 7 g
Protein: . . . . 10 g
Fat:. . . . . 7 g

Exchanges: 1 vegetable
1 medium-fat meat
½ fat
Carbohydrate choices: ½

Saturated fat: . . . . 1 g
Cholesterol: . . . . trace
Dietary fiber: . . . . 2 g
Sodium:. . . . . 45 mg

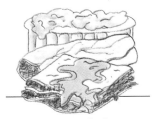

Layered black beans and tortillas

Sometimes called "Mexican Lasagna," this dish will soon become a favorite of you and your family.

Nonfat cooking spray
2 cups chopped onion
2 cloves garlic, minced
1 green bell pepper, chopped
1 red bell pepper, chopped
¾ cup bottled picante sauce
1½ teaspoons ground cumin
2 cans (15 ounces each) black beans, drained
1 can (14 ½ ounces) no-salt-added chopped tomatoes
12 six-inch corn tortillas
1 cup shredded reduced-fat Cheddar cheese
1½ cups lettuce, shredded
1 cup chopped fresh tomato
6 tablespoons fat-free sour cream

216

1. Preheat oven to 350°F. Coat a large skillet with cooking spray. Place over medium heat and add onion and garlic; sauté until tender. Add green and red peppers and sauté 3 minutes more, until tender. Add picante sauce, cumin, beans, and tomatoes; cook 5 minutes, stirring occasionally. Remove from heat and set aside.

2. Coat a 13" × 9" baking dish with cooking spray. Spoon 1 cup of bean mixture into dish. Arrange 6 tortillas in a single layer over the bean mixture and top with ½ cup cheese. Spoon 2½ cups bean mixture over cheese. Arrange 6 remaining tortillas over the beans; top with remaining beans. Cover and bake 30 minutes.

3. Uncover and top with remaining ½ cup cheese; bake 5 minutes more, or until cheese melts. Let stand 5 minutes more before serving. Cut into 6 equal servings. Top each with lettuce, tomato, and 1 tablespoon fat-free sour cream.

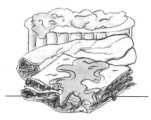

Preparation time: 25 minutes
Cooking time: 35 minutes

Yield: 8 servings
Serving size: about 1 cup

Exchanges: 3 starch
          1 vegetable
          1 very lean meat
Carbohydrate choices: 3

Nutrition per serving:
Calories: 283
Carbohydrate:. . . . . 47 g
Protein: . . . . 15 g
Fat:. . . . . 5 g

Saturated fat: . . . . 2 g
Cholesterol: . . . . 10 mg
Dietary fiber: . . . . 7 g
Sodium:. . . . . 320 mg

Vegetable frittata

2 teaspoons olive oil
½ cup chopped broccoli, asparagus, or green beans
½ cup chopped celery
2 green onions, chopped
1 cup liquid egg substitute (or 4 eggs)
1 tablespoon minced fresh parsley
½ teaspoon dried oregano
¼ teaspoon garlic powder (optional)
¼ teaspoon freshly ground black pepper
1 tablespoon water

What exactly is a frittata? Simply put, it's the Italian version of an omelet. Use whatever vegetables you like in this recipe, but keep in mind that fresher vegetables produce a better flavor.

217

1. Warm oil in a heavy frying pan over medium heat. Add the broccoli, celery, and onion and cook, stirring, 4–5 minutes, until crisp-tender.
2. In a mixing bowl, beat the egg substitute (or eggs), herbs, seasonings, and 1 tablespoon of water. Pour the egg mixture over the vegetables in the frying pan and cook about 30 seconds.
3. Cover the pan and continue cooking 2–3 more minutes, or until set. Cut frittata in half and slide out onto warmed plates.

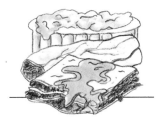

Preparation time: 15 minutes
Cooking time: 10 minutes

Yield: 2 servings
Serving size: ½ frittata

Nutrition per serving:

With egg substitute	**With eggs**
Exchanges: 1 vegetable	Exchanges: 1 vegetable
1 very lean meat	2 medium-fat meat
1 fat	1 fat
Carbohydrate choices: ½	Carbohydrate choices: ½
Calories: 116	Calories: 224
Carbohydrate:. . . . . 7 g	Carbohydrate:. . . . . 6 g
Protein: . . . . 11 g	Protein: . . . . 14 g
Fat:. . . . . 5 g	Fat:. . . . . 16 g
Saturated fat: . . . . 1 g	Saturated fat: . . . . 5 g
Cholesterol:. . . . . 0 mg	Cholesterol: . . . . 548 mg
Dietary fiber: . . . . 2 g	Dietary fiber: . . . . 2 g
Sodium:. . . . . 194 mg	Sodium:. . . . . 172 mg

218

Black bean and vegetable enchiladas

The black beans and corn tortillas combine to make this dish an excellent source of fiber—and it tastes great!

Nonfat cooking spray

2 cans (16 ounces each) black beans, rinsed and drained, divided in half

1 cup chopped onion

1 green pepper, chopped

2 tablespoons vegetable broth

2 cups picante sauce, divided in half

12 six-inch corn tortillas

1 cup chopped tomatoes

½ cup reduced-fat shredded Cheddar cheese

½ cup reduced-fat shredded mozzarella cheese

3 cups shredded lettuce

Fat-free sour cream (optional)

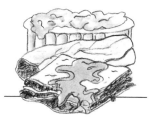

1. Preheat oven to 350°F and coat a 9" × 13" baking pan with cooking spray. Mash one can of the beans with a spoon or in a blender or food processor; set aside.

2. Sauté the onion and green pepper in the vegetable broth until tender, about 2–3 minutes. Add 1 cup picante sauce, the mashed beans, and the can of whole beans. Stir the mixture and heat thoroughly.

3. Spoon about ⅓ cup of the bean mixture down the center of each tortilla and roll it up. Place the tortillas seam-side down in the baking pan. Combine the remaining picante sauce and tomatoes; spoon over enchiladas. Cover with foil and bake 15 minutes.

4. Uncover and sprinkle with cheeses, and bake, uncovered, for 5 more minutes. To serve, place ½ cup lettuce on each plate and top with two enchiladas. Garnish with sour cream, if desired.

219

Preparation time: 15 minutes
Baking time: 20 minutes

Yield: 6 servings
Serving size: 2 enchiladas

Exchanges: 3½ starch
      1 lean meat
Carbohydrate choices: 3½

Nutrition per serving:

Calories: 336	Saturated fat: . . . . 2 g
Carbohydrate: . . . . 56 g	Cholesterol: . . . . 12 mg
Protein: . . . . 19 g	Dietary fiber: . . . . 13 g
Fat: . . . . 5 g	Sodium: . . . . 711 mg

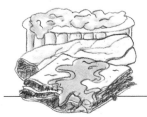

Hearty vegetable chili

There is one "secret" all great chilies have in common: slow cooking over low heat to intensify the flavors. This recipe recommends at least 30 minutes of simmering, but don't be afraid to let it sit longer. Just stir occasionally and add ½ cup water if it looks like your chili is drying out.

1 tablespoon olive or canola oil
1½ cups chopped onion
2 large cloves garlic, chopped
1 medium green pepper, chopped
2 tablespoons drained, canned mild chili peppers, chopped
1 can (28 ounces) whole tomatoes
⅛ teaspoon ground cloves
¼ teaspoon ground allspice
2 tablespoons chili powder
2 teaspoons oregano
2 tablespoons brown sugar
1 cup drained, cooked or canned kidney beans
1 cup drained, cooked or canned pinto beans

Heat oil in a large, heavy saucepan. Add chopped onion, garlic, green pepper, and chili peppers and sauté until soft. Add the tomatoes, spices, oregano, and sugar. Gently stir in beans. Bring mixture to a boil. Reduce heat, cover, and simmer for at least 30 minutes.

220

Preparation time: 10 minutes
Cooking time: 35 minutes

Exchanges: 3 carbohydrate
Carbohydrate choices: 3

Yield: 4 servings
Serving size: 1 cup

Nutrition per serving:
Calories: 237
Carbohydrate:. . . . . 44 g
Protein: . . . . 10 g
Fat:. . . . . 4 g

Saturated fat: . . . . 1 g
Cholesterol:. . . . . 0 mg
Dietary fiber: . . . . 10 g
Sodium:. . . . . 740 mg

Spinach lasagna

¼ **cup skim milk**

1 **container (15 ounces) light ricotta cheese**

1 **jar (about 32 ounces) meatless spaghetti sauce**

7 **lasagna noodles, cooked and drained**

1 **bunch (1 pound) fresh spinach, washed, dried, and torn into pieces**

½ **cup grated Parmesan cheese**

½ **cup sliced almonds**

2 **cups shredded reduced-fat mozzarella cheese**

1. Preheat oven to 350°F. Mix the milk and ricotta cheese in a small bowl; set aside.

2. Cover the bottom of a 9" × 13" baking pan with half the sauce. Follow with layers of half the noodles, half the spinach pieces, half the ricotta mixture, half the Parmesan cheese, half the almonds, and half the mozzarella cheese. Repeat the layers, reserving a little sauce and some almonds to sprinkle on top.

3. Bake for 30 minutes; let sit 10 minutes before cutting into 8 squares. Serve warm.

Fresh spinach and gooey mozzarella cheese makes this vegetarian lasagna a delicious dish. It might just become your favorite.

221

Preparation time: 15 minutes
Baking time: 30 minutes

Yield: 8 servings
Serving size: ⅛ recipe

Exchanges: 2 starch
    1 vegetable
    2 lean meat
    2 fat
Carbohydrate choices: 2½

Nutrition per serving:
Calories: 384
Carbohydrate: . . . . 37 g
Protein: . . . . 21 g
Fat: . . . . 18 g

Saturated fat: . . . . 7 g
Cholesterol: . . . . 42 mg
Dietary fiber: . . . . 6 g
Sodium: . . . . 860 mg

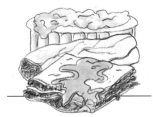

Noodles Romanoff

Think of this as a low-fat version of a fettuccine Alfredo. These noodles make a great side dish when you want to increase the protein in a meal.

1 cup low-fat cottage cheese
½ cup skim milk
¼ cup grated Parmesan cheese
2 green onions, chopped
1 tablespoon chopped fresh dill
or minced fresh parsley
½ teaspoon salt (optional)
¼ teaspoon black pepper
6 ounces whole wheat noodles

1. In a mixing bowl or food processor, blend the cottage cheese and milk until smooth. Add the Parmesan, onions, herbs, and seasonings; mix well.
2. Cook the noodles in lightly salted boiling water just until tender; drain. Return the noodles to the saucepan and fold in the cheese mixture. Stir gently over low heat until hot and bubbly. Serve immediately, sprinkled with extra grated cheese, if desired.

222

Preparation time: 10 minutes
Cooking time: 10 minutes

Yield: 8 servings
Serving size: ½ cup

Exchanges: 1 starch
  1 lean meat
Carbohydrate choices: 1

Nutrition per serving:
Calories: 121
Carbohydrate:. . . . . 17 g
Protein: . . . . 10 g
Fat:. . . . . 2 g

Saturated fat: . . . . 1 g
Cholesterol:. . . . . 4 mg
Dietary fiber: . . . . 3 g
Sodium:. . . . . 164 mg

Stuffed manicotti shells

1 pound firm tofu, mashed
6 ounces shredded mozzarella cheese
½ cup fresh parsley
1 tablespoon onion powder
1 teaspoon garlic powder
½ teaspoon dried basil
1 jar (about 30 ounces) spaghetti sauce
10 jumbo manicotti shells, cooked
¼ cup grated Parmesan cheese

Healthy and protein-rich tofu takes the place of fattening ricotta cheese in this updated version of a family favorite.

1. Preheat oven to 350°F. In a medium bowl, combine the tofu, mozzarella cheese, parsley, onion powder, garlic powder, and basil; set the mixture aside.
2. Spread 2 cups of spaghetti sauce in the bottom of a 9" × 9" pan. Spoon ⅓ cup of the tofu mixture into each cooked shell. Arrange the shells on the sauce and spoon remaining sauce over them. Sprinkle the shells with Parmesan cheese. Bake 25–30 minutes until lightly browned and bubbly.

223

Preparation time: 10 minutes
Baking time: 30 minutes

Yield: 10 servings
Serving size: 1 shell

Exchanges: 1 starch
         1 medium-fat meat
Carbohydrate choices: 1

Nutrition per serving:
Calories: 150
Carbohydrate: . . . . 18 g
Protein: . . . . 9 g
Fat: . . . . 6 g

Saturated fat: . . . . 2 g
Cholesterol: . . . . 12 mg
Dietary fiber: . . . . 2 g
Sodium: . . . . 625 mg

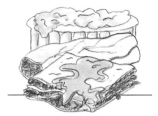

Macaroni, cheese, and tomatoes

Here's a classic recipe that is perfectly suited for a busy night. You can cut your cooking time to 15 minutes by zapping this casserole in the microwave.

1 cup elbow macaroni
1 can (16 ounces) whole tomatoes
1 tablespoon minced fresh parsley
 or chopped fresh dill
½ teaspoon Dijon mustard
¼ teaspoon freshly ground black pepper
1 cup shredded low-fat Cheddar cheese
2 tablespoons cracker crumbs or crushed corn flakes

1. Preheat the oven to 350°F. Cook the macaroni in lightly salted boiling water according to package directions. Drain.
2. Break up the tomatoes in their juice. Stir in the herbs and seasonings. Combine the cooked macaroni, cheese, and tomato mixture; mix lightly.
3. Spoon the mixture into a lightly oiled 6-cup casserole. Sprinkle with crumbs. Bake until the crumbs are brown and the mixture is bubbly, about 30 minutes. (Or MICROWAVE on High, uncovered, 4–5 minutes.)

224

Preparation time: 10 minutes
Cooking time: 40 minutes

Yield: 5 servings
Serving size: 1 cup

Nutrition per serving:
Calories: 173
Carbohydrate: . . . . 21 g
Protein: . . . . 9 g
Fat: . . . . 5 g

Exchanges: 1 starch
 1 vegetable
 1 medium-fat meat
Carbohydrate choices: 1½

Saturated fat: . . . . 1 g
Cholesterol: . . . . trace
Dietary fiber: . . . . 5 g
Sodium: . . . . 418 mg

Creamy macaroni and cheese

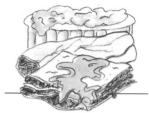

1¼ cups elbow macaroni
2 teaspoons margarine
2 tablespoons all-purpose flour
2 cups skim milk
½ teaspoon salt (optional)
¼ teaspoon ground black pepper
1 tablespoon minced onion (optional)
2–3 drops hot pepper (or Tabasco) sauce
1½ cups shredded low-fat Cheddar cheese
2 tablespoons dry bread crumbs

Good, old-fashioned macaroni and cheese can be made tangier with extra-sharp Cheddar and a few extra drops of hot pepper sauce.

1. Preheat the oven to 350°F. Cook the macaroni in lightly salted boiling water according to package directions. Drain.
2. In a medium saucepan, melt the margarine; whisk in the flour, milk, salt (optional), pepper, onion (optional), and hot pepper sauce. Whisk over medium heat until smooth and thickened.
3. In a lightly oiled 6-cup casserole, layer the macaroni, cheese, and sauce two times, reserving 2 tablespoons of cheese for the top.
4. Combine the bread crumbs and reserved cheese and sprinkle over the top. Bake until lightly browned and mixture is bubbly, about 30 minutes. (Or MICROWAVE on High, uncovered, 4–5 minutes.)

225

Preparation time: 10 minutes
Cooking time: 40 minutes

Yield: 4 servings
Serving size: 1 cup

Exchanges: 2 starch
          2 medium-fat meat
          ½ fat
Carbohydrate choices: 2

Nutrition per serving:
Calories: 329
Carbohydrate:. . . . . 35 g
Protein: . . . . 19 g
Fat:. . . . . 12 g

Saturated fat: . . . . 3 g
Cholesterol:. . . . . 2 mg
Dietary fiber: . . . . 5 g
Sodium:. . . . . 840 mg
(omitting salt) . . . . 573 mg

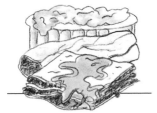

Tangy cheese tortellini

Sun-dried tomatoes give any dish a powerful, concentrated flavor. You will especially love them with tortellini. If you can't find freshly made tortellini, use frozen tortellini from your supermarket.

¼ cup sun-dried tomatoes (not oil-packed)
½ cup hot water
1 tablespoon olive oil
2 large cloves garlic, peeled and minced
½ cup chopped red pepper
1 teaspoon dried oregano
1 small zucchini, chopped
1 package (9 ounces) low-fat fresh cheese tortellini
1 tablespoon fresh grated Parmesan cheese

1. Combine tomatoes and hot water in a small bowl; allow tomatoes to soak for 15 minutes. Drain and finely chop the tomatoes. Set aside.
2. Heat oil in a nonstick skillet. Add the garlic, pepper, and oregano, sautéing 2–3 minutes. Stir in zucchini and sauté an additional 2 minutes. Stir in tomatoes and keep mixture warm.
3. Cook the tortellini according to the package directions. Drain. Mix in warm tomato mixture. Sprinkle with Parmesan cheese and serve.

226

Preparation time: 15 minutes
Cooking time: 15 minutes

Yield: 4 servings
Serving size: ¼ recipe

Exchanges: 1½ starch
 1½ fat
Carbohydrate choices: 1½

Nutrition per serving:
Calories: 185
Carbohydrate:. . . . . 24 g
Protein: . . . . 8 g
Fat:. . . . . 7 g

Saturated fat: . . . . 2 g
Cholesterol: . . . . 21 mg
Dietary fiber: . . . . 3 g
Sodium:. . . . . 260 mg

Penne with tomato sauce

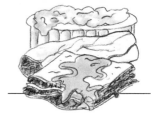

¾ **pound penne**

1 can (28 ounces) whole plum tomatoes

½ **cup loosely packed fresh basil leaves,
cleaned and patted dry**

2 cloves garlic, chopped

1 cup part-skim ricotta cheese

¼ **cup Parmesan cheese**

Chopped fresh basil for garnish (optional)

1. Prepare pasta according to package directions. While pasta is cooking, combine tomatoes, basil, and garlic in a blender or food processor. Blend at low speed until tomatoes are pureed. Pour mixture into large saucepan. Heat to boiling, reduce heat, cover, and simmer 5 minutes.

2. Drain pasta when done, return to cooking pot, and add tomato sauce; stir until pasta is completely coated with sauce. Remove pot from heat and stir in ricotta and Parmesan cheese. Divide onto serving plates and top with fresh basil, if desired.

The sauce in this recipe can be made ahead of time and kept in the refrigerator for up to 3 weeks. Use it in all your pasta dishes.

227

Preparation time: 10 minutes
Cooking time: 10 minutes

Yield: about 8 servings
Serving size: 1⅓ cups

Exchanges: 2½ starch
　　　　　　1 lean meat
Carbohydrate choices: 2½

Nutrition per serving:
Calories: 245
Carbohydrate: . . . . 40 g
Protein: . . . . 11 g
Fat: . . . . 4 g

Saturated fat: . . . . 2 g
Cholesterol: . . . . 12 mg
Dietary fiber: . . . . 3 g
Sodium: . . . . 417 mg

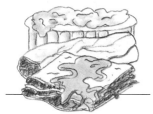

Bean-stuffed cabbage rolls

Black-eyed peas are really beans. They have a smoky flavor that will remind you of the traditional ground beef filling that normally goes into these cabbage rolls.

228

16 medium cabbage leaves (about 1 medium head)
2 cups cooked (or canned) black-eyed peas, mashed
1 cup cooked barley
1 cup finely chopped celery
½ cup minced onion
1 teaspoon salt (optional)
1 tablespoon minced fresh basil
   or 1 teaspoon dried basil
½ teaspoon dried oregano
½ teaspoon dried leaf thyme
2–3 drops hot pepper (or Tabasco) sauce
2 cups tomato juice

1. Core the cabbage, wrap in plastic wrap, and freeze overnight to wilt the leaves. To separate leaves, run warm water into the core of the frozen head. Trim the center rib on each of the 16 leaves to give them a uniform thickness, but do not remove the ribs.

2. In a mixing bowl, mash the black-eyed peas and barley together. Add the celery, onion, salt (optional), basil, oregano, thyme, and hot pepper sauce. Work together with your hands until well blended. Preheat the oven to 350°F.

3. Place about ¼ cup of the black-eyed pea mixture on the rib end of a cabbage leaf. Roll up, tucking in the sides. Repeat with all of the leaves. Pack the cabbage rolls tightly into a 2-quart casserole.

4. Pour the tomato juice over the rolls. Cover tightly and bake 1 hour. (Or MICROWAVE on High, covered, for 15 minutes.)

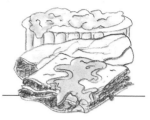

Preparation time: 20 minutes
Cooking time: 1 hour

Yield: 16 servings
Serving size: 1 cabbage roll

Exchanges: ½ starch
          1 vegetable
Carbohydrate choices: ½

Nutrition per serving:
Calories: 53
Carbohydrate:. . . . . 10 g
Protein: . . . . 2 g
Fat: . . . . trace

Saturated fat: . . . . 0 g
Cholesterol:. . . . . 0 mg
Dietary fiber: . . . . 3 g
Sodium:. . . . . 255 mg
(omitting salt) . . . . 121 mg

No-egg salad

1 can (about 15 ounces) chickpeas, rinsed and drained
¼ cup Cider Vinegar Dressing (recipe, p. 115)
¼ cup chopped celery
¼ teaspoon curry powder (or more to taste)
⅛ teaspoon garlic powder

Combine all of the ingredients in a food processor and process, pulsing on and off, until coarsely chopped (or mash by hand). Do not overprocess; a coarse texture is more like a real egg salad.

Real egg salad contains a lot of cholesterol because of the egg yolks. This version provides the egg salad taste, texture, and protein with almost no fat. And it contains a good amount of fiber.

229

Preparation time: 10 minutes

Yield: 6 servings
Serving size: ⅓ cup

Exchanges: 1 starch
Carbohydrate choices: 1

Nutrition per serving:
Calories: 86
Carbohydrate:. . . . . 15 g
Protein: . . . . 5 g
Fat: . . . . trace

Saturated fat: . . . . trace
Cholesterol:. . . . . 5 mg
Dietary fiber: . . . . 4 g
Sodium:. . . . . 25 mg

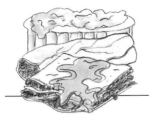

Spanish bulgur

Soy nuts are cooked, roasted soybeans, and they make a wonderful addition to this recipe. You can also serve this in smaller portions as a side dish to another main course.

2 tablespoons olive oil
1 cup thinly sliced carrot
½ cup coarsely chopped onion
1 clove garlic, minced
1¼ cups bulgur (cracked wheat)
3 cups low-sodium chicken or beef broth
1 can (16 ounces) whole tomatoes, chopped
2 teaspoons paprika
1 teaspoon dried tarragon
1 teaspoon salt (optional)
¼ teaspoon freshly ground black pepper
1 cup coarsely chopped celery
1 cup coarsely chopped green bell pepper
1 cup cooked (or canned) garbanzo beans (chickpeas), drained
½ cup coarsely chopped soy nuts

1. Heat oil in a frying pan; add the carrot, onion, and garlic, and stir-fry over medium heat 4–5 minutes. Add the bulgur and continue to cook, stirring, about 3 minutes.
2. Add the broth, tomatoes, paprika, tarragon, salt (optional), and pepper. Bring to a boil, reduce heat, cover, and simmer 30 minutes.
3. Stir in the celery, green pepper, garbanzo beans, and soy nuts. Cover and simmer 15 minutes longer. Turn off heat and let stand, covered, 10 minutes. Fluff with a fork and serve.

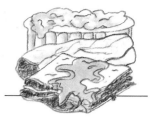

Preparation time: 15 minutes
Cooking time: 55 minutes

Yield: 8 servings
Serving size: 1 cup

Nutrition per serving:
Calories: 211
Carbohydrate:. . . . . 31 g
Protein: . . . . 8 g
Fat:. . . . . 6 g

Exchanges: 2 starch
            1 lean meat
Carbohydrate choices: 2

Saturated fat: . . . . 1 g
Cholesterol:. . . . . 3 mg
Dietary fiber: . . . . 6 g
Sodium:. . . . . 421 mg
(omitting salt) . . . . 154 mg

Mushroom omelet

1 teaspoon vegetable oil
1 small onion, chopped
½ pound mushrooms, cleaned and sliced
1 cup liquid egg substitute (or 4 eggs)
¼ cup shredded low-fat Swiss cheese
1 tablespoon minced fresh basil or parsley
½ teaspoon salt (optional)
¼ teaspoon ground white pepper

1. Heat the oil in an omelet or frying pan. Sauté the onion, stirring, about 2 minutes. Add the mushrooms and sauté about 3 more minutes.
2. In a mixing bowl, beat the egg substitute (or eggs) with the cheese, herbs, and seasonings. Pour the egg mixture over the mushrooms and cook over medium heat 3–4 minutes, or until the mixture is set on top and golden brown on the bottom.
3. Run a spatula around the inside of the frying pan to loosen the omelet. Fold the omelet in half and turn it out onto a warm serving platter.

An omelet doesn't have to be just for breakfast anymore. For an unusual but delightful afternoon or evening treat, serve this with an Asian dipping sauce: ¼ cup chicken broth, 2 tablespoons soy sauce, 1 teaspoon sugar, a pinch of garlic powder, and a pinch of ground ginger.

231

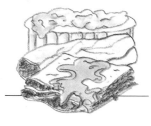

Preparation time: 10 minutes
Cooking time: 10 minutes

Yield: 2 servings
Serving size: ½ omelet

Nutrition per serving:

With egg substitute
Exchanges: 2 vegetable
           2 lean meat
           ½ fat
Carbohydrate choices: ½

Calories: 179
Carbohydrate:. . . . . 10 g
Protein: . . . . 15 g
Fat: . . . . 8 g
Saturated fat: . . . . 1 g
Cholesterol: . . . . 3 mg
Dietary fiber: . . . . 2 g
Sodium: . . . . 880 mg
(omitting salt) . . . . . . 347 mg

With eggs
Exchanges: 2 vegetable
           2 medium-fat meat
           2 fat
Carbohydrate choices: ½

Calories: 287
Carbohydrate:. . . . . 9 g
Protein: . . . . 18 g
Fat: . . . . 19 g
Saturated fat: . . . . 5 g
Cholesterol: . . . . 551 mg
Dietary fiber: . . . . 2 g
Sodium: . . . . 858 mg
(omitting salt) . . . . . . 325 mg

Orzo stuffed peppers

Stuffed peppers are not only easy to make, they are incredibly versatile. Use your imagination to create whatever stuffing you want. Instead of orzo, try couscous, rice, or even polenta.

8 ounces orzo (or other small pasta shape)

2 teaspoons oil

2 cloves garlic, minced

1 medium onion, chopped

1 celery stalk, diced

½ teaspoon thyme

1 tablespoon chopped fresh parsley

½ cup grated Parmesan cheese

1½ plus ½ cups low-sodium chicken broth

3 ounces reduced-fat provolone cheese, grated and divided in half

6 red bell peppers

3 teaspoons Seasoned Bread Crumbs (recipe, p. 363) or commercial bread crumbs

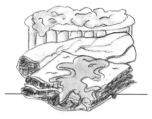

1. Preheat oven to 350°F. Prepare pasta according to package directions; drain and set aside.

2. Heat oil in medium saucepan; add garlic, onion, and celery. Cover and cook until vegetables are soft. Remove from heat. Stir in pasta, thyme, parsley, Parmesan cheese, ½ cup of the chicken broth, and half the provolone cheese. Set aside.

3. Cut tops off the peppers and remove and discard seeds and membranes. If you have to, cut a small piece off the bottoms so the peppers will stand upright. Spoon the pasta mixture into each pepper and set in baking dish. Sprinkle each pepper with ½ teaspoon bread crumbs. Sprinkle the remaining half of the provolone cheese on top of the peppers. Pour the remaining 1½ cups of chicken broth around the peppers. Bake 45 minutes until lightly browned on top and tender. Serve immediately.

233

Preparation time: 25 minutes
Baking time: 45 minutes

Yield: 6 servings
Serving size: 1 pepper

Exchanges: 2 starch
1 vegetable
1 lean meat
½ fat
Carbohydrate choices: 2½

Nutrition per serving:
Calories: 272
Carbohydrate: . . . . 38 g
Protein: . . . . 14 g
Fat: . . . . 7 g
Saturated fat: . . . . 3 g
Cholesterol: . . . . 17 mg
Dietary fiber: . . . . 3 g
Sodium: . . . . 383 mg

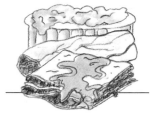

Lentil burgers

Vegetarian burgers have become very popular lately; you can find a wide variety in the frozen foods section of your supermarket. But why pay high prices when you can make this tasty, protein-rich burger at home?

1 can (about 19 ounces) brown lentils, rinsed and drained
2/3 cup bread crumbs
1/4 cup minced onion
1/4 cup minced celery
1 teaspoon Worcestershire sauce
1/2 teaspoon salt (optional)
1/2 teaspoon freshly ground black pepper
1/3 cup cold water
1 tablespoon vegetable oil
2 slices low-fat processed cheese, cut in halves

1. In a mixing bowl, mash the lentils. Add the bread crumbs, onion, celery, Worcestershire, salt (optional), pepper, and 1/3 cup water. Mix well.
2. Form lentil mixture into 4 burgers, each about 1/2 inch thick. Heat the oil in a heavy frying pan and brown the burgers on both sides, about 4–5 minutes each side. Top each with a half-slice of cheese and serve.

234

Preparation time: 15 minutes
Cooking time: 10 minutes

Yield: 4 servings
Serving size: 1 burger

Nutrition per serving:
Calories: 267
Carbohydrate: . . . . 37 g
Protein: . . . . 14 g
Fat: . . . . 7 g

Exchanges: 2½ starch
1 very lean meat
1 fat
Carbohydrate choices: 2½

Saturated fat: . . . . 2 g
Cholesterol: . . . . 7 mg
Dietary fiber: . . . . 4 g
Sodium: . . . . 607 mg
(omitting salt) . . . . 340 mg

Baked cheesy vegetable pie

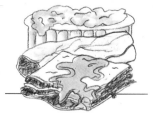

Nonfat cooking spray
4 cups frozen shredded potatoes, thawed
1 cup shredded reduced-fat Cheddar cheese
1 cup mixed vegetables, cut into bite-size pieces
¾ cup skim milk
¾ cup liquid egg substitute
½ teaspoon salt
¼ teaspoon pepper

Make this delicious pie for either breakfast or dinner. You can use whatever vegetables you happen to have on hand.

1. Preheat oven to 350°F and coat a 9-inch pie plate with cooking spray. Combine the potatoes, cheese, vegetables, skim milk, egg substitute, salt, and pepper in a large mixing bowl and stir well. Pour the mixture into the pie plate.
2. Bake, uncovered, for 45 minutes, or until a knife inserted in the center comes out clean. Let stand 10 minutes before slicing into 4 wedges.

235

Preparation time: 5 minutes
Baking time: 45 minutes

Yield: 4 servings
Serving size: 1 wedge

Exchanges: 2 starch
2 lean meat
Carbohydrate choices: 2

Nutrition per serving:
Calories: 269
Carbohydrate:. . . . . 33 g
Protein: . . . . 20 g
Fat:. . . . . 7 g

Saturated fat: . . . . 4 g
Cholesterol: . . . . 21 mg
Dietary fiber: . . . . 4 g
Sodium:. . . . . 641 mg

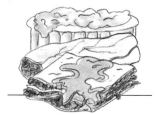

California veggie wraps

Veggie wraps are a perfect low-calorie alternative to tacos or burritos. For extra zing, add ½ teaspoon of packaged taco hot sauce to the inside filling of each wrap.

1 tablespoon olive oil

2 cups broccoli florets

1 cup sliced fresh mushrooms

1 red bell pepper, thinly sliced

½ cup sliced green onions

8 six-inch corn tortillas

1 cup shredded reduced-fat Cheddar
  or Monterey Jack cheese

Nonfat sour cream (optional)

Salsa (optional)

1. Preheat oven to 375°F. Heat oil in a large nonstick skillet. Add broccoli, mushrooms, red pepper, and onions. Cook 2–3 minutes until crisp-tender. Set aside.

2. Warm the tortillas according to package directions. Divide the vegetable mixture evenly among the tortillas, placing it in a line along the center of each. Top each tortilla with 2 tablespoons of cheese. Fold tortillas in half or roll them up to enclose the filling.

3. Place the tortillas on an ungreased baking sheet and bake 3–5 minutes until the cheese is melted. Serve immediately with sour cream and salsa, if desired.

236

Preparation time: 10 minutes
Cooking time: 10 minutes

Yield: 8 servings
Serving size: 1 tortilla

Exchanges: ½ starch
              1 vegetable
              1 fat
Carbohydrate choices: 1

Nutrition per serving:
Calories: 109
Carbohydrate:. . . . . 12 g
Protein: . . . . 6 g
Fat:. . . . . 5 g

Saturated fat: . . . . 2 g
Cholesterol:. . . . . 10 mg
Dietary fiber: . . . . 2 g
Sodium:. . . . . 112 mg

Chapter 10

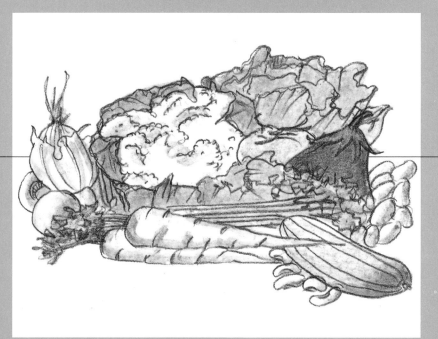

VEGETABLES

*V*egetables are among the most flexible foods on the planet. They can be boiled, baked, sautéed, grilled, poached, or, in many cases, eaten raw. Vegetables can be incorporated into a main dish, as is the case with many casseroles, or they can be served on the side to help round out the flavor, texture, and nutritional value of a meal. All this, and they are abundantly healthy for us; vegetables contain valuable vitamins and minerals, have little or no fat, and have very few calories.

When shopping for vegetables, choose those that are firm to the touch and bright in color. Most vegetables will keep fresh in the refrigerator for 5–7 days. Vegetables that should not be refrigerated are potatoes, sweet potatoes, onions, and winter squash. These are best stored in a cool, dark location such as the basement or a cupboard away from the oven and stove.

The recipes included in this chapter encompass over a dozen different vegetables and almost every method of cooking imaginable. Several of these recipes are microwavable. Enjoy!

Roasted broccoli and cauliflower

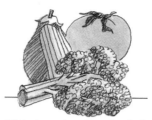

2 cups fresh broccoli florets
2 cups fresh cauliflower florets
2 garlic cloves, minced
1 tablespoon olive oil
⅛ teaspoon salt
¼ teaspoon pepper
Nonfat cooking spray
¼ cup slivered almonds

This is a simple side dish to throw together when you have a more complicated main course. In fact, you can slide this vegetable dish into the oven along with your roast or casserole.

Preheat oven to 400°F. Combine broccoli, cauliflower, and garlic. Add olive oil, salt, and pepper, stirring well to coat. Place mixture in a baking dish coated with nonfat cooking spray. Bake for 20 minutes or until tender and lightly browned, stirring every 5 minutes. Sprinkle almond slivers on top and bake 5 minutes longer, being careful not to let the almonds burn.

239

Preparation time: 5 minutes
Baking time: 25 minutes

Yield: 8 servings
Serving size: ½ cup

Exchanges: 1 vegetable
½ fat
Carbohydrate choices: 0

Nutrition per serving:
Calories: 49
Carbohydrate:. . . . . 4 g
Protein: . . . . 2 g
Fat:. . . . . 3 g

Saturated fat: . . . . trace
Cholesterol:. . . . . 0 mg
Dietary fiber: . . . . 2 g
Sodium:. . . . . 43 mg

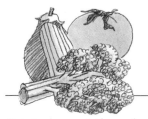

Mixed mashed vegetables

Potatoes aren't the only vegetables that can be served mashed. These root vegetables make a wonderful side dish.

1½ cups peeled, chopped turnip or rutabaga
1½ cups peeled, chopped carrot
1 cup peeled, chopped sweet potato
½ cup part-skim ricotta cheese
2 teaspoons margarine
½ teaspoon salt (optional)
¼ teaspoon ground white pepper

1. In a medium saucepan, combine the turnip (or rutabaga), carrot, and sweet potato. Cover with cold water, bring to a boil, lower heat, and cook until the vegetables are very tender, about 20 minutes. (Or MICROWAVE on High, covered, in a microwave-safe dish until tender, about 15 minutes.)
2. Drain the vegetables; add the ricotta cheese and mash, whip, or press through a strainer into a mixing bowl. Stir in the margarine and season to taste with salt (optional) and pepper.

240

Preparation time: 10 minutes
Cooking time: 20 minutes

Yield: 4 servings
Serving size: ½ cup

Nutrition per serving:
Calories: 164
Carbohydrate:. . . . . 19 g
Protein: . . . . 8 g
Fat:. . . . . 7 g

Exchanges: 1 starch
          1 vegetable
          1½ fat
Carbohydrate choices: 1

Saturated fat: . . . . 3 g
Cholesterol: . . . . 10 mg
Dietary fiber: . . . . 4 g
Sodium: . . . . 424 mg
(omitting salt) . . . . 157 mg

Asparagus with mustard vinaigrette

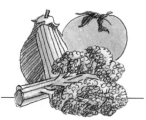

1 pound fresh asparagus
2 teaspoons Dijon mustard
3 tablespoons red wine vinegar
1 teaspoon granulated sugar
¼ teaspoon salt (optional)
¼ teaspoon black pepper
1 tablespoon minced fresh parsley
2 tablespoons olive oil

1. Wash asparagus and trim the ends. If stems are tough, remove the outer layer with a vegetable peeler. Drop asparagus into boiling water and cook until desired texture is reached; drain.

2. Meanwhile, whisk together mustard, vinegar, sugar, salt (optional), pepper, and parsley. Slowly whisk in olive oil until mixture is well blended. Pour over cooked asparagus and serve immediately.

How can you tell when asparagus has been cooked enough? It's a matter of personal taste. Some people think this pungent vegetable is ready to eat as soon as it changes to a bright green color and is still crispy, about 5 minutes. Others boil asparagus until it is completely wilted and very tender, about 10 minutes.

241

Preparation time: 5 minutes
Cooking time: 5–10 minutes

Yield: 6 servings
Serving size: ½ cup

Exchanges: 1 vegetable
1 fat
Carbohydrate choices: 0

Nutrition per serving:
Calories: 56
Carbohydrate: . . . . 3 g
Protein: . . . . 1 g
Fat: . . . . 5 g

Saturated fat: . . . . <1 g
Cholesterol: . . . . 0 mg
Dietary fiber: . . . . 1 g
Sodium: . . . . 121 mg
(omitting salt) . . . . 32 mg

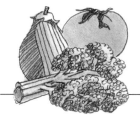

Lentil-stuffed tomatoes

Lentils, unlike other beans, don't take very long to cook, so you can use the dried variety and start from scratch. If you're pressed for time, however, canned lentils work fine in these delicious stuffed tomatoes.

242

4 firm, medium-size tomatoes
¼ cup chopped celery
¼ cup minced onion
2 tablespoons chopped green bell pepper
½ teaspoon curry powder, or more to taste
¼ teaspoon salt (optional)
1 cup cooked brown lentils, drained
1 tablespoon freshly grated Parmesan cheese

1. Preheat oven to 400°F. Core the tomatoes, then cut a slice off the top to allow you to insert a spoon. Scoop the pulp and juice into a bowl and mash. Place the tomato shells cut side down on paper towels to drain.
2. In a medium saucepan, place the tomato pulp–juice mixture, celery, onion, pepper, curry, and salt (optional). Cook, stirring, over medium heat until the vegetables are tender, about 5 minutes.
3. Add the lentils and continue cooking until the mixture is thick and the lentils are quite soft. Divide the mixture evenly into the 4 tomato shells, sprinkle with Parmesan cheese, and place tomatoes into muffin cups set or on a baking sheet. Bake until heated through, about 10–15 minutes.

Preparation time: 15 minutes
Cooking time: 20 minutes

Yield: 4 servings
Serving size: 1 stuffed tomato

Exchanges: 1 carbohydrate
Carbohydrate choices: 1

Nutrition per serving:
Calories: 92
Carbohydrate:. . . . . 16 g
Protein: . . . . 5 g
Fat:. . . . . 1 g
Saturated fat: . . . . trace
Cholesterol: . . . . trace
Dietary fiber: . . . . 4 g
Sodium:. . . . . 174 mg
(omitting salt) . . . . 41 mg

Scalloped tomatoes

1 can (about 16 ounces) tomatoes
¼ cup chopped onion
¼ cup diced green or red bell pepper
2 tablespoons minced fresh parsley
½ cup Seasoned Bread Crumbs (recipe, p. 363)
   or commercial bread crumbs
¼ teaspoon salt (optional)
¼ teaspoon freshly ground black pepper

Make this easy vegetable side dish when you need a change from routine vegetables. It takes just a few minutes to prepare.

1. Drain the juice from the tomatoes into a nonreactive frying pan; reserve the tomatoes. Add the onion, bell pepper, and parsley to the tomato juice and cook, stirring, until the vegetables are tender and the liquid is nearly evaporated.
2. Roughly chop the reserved tomatoes and add them, together with all but 1 tablespoon of the bread crumbs, to the tomato juice mixture. Cook, stirring occasionally, until heated through, about 5 minutes. Add salt (optional) and pepper. Pour into a serving dish and sprinkle with reserved crumbs.

243

Preparation time: 5 minutes
Cooking time: 10 minutes

Exchanges: 1 carbohydrate
Carbohydrate choices: 1

Yield: 4 servings
Serving size: ½ cup

Nutrition per serving:
Calories: 71
Carbohydrate:. . . . . 13 g
Protein: . . . . 2 g
Fat:. . . . . 1 g
Saturated fat:. . . . . trace
Cholesterol: . . . . trace
Dietary fiber: . . . . 2 g
Sodium:. . . . . 352 mg
(omitting salt) . . . . 219 mg

Skinny scalloped potatoes

Don't peel your potatoes! Not only do you spend extra time, but you end up throwing away much of the flavor and minerals along with the peel. After this creamy potato dish, we are certain you will never peel again.

Nonfat cooking spray
2 cups Basic White Sauce (recipe, p. 354)
4 medium baking potatoes, scrubbed well
 and cut crosswise into ⅛-inch slices
2 medium onions, peeled and sliced thin

1. Preheat oven to 350°F. Coat a 6-cup shallow casserole with cooking spray. Layer half the sauce, half the potatoes, all of the onions, the remaining potatoes, and end with the remaining sauce in the casserole.
2. Cover and bake 40 minutes. Uncover and bake until golden brown and bubbly, about 20 more minutes.

244

Preparation time: 10 minutes
Baking time: 1 hour

Exchanges: 1½ carbohydrate
Carbohydrate choices: 1½

Yield: 9 servings
Serving size: ½ cup

Nutrition per serving:
Calories: 121
Carbohydrate:. . . . . 25 g
Protein: . . . . 4 g
Fat:. . . . . 1 g
Saturated fat:. . . . . trace
Cholesterol: . . . . trace
Dietary fiber: . . . . 2 g
Sodium:. . . . . 41 mg

Baked stuffed potatoes

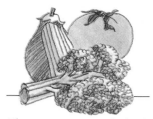

4 small baking potatoes, scrubbed (unpeeled)
½ cup low-fat cottage cheese
⅓ cup cold water
2 tablespoons chopped fresh parsley, chives, or dill
2 tablespoons freshly grated Parmesan cheese
Pepper and paprika (optional)

These tasty, twice-baked potatoes can be prepared ahead of time for convenience. For softer skins, wrap these potatoes in aluminum foil the first time you bake them.

1. Preheat the oven to 400°F. Prick the potatoes with a fork or sharp, thin knife. Bake the potatoes until cooked through (test with a sharp knife), about 35–40 minutes. Remove from the oven. (Or MICROWAVE on High, wrapped individually in microwave-safe paper toweling, for 20 minutes. Remove from microwave oven, wrap individually in aluminum foil, and let rest 5 minutes before proceeding.)
2. Cut a slice off the top of each potato. Scoop out the insides of each potato, reserving the shells. In a mixing bowl, combine the potato, cottage cheese, ⅓ cup water, herbs, cheese, and seasonings; mash until smooth.
3. Spoon the potato mixture back into the potato shells. Place on a baking sheet. Sprinkle with paprika and pepper, if desired. Bake in a 400°F oven until golden brown and heated through, about 15–20 minutes.

245

Preparation time: 15 minutes
Cooking time: 1 hour

Yield: 4 servings
Serving size: 1 stuffed potato

Exchanges: 1 starch
       1 very lean meat
Carbohydrate choices: 1

Nutrition per serving:
Calories: 103
Carbohydrate: . . . . 18 g
Protein: . . . . 6 g
Fat: . . . . 1 g

Saturated fat: . . . . trace
Cholesterol: . . . . 3 mg
Dietary fiber: . . . . 2 g
Sodium: . . . . 144 mg

Colorful vegetable casserole

The wine, chicken broth granules, garlic, and margarine lend these vegetables a savory flavor. This is definitely a dish to make for the holidays!

Nonfat cooking spray

1 package (16 ounces) frozen Italian-mix vegetables

1 large green pepper, cut into strips

1 pound baby carrots, halved

1 medium zucchini, unpeeled, cut into ½-inch slices

4 medium tomatoes, quartered

1 cup celery, sliced

2 tablespoons margarine

1½ cups chopped onion

2 large garlic cloves, minced

2 teaspoons instant reduced-sodium chicken broth granules

2 tablespoons cooking wine

½ teaspoon salt (optional)

½ teaspoon pepper

246

1. Preheat oven to 325°F. Spray a 3-quart casserole or Dutch oven with cooking spray. Spread frozen vegetables in an even layer in the casserole. Follow with layers of green pepper strips, baby carrots, zucchini slices, tomato pieces, and celery.

2. Melt the margarine in a skillet. Add onion and garlic, sautéing until tender. Stir in broth granules, wine, salt (optional), and pepper. Pour skillet mixture over vegetables.

3. Cover casserole and bake for approximately 1 hour until vegetables are crisp-tender.

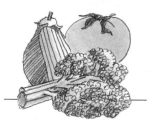

Preparation time: 20 minutes
Baking time: 1 hour

Yield: 10–12 servings
Serving size: 1 cup

Exchanges: 3 vegetable
½ fat
Carbohydrate choices: 1

Nutrition per serving:
Calories: 88
Carbohydrate:. . . . . 15 g
Protein: . . . . 3 g
Fat:. . . . . 3 g

Saturated fat: . . . . <1 g
Cholesterol:. . . . . 0 mg
Dietary fiber: . . . . 4 g
Sodium:. . . . . 227 mg
(omitting salt) . . . . 130 mg

Baked carrots

10 medium carrots, peeled and shredded
1 tablespoon sugar
½ teaspoon salt (optional)
¼ teaspoon ground black pepper
2 tablespoons reduced-fat margarine

This wonderfully simple cooking method can also be used with other hard vegetables, such as turnips, beets, parsnips, and potatoes.

247

Preheat oven to 350°F. Combine carrots, sugar, salt (optional), and pepper in a deep casserole. Cut margarine into small pieces and sprinkle on top. Cover and bake for 1 hour or until vegetables are tender.

Preparation time: 10 minutes
Baking time: 1 hour

Yield: 6 servings
Serving size: ¾ cup

Exchanges: 1 carbohydrate
Carbohydrate choices: 1

Nutrition per serving:
Calories: 76
Carbohydrate:. . . . . 14 g
Protein: . . . . 1 g
Fat:. . . . . 2 g

Saturated fat: . . . . trace
Cholesterol:. . . . . 0 mg
Dietary fiber: . . . . 3 g
Sodium:. . . . . 280 mg
(omitting salt) . . . . 102 mg

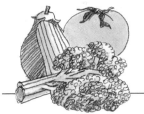

Spinach "pie"

This spinach pie makes a great side dish or a wonderful breakfast. Add cooked Russet potatoes to the egg mixture for a heartier pie.

10 ounces fresh spinach, washed, stemmed, and patted dry, or one 10-ounce package frozen spinach, thawed and drained

2 eggs, well beaten (or ½ cup liquid egg substitute)

1 cup skim milk

⅓ cup chopped celery

¼ cup minced onion

2 tablespoons freshly grated Parmesan cheese

½ teaspoon freshly grated nutmeg

½ teaspoon salt (optional)

½ teaspoon freshly ground black pepper

1. Preheat oven to 375°F. Place fresh spinach in a heavy saucepan; cover and cook over low heat until just wilted. (Or MICROWAVE on High, uncovered, about 4 minutes.) Drain well and chop coarsely. (If using frozen spinach, simply drain well and chop.)

2. In a mixing bowl, combine the eggs (or egg substitute), milk, celery, onion, Parmesan, salt (optional), and pepper. Fold the spinach into the egg mixture, then pour into a lightly oiled 9-inch pie plate. Bake until set (a knife inserted in the center should come out clean), about 35–40 minutes.

248

Preparation time: 10 minutes
Cooking time: 45 minutes

Yield: 6 servings
Serving size: ⅙ pie

Exchanges: 1 vegetable
          1 very lean meat
Carbohydrate choices: ½

Nutrition per serving:

With egg		**With egg substitute**	
Calories:	63	Calories:	45
Carbohydrate:	8 g	Carbohydrate:	5 g
Protein:	5 g	Protein:	5 g
Fat:	3 g	Fat:	1 g
Saturated fat:	1 g	Saturated fat:	trace
Cholesterol:	93 mg	Cholesterol:	trace
Dietary fiber:	2 g	Dietary fiber:	2 g
Sodium:	302 mg	Sodium:	306 mg
(omitting salt)	124 mg	(omitting salt)	128 mg

Confetti peas

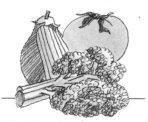

½ **cup diced red bell pepper**
½ **cup diced celery**
⅓ **cup chopped onion**
½ **cup low-sodium chicken broth**
1½ **cups frozen peas**
Freshly ground black pepper to taste (optional)

In a medium saucepan with a tight-fitting lid, combine all of the ingredients. Bring to a boil, lower heat, cover, and cook until the peas are tender, about 5 minutes. Season with black pepper, if desired.

Here's a simple way to add zest to plain green peas.

249

Preparation time: 10 minutes
Cooking time: 10 minutes

Exchanges: 1 starch
Carbohydrate choices: 1

Yield: 4 servings
Serving size: ½ cup

Nutrition per serving:
Calories: 74
Carbohydrate:. . . . . 13 g
Protein: . . . . 4 g
Fat: . . . . trace

Saturated fat: . . . . trace
Cholesterol: . . . . trace
Dietary fiber: . . . . 4 g
Sodium:. . . . . 91 mg

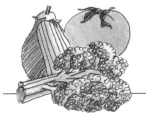

Asparagus risotto

3 cups low-sodium chicken broth

2 tablespoons olive oil

½ pound fresh thin asparagus, washed, trimmed, and cut into ½-inch pieces

1 small onion, chopped

1 cup white rice, preferably Italian Arborio, uncooked

2 tablespoons freshly grated Parmesan cheese

½ teaspoon salt (optional)

¼ teaspoon freshly ground black pepper

1. In a saucepan, bring the broth to a boil, then lower to a simmer. In another saucepan, heat the oil. Add the asparagus pieces (reserving the tips) and onion; cook, stirring, until the onion is wilted, about 4 minutes. Add the rice and stir over low heat until all kernels are well coated with oil.

2. Add the hot broth to the rice mixture about ½ cup at a time, and cook over medium heat, stirring continually. Wait until the rice absorbs the broth before adding another ½ cup. Repeat until the rice is cooked; this entire process should take 15–20 minutes. If using Arborio rice, the consistency should be creamy, somewhat like that of rice pudding.

3. With the addition of the last ½ cup or so of broth, add the asparagus tips and cook 3–5 more minutes. Stir in the cheese and season to taste.

To make risotto in the MICROWAVE: Do not preheat the broth. Combine the oil and onion in a 10-inch quiche or deep pie dish; cook on High, uncovered, 4 minutes. Add the asparagus and rice, stir well, and cook on High, uncovered, 4 more minutes. Add the broth all at once. Cook on High, uncovered, 9 minutes. Stir well. Cook on High 9 more minutes. Add the asparagus tips, cheese, and seasoning. Allow to stand, uncovered, 5 minutes before serving.

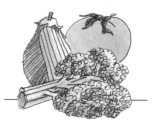

Preparation time: 10 minutes
Cooking time: 35 minutes

Yield: 6 servings
Serving size: ¾ cup

Exchanges: 1 starch
      1 vegetable
      1 fat
Carbohydrate choices: 1

Nutrition per serving:

Calories: 156
Carbohydrate: . . . . 20 g
Protein: . . . . 4 g
Fat: . . . . 6 g

Saturated fat: . . . . 1 g
Cholesterol: . . . . 5 mg
Dietary fiber: . . . . 1 g
Sodium: . . . . 267 mg
(omitting salt) . . . . 89 mg

Zesty Harvard beets

1 can (about 16 ounces) diced or sliced beets
2 teaspoons white wine vinegar
1 teaspoon grated orange zest
1 teaspoon cornstarch
1 tablespoon orange juice

Orange zest and juice bring a bright, sweet note to these colorful beets.

251

In a saucepan, combine the beets, their juice, the vinegar, and orange zest. In a small bowl, stir the cornstarch and orange juice together until smooth and add to the beets. Cook the beets until the sauce is smooth and thickened, about 3–5 minutes. Serve warm or at room temperature.

Preparation time: 5 minutes
Cooking time: 5 minutes

Yield: 4 servings
Serving size: ½ cup

Exchanges: 1 vegetable
Carbohydrate choices: ½

Nutrition per serving:

Calories: 34
Carbohydrate: . . . . 8 g
Protein: . . . . 1 g
Fat: . . . . trace

Saturated fat: . . . . trace
Cholesterol: . . . . trace
Dietary fiber: . . . . 2 g
Sodium: . . . . 224 mg

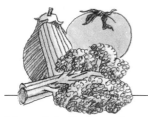

Green beans
with water chestnuts

The subtle flavors of garlic and soy sauce mingle in this Asian-inspired dish. For some extra spice, add 1 tablespoon of chili garlic sauce to the recipe in Step 1.

½ cup low-sodium chicken broth
1 teaspoon minced, fresh ginger root
1 clove garlic, minced
1 green onion, sliced diagonally
12 ounces fresh green beans, washed, ends trimmed, and cut in half lengthwise
⅓ cup water chestnuts, sliced thin
1 teaspoon soy sauce
Freshly ground black pepper to taste

1. In a wok or frying pan, combine the broth, ginger, garlic, and green onion; bring to a boil. Add the green beans and water chestnuts; sprinkle with soy sauce.
2. Cover tightly and cook until the beans are crisp-tender, about 4–5 minutes. Uncover, raise the heat, and stir-fry briefly to evaporate any remaining liquid. Season to taste. Serve hot.

252

Preparation time: 10 minutes
Cooking time: 10 minutes

Yield: 6 servings
Serving size: ½ cup

Exchanges: 1 vegetable
Carbohydrate choices: 0

Nutrition per serving:
Calories: 26
Carbohydrate: . . . . 5 g
Protein: . . . . 1 g
Fat: . . . . trace
Saturated fat: . . . . trace
Cholesterol: . . . . trace
Dietary fiber: . . . . 2 g
Sodium: . . . . 60 mg

Green bean and red pepper sauté

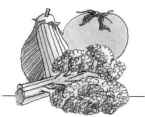

1 pound fresh green beans, ends trimmed
2 tablespoons olive oil
1 large red bell pepper, cut into strips
1 teaspoon lemon juice
¼ cup chopped salted cashews
Freshly ground black pepper (to taste)

1. In a large saucepan, bring 3 quarts water to a boil. Add green beans and return water to a boil. Cook, uncovered, for 8–10 minutes until crisp-tender, then drain. Plunge beans into cold water to stop cooking. Beans may be covered and refrigerated overnight at this point.
2. Heat oil in a large saucepan or wok until hot. Sauté red pepper over medium heat for 2–3 minutes. Stir in beans, lemon juice, cashews, and pepper. Cook and stir gently until thoroughly heated, about 6–8 minutes. Transfer to a serving platter and serve immediately.

If you are used to cooking green beans for a long period of time, you will be thrilled at the taste of these crispy beans. To save time in the cooking process, you can cut the beans and red pepper strips into 1-inch pieces before cooking.

253

Preparation time: 5 minutes
Cooking time: 20 minutes

Yield: 6 servings
Serving size: ½ cup

Exchanges: 1 vegetable
1½ fat
Carbohydrate choices: ½

Nutrition per serving:
Calories: 94
Carbohydrate: . . . . 7 g
Protein: . . . . 2 g
Fat: . . . . 7 g
Saturated fat: . . . . 1 g
Cholesterol: . . . . 0 mg
Dietary fiber: . . . . 2 g
Sodium: . . . . 40 mg

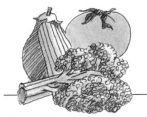

German cabbage

The mild and mellow flavor of this classic dish will delight your taste buds. For variety, use red cabbage or a combination of red and green.

254

⅓ cup low-sodium chicken broth
⅓ cup dry white wine (not "cooking wine")
2–4 whole allspice berries
   or ¼ teaspoon ground allspice
1 teaspoon caraway seeds
4 cups shredded cabbage
1 onion, peeled and thinly sliced
1 tart apple, peeled and thinly sliced

1. In a heavy saucepan or casserole with a tight-fitting lid, combine the broth, wine, allspice, and caraway seeds. Bring to a boil.
2. Toss together the cabbage, onion, and apple, and add to the saucepan.
3. Cover and cook over low heat until the cabbage is very tender, about 1–1½ hours, or bake in a 400°F oven for the same length of time. (Or MICROWAVE on High, covered, 12–14 minutes.)

Preparation time: 10 minutes
Cooking time: 1–1½ hours

Exchanges: 1 vegetable
Carbohydrate choices: 0

Yield: 5 servings
Serving size: ½ cup

Nutrition per serving:
Calories: 27
Carbohydrate:. . . . . 5 g
Protein: . . . . 1 g
Fat: . . . . trace

Saturated fat: . . . . trace
Cholesterol: . . . . trace
Dietary fiber: . . . . 2 g
Sodium:. . . . . 15 mg

Zucchini with tomato sauce and cheese

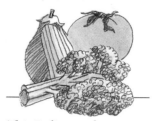

1 tablespoon olive oil

¼ cup minced onion

1–2 cloves garlic, minced

1 tablespoon all-purpose flour

¼ teaspoon salt (optional)

¼ teaspoon freshly ground black pepper

¾ cup tomato juice

1 tablespoon minced fresh basil
   or 1 teaspoon dried basil

4 small zucchini, well washed, ends trimmed,
   and cut in half lengthwise

1 cup shredded part-skim mozzarella cheese

This Italian-style zucchini works well over noodles or rice. Be sure not to overcook the zucchini—it's best when still crispy.

1. Heat the oil in a small saucepan and sauté the onion and garlic over medium-low heat until soft but not brown. Stir in the flour, salt (optional), and pepper, and cook, stirring, until smooth. Add the tomato juice and basil and cook, stirring, until thickened, 3–4 minutes.
2. Drop the zucchini halves into salted boiling water and cook until crisp-tender, about 2–3 minutes. Drain well.
3. Place the zucchini cut side up in a warm ovenproof dish. Drizzle the tomato sauce over the zucchini, and sprinkle with mozzarella cheese. Place under the broiler or bake in a hot oven just long enough for the cheese to melt.

255

Preparation time: 15 minutes
Cooking time: 20 minutes

Yield: 4 servings
Serving size: 2 zucchini halves
   with sauce

Exchanges: 1 lean meat
   1 vegetable
   1 fat
Carbohydrate choices: ½

Nutrition per serving:
Calories: 133
Carbohydrate: . . . . 8 g
Protein: . . . . 8 g
Fat: . . . . 8 g

Saturated fat: . . . . 3 g
Cholesterol: . . . . 16 mg
Dietary fiber: . . . . 2 g
Sodium: . . . . 500 mg
(omitting salt) . . . . 367 mg

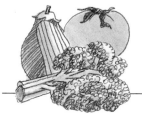

Crispy baked parsnips

Parsnips, which resemble white or pale-colored carrots, have a taste similar to sweet potatoes. When purchasing parsnips, buy the smaller variety; larger parsnips may have tough cores. Also avoid any parsnips that are limp or have brown spots.

**1 pound parsnips, peeled
and cut into 2½-inch julienne sticks**
2 tablespoons skim milk
1 teaspoon vegetable oil
¼ cup dry bread crumbs
¼ teaspoon salt (optional)
¼ teaspoon ground white pepper

1. Steam or cook the parsnip sticks in a small amount of boiling water until crisp-tender, about 10 minutes. (Or MICROWAVE on High, covered, with 1 cup water, about 8 minutes.) Cool slightly. Preheat the oven to 425°F.
2. Mix the milk and oil in a small bowl. Dip the parsnip sticks into the milk mixture, then coat individually with bread crumbs. Season with salt (optional) and pepper.
3. Place the breaded parsnip sticks on a lightly oiled baking sheet and bake until crisp and golden brown, about 15–20 minutes.

Preparation time: 10 minutes
Cooking time: 30 minutes

Yield: 4 servings
Serving size: ½ cup

Exchanges: 1 starch
Carbohydrate choices: 1

Nutrition per serving:
Calories: 95
Carbohydrate:. . . . . 17 g
Protein: . . . . 2 g
Fat:. . . . . 2 g
Saturated fat: . . . . trace
Cholesterol: . . . . trace
Dietary fiber: . . . . 5 g
Sodium:. . . . . 195 mg
(omitting salt) . . . . 62 mg

Easy cheesy vegetable casserole

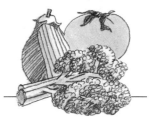

This veggie casserole is high in fiber and great taste—and it's hearty enough to eat as a main course.

1½ cups water
4 medium white or yellow potatoes,
   peeled and sliced ½-inch thick
1 cup bite-size raw cauliflower florets
1 cup bite-size raw broccoli florets
4 medium carrots, peeled and sliced into ¼-inch coins
1 medium onion, chopped
2 cups frozen, cut green beans
Nonfat cooking spray
1 can (10¾ ounces) reduced-fat, reduced-sodium
   cream of chicken soup
½ cup skim milk
1 cup shredded reduced-fat Cheddar cheese

1. Preheat oven to 350°F. Bring water to a boil in a large pot over high heat. Add the potatoes and cook, covered, for 5 minutes. Add the cauliflower, broccoli, carrots, onion, and frozen green beans. Return water to a boil, cover, and cook 10–12 minutes until vegetables are tender. Drain.
2. Spray a 2-quart baking dish with cooking spray. Add cooked vegetables. Combine the canned soup and milk. Pour soup mixture over the vegetables, mixing gently. Cover and bake casserole for 20–25 minutes. Uncover and sprinkle with cheese. Bake 3–4 minutes longer, until cheese melts.

257

Preparation time: 20 minutes
Baking time: 30 minutes

Yield: 8 servings
Serving size: ⅛ recipe

Exchanges: 1 starch
   2 vegetable
   1 medium-fat meat
Carbohydrate choices: 2

Nutrition per serving:
Calories: 190
Carbohydrate:. . . . . 27 g
Protein: . . . . 9 g
Fat:. . . . . 5 g

Saturated fat: . . . . 3 g
Cholesterol:. . . . . 13 mg
Dietary fiber: . . . . 5 g
Sodium:. . . . . 475 mg

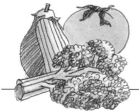

Stir-fried summer squash

Parslied garlic salt—garlic salt and dried parsley flakes combined—give this squash a fantastic flavor. Mix this seasoning and use it in other vegetable dishes or use it in place of regular salt at the table.

258

Nonfat cooking spray

1 teaspoon olive oil

4 small yellow squash (approximately 5 inches long), quartered and sliced ¼-inch thick (about 2 cups total)

2 medium zucchini (approximately 6–7 inches long), quartered and sliced ¼-inch thick (about 2 cups total)

1 cup thinly sliced onion, separated into rings

¾ teaspoon parslied garlic salt

Coat a nonstick wok or sauté pan with cooking spray. Preheat, then add oil. When the oil is hot, add the yellow squash, zucchini, and onion. Cook, stirring constantly, for 4–5 minutes, or until the squash is crisp-tender. Sprinkle with parslied garlic salt and toss to coat. Serve immediately.

Preparation time: 10 minutes
Cooking time: 5 minutes

Yield: 7 servings
Serving size: ½ cup

Exchanges: 1 vegetable
Carbohydrate choices: ½

Nutrition per serving:

Calories: 33	Saturated fat: . . . . <1 g
Carbohydrate:. . . . . 5 g	Cholesterol:. . . . . 0 mg
Protein: . . . . 1 g	Dietary fiber: . . . . 1 g
Fat:. . . . . 1 g	Sodium:. . . . . 222 mg

Chapter 11

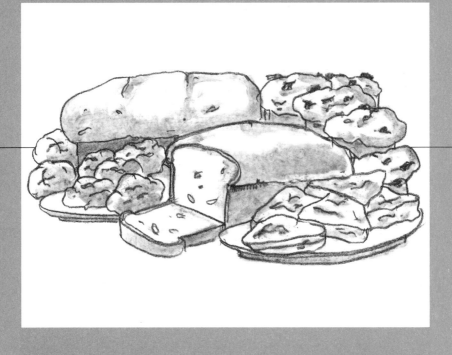

BREADS AND MUFFINS

*T*here's nothing quite like the smell, taste, and texture of homemade bread fresh from the oven. Store-bought loaves simply cannot compare.

This chapter contains a wonderful selection of healthful and delicious breads, rolls, biscuits, and muffins. Our Cheese Biscuits, Oatmeal Scones, and Jalapeño Cornbread will have you clamoring for more.

Breads and bread products are an especially important part of a balanced diet for people with diabetes. They are good sources of complex carbohydrates and fiber—and they are easy to keep on hand for snacking or meals! Make any of these recipes ahead of time and freeze it for later use. Never put bread products in the refrigerator, however, as this only makes them turn stale faster.

Healthful banana bread

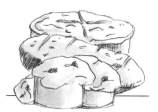

Nonfat cooking spray
1½ cups whole wheat flour
½ cup unsweetened shredded coconut
2 teaspoons baking powder
½ teaspoon baking soda
½ teaspoon salt (optional)
1 cup mashed ripe (or overripe) banana
3 tablespoons vegetable oil
2 tablespoons honey

1. Preheat oven to 350°F. Coat an 8" × 4" loaf pan with nonfat cooking spray.
2. In a mixing bowl, combine the flour, coconut, baking powder, baking soda, and salt (optional). In another mixing bowl, combine the banana, oil, and honey.
3. Stir the banana mixture into the dry ingredients until just combined. (Do not overmix.) The batter should be lumpy and stiff.
4. Spread the batter evenly into the prepared load pan and bake until a tester (toothpick) inserted in the center comes out clean, about 45–50 minutes. Allow the bread to cool in the pan about 10 minutes, then turn it out of the pan and cool completely on a baking rack.

Need to get rid of those brown-spotted bananas from last week? Don't throw them in the garbage; instead use them to create this classic bread.

261

Preparation time: 15 minutes
Baking time: 50 minutes

Yield: 14 servings
Serving size: one slice,
       ½-inch thick

Exchanges: 1 starch
       1 fat
Carbohydrate choices: 1

Nutrition per serving:
Calories: 112
Carbohydrate:. . . . . 13 g
Protein: . . . . 2 g
Fat:. . . . . 5 g
Saturated fat: . . . . 2 g
Cholesterol: . . . . trace
Dietary fiber: . . . . 2 g
Sodium:. . . . . 168 mg
(omitting salt) . . . . 92 mg

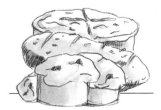

Orange nut bread

As with any recipe, the fresher the ingredients, the better the flavor. Try freshly squeezed orange juice instead of commercial brands or concentrate.

Nonfat cooking spray
1½ cups all-purpose flour
¼ cup sugar
2 teaspoons baking powder
½ teaspoon salt (optional)
⅓ cup chopped almonds or walnuts
¼ cup chopped raisins
2 tablespoons grated orange zest
1 egg, beaten (or ¼ cup liquid egg substitute)
½ cup orange juice
2 teaspoons vegetable oil

1. Preheat the oven to 350°F. Coat an 8" × 4" loaf pan with nonfat cooking spray.
2. In a mixing bowl, combine the flour, sugar, baking powder, and salt (optional). Stir in the nuts, raisins, and orange zest until well mixed.
3. In another mixing bowl, whisk together the egg (or egg substitute), orange juice, and oil. Pour this mixture into the dry ingredients and mix only until combined.
4. Turn the batter out into the prepared loaf pan and bake until a tester (toothpick) inserted into the center comes out clean, about 40 minutes. Cool in the pan 10 minutes, then turn out onto a rack to cool completely. Wrap well and store overnight before slicing.

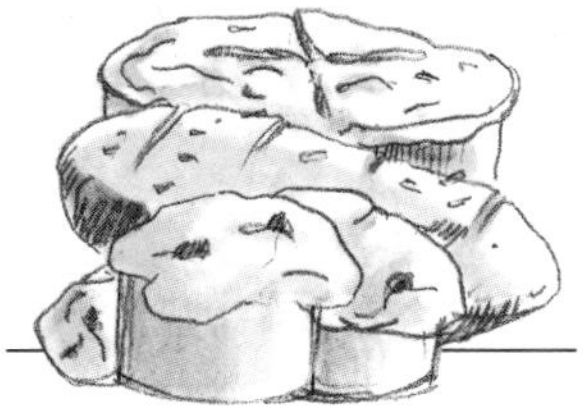

Preparation time: 10 minutes
Baking time: 40 minutes

Yield: 15 servings
Serving size: one slice,
            ½-inch thick

Exchanges: 1 starch
      ½ fat
Carbohydrate choices: 1

Nutrition per serving:

With egg

Calories: 94
Carbohydrate: . . . . 15 g
Protein: . . . . 2 g
Fat: . . . . 3 g
Saturated fat: . . . . trace
Cholesterol: . . . . 18 mg
Dietary fiber: . . . . 1 g
Sodium: . . . . 133 mg
(omitting salt) . . . . 62 mg

With egg substitute

Calories: 90
Carbohydrate: . . . . 15 g
Protein: . . . . 2 g
Fat: . . . . 2 g
Saturated fat: . . . . trace
Cholesterol: . . . . trace
Dietary fiber: . . . . 1 g
Sodium: . . . . 134 mg
(omitting salt) . . . . 63 mg

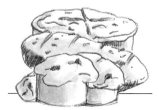

German rye bread

Caraway seeds give a great flavor and crunch to this traditional rye bread.

1 teaspoon sugar
½ cup warm water
1 package active dry yeast
1 tablespoon vegetable oil
1 teaspoon honey
¾ cup cold water
1 tablespoon caraway seeds (optional)
1 teaspoon salt
1 cup rye flour
1½ cups plus 1 cup all-purpose flour, plus additional
  as needed

1. Dissolve the sugar in ½ cup warm water. Stir in the yeast and allow to proof 5–10 minutes.
2. In a large mixing bowl, combine the oil and honey with ¾ cup water. Stir in the caraway seeds (optional), salt, rye flour, and 1 cup all-purpose flour. Beat 2–3 minutes, until smooth.
3. Work about 1½ cups all-purpose flour into the dough. Turn the dough out onto a floured work surface and knead until smooth, elastic, and no longer sticky, about 8 minutes, adding more all-purpose flour as necessary.
4. Place the dough in a lightly oiled bowl and turn it to coat all sides with oil. Cover the bowl with plastic wrap and allow to rise in a warm, draft-free place until doubled in volume, about 45–60 minutes.
5. Punch the dough down. Form it into a loaf and place in a lightly greased 9" × 5" loaf pan. Cover loosely and allow to rise until doubled in volume, about 45 minutes.
6. About 15 minutes before baking, preheat the oven to 375°F. Bake until the loaf is lightly browned and sounds hollow when tapped on bottom, about 30–35 minutes. Cool on a rack.

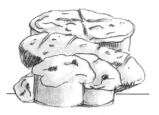

Preparation time: 20 minutes
Rising time: 1½ hours
Baking time: 35 minutes

Exchanges: 1 starch
Carbohydrate choices: 1

Yield: 20 servings
Serving size: 1 slice

Nutrition per serving:
Calories: 85
Carbohydrate: . . . . 17 g
Protein: . . . . 2 g
Fat: . . . . 1 g
Saturated fat: . . . . trace
Cholesterol: . . . . trace
Dietary fiber: . . . . 1 g
Sodium: . . . . 107 mg

265

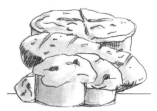

Dinner rolls

If you need a warm, draft-free place to let your dough rise, look no farther than your very own oven. Make sure the oven is off before you set the dough inside.

266

2 teaspoons honey
½ cup warm water
2 packages active dry yeast
1 cup low-fat cottage cheese
¼ cup orange juice
1 egg, beaten (or ¼ cup liquid egg substitute)
2½ cups all-purpose flour, plus additional as needed (approximately 4 cups total)
1 teaspoon salt
½ teaspoon aniseed, caraway seed, or dillweed (optional)

1. Dissolve the honey in ½ cup warm water. Sprinkle the yeast over the water and allow to proof, about 10 minutes. Stir well.
2. In a small saucepan, combine the cottage cheese, orange juice, and egg (or egg substitute); stir over very low heat until just warm to the touch. Set aside.
3. In a large mixing bowl, combine 2½ cups flour, the salt, and aniseed (optional). Add the yeast and cottage cheese mixtures and beat well. Stir in enough remaining flour to make a soft dough that leaves the sides of the bowl.
4. Turn the dough out onto a floured surface and knead 8–10 minutes, until the dough is smooth, elastic, and no longer sticky. Place in a lightly oiled bowl and turn to oil on all sides.
5. Cover with plastic wrap and allow to rise in a warm, draft-free place until doubled in volume, about 1–1½ hours. Punch down. Shape into 24 rolls, or form into a loaf or braid, and place on a lightly-oiled baking sheet.

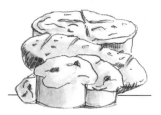

6. Cover loosely with plastic wrap and allow to rise in a warm, draft-free place until doubled in volume, about 45–60 minutes.

7. About 15 minutes before baking, preheat the oven to 375°F. Bake the rolls until golden brown, about 20–25 minutes. (If you make the loaf or braid, bake until it is golden brown and sounds hollow when you tap the bottom, about 40–45 minutes.) Cool on racks.

Preparation time: 35 minutes
Rising time: 1¾–2½ hours
Baking time: 25 minutes

Yield: 24 rolls or 1 loaf
Serving size: 1 roll or 1 slice

Exchanges: 1 starch
Carbohydrate choices: 1

Nutrition per serving:

With egg
Calories: 82
Carbohydrate: . . . . 16 g
Protein: . . . . 4 g
Fat: . . . . 1 g
Saturated fat: . . . . trace
Cholesterol: . . . . 12 mg
Dietary fiber: . . . . <1 g
Sodium: . . . . 89 mg

With egg substitute
Calories: 79
Carbohydrate: . . . . 16 g
Protein: . . . . 4 g
Fat: . . . . trace
Saturated fat: . . . . trace
Cholesterol: . . . . trace
Dietary fiber: . . . . <1 g
Sodium: . . . . 89 mg

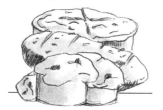

Cottage casserole bread

Cottage cheese adds protein to this easy casserole bread. For those who dislike poppy seeds, try sesame seeds instead.

268

3 teaspoons plus 1 teaspoon sugar
¼ cup warm water
1 package active dry yeast
1¼ cups low-fat cottage cheese
1½ cups plus 1 cup all-purpose flour
1 tablespoon poppy seeds
½ teaspoon salt
½ teaspoon baking soda
1 egg, well beaten

1. Dissolve 1 teaspoon of the sugar in ¼ cup warm water. Stir in the yeast and allow to proof 5–10 minutes. Meanwhile, heat the cottage cheese very gently in a saucepan until warm.
2. In a large mixing bowl, combine 1 cup of the flour, the remaining 3 teaspoons sugar, poppy seeds, salt, and baking soda. Stir in the warmed cottage cheese, the egg, and the yeast mixture. Beat the mixture about 3 minutes.
3. Stir in 1–1½ cups of the remaining flour to form a stiff dough. Cover the bowl with plastic wrap and allow to rise in a warm, draft-free place until doubled in volume, about 1 hour.
4. Stir dough down. Turn into an oiled 6-cup casserole. Cover and allow to rise in a warm place about 30–45 minutes.
5. About 15 minutes before baking, preheat the oven to 350°F. Bake until golden brown, 30–35 minutes. Cut into 12 wedges.

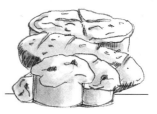

Preparation time: 15 minutes
Rising time: 1¾ hours
Baking time: 35 minutes

Yield: 12 servings
Serving size: 1 wedge

Nutrition per serving:

Calories: 114
Carbohydrate:. . . . . 20 g
Protein: . . . . 6 g
Fat:. . . . . 1 g

Exchanges: 1½ starch
Carbohydrate choices: 1½

Saturated fat: . . . . trace
Cholesterol:. . . . . 24 mg
Dietary fiber: . . . . <1 g
Sodium:. . . . . 206 mg

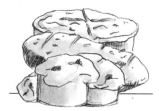

Harvest rolls

Here's a traditional recipe that is perfect for holidays or every day. The molasses gives these rolls their distinctive taste.

1 teaspoon sugar
½ cup warm water
1 package dry yeast
1 cup skim milk
1 teaspoon molasses
½ teaspoon salt
3 cups whole wheat flour
¾ cup all-purpose flour

1. Dissolve the sugar in ½ cup warm water. Stir in the yeast and allow to proof 5–10 minutes.
2. In a large mixing bowl, combine the milk, molasses, and salt. Stir in the whole wheat flour and yeast mixture; mix well.
3. Place ¼ cup all-purpose flour on a board. Turn the dough out onto the floured work surface and knead until smooth, elastic, and no longer sticky, about 8 minutes, adding more of the all-purpose flour as necessary.
4. Place the dough in a lightly oiled bowl and turn it to coat all sides with oil. Cover the bowl with plastic wrap and allow to rise in a warm, draft-free place until doubled in volume, about 1–1½ hours.

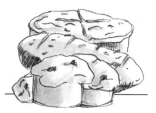

5. Punch down the dough. Divide it into 24 equal portions and form each portion into a roll. Place the rolls 2 inches apart on a baking sheet that has been lightly greased, lined with parchment, or coated with nonfat cooking spray. Cover loosely and allow to rise until doubled in volume, about 1 hour.

6. About 15 minutes before baking, preheat the oven to 400°F. Bake the rolls until brown, about 12–15 minutes. Cool on a rack.

271

Preparation time: 30 minutes
Rising time: 2–2½ hours
Baking time: 15 minutes

Yield: 24 servings
Serving size: 1 roll

Exchanges: 1 starch
Carbohydrate choices: 1

Nutrition per serving:
Calories: 69
Carbohydrate:. . . . . 14 g
Protein: . . . . 3 g
Fat: . . . . trace

Saturated fat: . . . . trace
Cholesterol: . . . . trace
Dietary fiber: . . . . 2 g
Sodium:. . . . . 51 mg

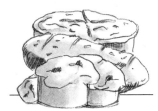

Whole wheat biscuits

1½ cups whole wheat flour
½ cup all-purpose flour
1 tablespoon baking powder
½ teaspoon salt (optional)
2 tablespoons margarine
1 cup skim milk

1. Preheat the oven to 425°F. In a mixing bowl, combine the flours, baking powder, and salt (optional).
2. Cut in the margarine with a pastry blender or 2 knives. Add the milk and mix it quickly into the dry ingredients.
3. Turn the dough out onto a floured work surface and knead briefly, 6–8 strokes. With a rolling pin, flatten the dough to ¾-inch thickness.
4. Cut into 12 round, 2-inch biscuits or into 12 wedges or squares. Place on a lightly greased or parchment-lined baking sheet and bake until lightly browned, 12–15 minutes.

272

Preparation time: 10 minutes
Baking time: 15 minutes

Yield: 12 servings
Serving size: 1 biscuit

Nutrition per serving:
Calories: 97
Carbohydrate:. . . . . 15 g
Protein: . . . . 3 g
Fat:. . . . . 3 g

Exchanges: 1 starch
            ½ fat
Carbohydrate choices: 1

Saturated fat: . . . . 1 g
Cholesterol: . . . . trace
Dietary fiber: . . . . 2 g
Sodium:. . . . . 230 mg
(omitting salt) . . . . 141 mg

Herb biscuits

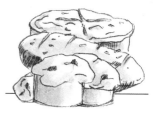

Combine ½ teaspoon each of dried thyme, rosemary, and basil, and add to the dry ingredients before proceeding to Step 2 above.

Cheese biscuits

Add ½ cup shredded low-fat Cheddar cheese and ¼ cup grated Parmesan cheese to the dry ingredients before proceeding to Step 2 above.

Yield: 12 servings
Serving size: 1 biscuit

Exchanges: 1 starch
         1 fat
Carbohydrate choices: 1

Nutrition per serving:
Calories: 128
Carbohydrate: . . . . 15 g
Protein: . . . . 6 g
Fat: . . . . 5 g

Saturated fat: . . . . 2 g
Cholesterol: . . . . 7 mg
Dietary fiber: . . . . 2 g
Sodium: . . . . 311 mg
(omitting salt) . . . . 222 mg

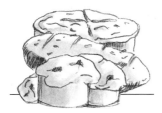

Oatmeal scones

Scones are an easy-to-make Saturday morning treat. Serve them topped with a teaspoon of all-fruit jam or preserves.

1¾ cups quick-cooking (not instant) rolled oats
1½ cups all-purpose flour
¼ cup sugar
1 tablespoon baking powder
½ teaspoon salt (optional)
½ cup margarine, melted
⅓ cup skim milk
1 egg (or ¼ cup liquid egg substitute)

1. Preheat oven to 425°F. In a large mixing bowl, combine the oats, flour, sugar, baking powder, and salt (optional).
2. In another mixing bowl, whisk together the margarine, milk, and egg (or egg substitute). Stir the liquid ingredients into the dry ingredients just until combined. (Do not overmix.)
3. Turn the dough out onto a lightly floured surface and pat or roll it into a 9" × 12" rectangle. Cut into 9 rectangles, then cut each again diagonally to form 18 triangles.
4. Place the triangles on a lightly greased baking sheet and bake until golden brown, about 12–14 minutes. Serve warm.

274

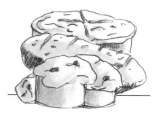

Preparation time: 15 minutes
Baking time: 15 minutes

Yield: 18 servings
Serving size: 1 scone

Nutrition per serving:
With egg
Calories: 120
Carbohydrate: . . . . 16 g
Protein: . . . . 3 g
Fat: . . . . 5 g
Saturated fat: . . . . 1 g
Cholesterol: . . . . 15 mg
Dietary fiber: . . . . 1 g
Sodium: . . . . 179 mg
(omitting salt) . . . . 120 mg

Exchanges: 1 starch
      1 fat
Carbohydrate choices: 1

With egg substitute
Calories: 117
Carbohydrate: . . . . 16 g
Protein: . . . . 3 g
Fat: . . . . 5 g
Saturated fat: . . . . 1 g
Cholesterol: . . . . trace
Dietary fiber: . . . . 1 g
Sodium: . . . . 180 mg
(omitting salt) . . . . 121 mg

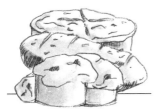

Best bran muffins

276

Nonfat cooking spray (optional)
1 cup all-purpose flour
1 cup unprocessed or miller's bran
¼ cup packed brown sugar
2½ teaspoons baking powder
1 teaspoon cinnamon
½ teaspoon salt (optional)
1 cup skim milk
¼ cup vegetable oil
1 egg (or ¼ cup liquid egg substitute)

1. Preheat the oven to 400°F. Line 12 muffin cups with paper liners or coat with nonfat cooking spray.
2. In a mixing bowl, combine the flour, bran, brown sugar, baking powder, cinnamon, and salt (optional). In another bowl, whisk together the milk, oil, and egg (or egg substitute).
3. Stir the milk mixture into the dry ingredients just until combined. (Do not overmix.) The mixture should be lumpy.
4. Fill each muffin cup ⅔ full. Bake until golden brown, about 20–22 minutes.

Preparation time: 15 minutes
Baking time: 20 minutes

Yield: 12 servings
Serving size: 1 muffin

Exchanges: 1 starch
　　　　　　1 fat
Carbohydrate choices: 1

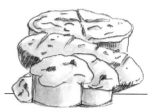

Nutrition per serving:

With egg
Calories: 123
Carbohydrate: . . . . 16 g
Protein: . . . . 3 g
Fat: . . . . 5 g
Saturated fat: . . . . 1 g
Cholesterol: . . . . 23 mg
Dietary fiber: . . . . 2 g
Sodium: . . . . 196 mg
(omitting salt) . . . . . . 107 mg

With egg substitute
Calories: 119
Carbohydrate: . . . . 16 g
Protein: . . . . 3 g
Fat: . . . . 5 g
Saturated fat: . . . . 1 g
Cholesterol: . . . . trace
Dietary fiber: . . . . 2 g
Sodium: . . . . 197 mg
(omitting salt) . . . . . . 108 mg

Fruit and nut bran muffins

Add about 2 tablespoons each chopped raisins and chopped nuts to the flour mixture (step 2) and proceed as outlined above.

VARIATION

Yield: 12 servings
Serving size: 1 muffin

Exchanges: 1 starch
       1 fat
Carbohydrate choices: 1

Nutrition per serving:

With egg
Calories: 134
Carbohydrate: . . . . 17 g
Protein: . . . . 3 g
Fat: . . . . 6 g
Saturated fat: . . . . 1 g
Cholesterol: . . . . 23 mg
Dietary fiber: . . . . 3 g
Sodium: . . . . 196 mg
(omitting salt) . . . . . . 107 mg

With egg substitute
Calories: 129
Carbohydrate: . . . . 17 g
Protein: . . . . 3 g
Fat: . . . . 6 g
Saturated fat: . . . . 1 g
Cholesterol: . . . . trace
Dietary fiber: . . . . 3 g
Sodium: . . . . 197 mg
(omitting salt) . . . . . . 108 mg

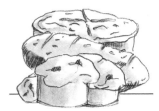

Nutty bran muffins

Add ¼ cup chopped walnuts to the flour mixture (step 2) and proceed as outlined above.

Yield: 12 servings
Serving size: 1 muffin

Exchanges: 1 starch
1 fat
Carbohydrate choices: 1

Nutrition per serving:

With egg		*With egg substitute*	
Calories:	137	Calories:	132
Carbohydrate:	16 g	Carbohydrate:	16 g
Protein:	3 g	Protein:	3 g
Fat:	7 g	Fat:	6 g
Saturated fat:	1 g	Saturated fat:	1 g
Cholesterol:	23 mg	Cholesterol:	trace
Dietary fiber:	3 g	Dietary fiber:	3 g
Sodium:	196 mg	Sodium:	197 mg
(omitting salt)	107 mg	(omitting salt)	108 mg

278

Cornmeal muffins

Skim milk and liquid egg substitute can turn this family favorite into a healthy accompaniment to any meal. Serve this with breakfast or with a chili or stew.

Nonfat cooking spray (optional)

1 cup skim milk

1 cup cornmeal

1¼ cups all-purpose flour

2–4 teaspoons sugar (to taste)

4 teaspoons baking powder

1 teaspoon salt (optional)

2 eggs, beaten (or ½ cup liquid egg substitute)

3 tablespoons vegetable oil

1. Preheat the oven to 400°F. Line 12 muffin cups with paper liners or coat with nonfat cooking spray. In a mixing bowl, stir the milk into the cornmeal and let stand 10 minutes.

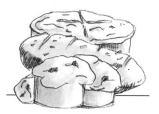

2. In a mixing bowl, combine the flour, sugar, baking powder, and salt (optional). Add the eggs (or egg substitute) and oil to the cornmeal mixture. Stir in the flour mixture until just combined.

3. Fill each muffin cup ⅔ full. Bake until golden brown, about 18–20 minutes. Serve warm.

Preparation time: 15 minutes
Baking time: 20 minutes

Yield: 12 servings
Serving size: 1 muffin

Exchanges: 1 starch
        1 fat
Carbohydrate choices: 1

Nutrition per serving:

With egg	*With egg substitute*
Calories: 135	Calories: 126
Carbohydrate: . . . . 19 g	Carbohydrate: . . . . 19 g
Protein: . . . . 4 g	Protein: . . . . 3 g
Fat: . . . . 5 g	Fat: . . . . 4 g
Saturated fat: . . . . 1 g	Saturated fat: . . . . 1 g
Cholesterol: . . . . 46 mg	Cholesterol: . . . . trace
Dietary fiber: . . . . 1 g	Dietary fiber: . . . . 1 g
Sodium: . . . . 342 mg	Sodium: . . . . 344 mg
(omitting salt) . . . . . . 164 mg	(omitting salt) . . . . 166 mg

279

Jalapeño cornmeal muffins

Fold in 3 tablespoons minced jalapeño pepper (about 3 small peppers) at the end of Step 2 above.

VARIATION
Try adding jalapeños to your cornmeal muffins for a Southwestern kick.

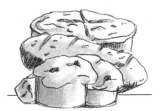

Popovers

Dust the tops of these popovers with cinnamon for a delicious, low-calorie dessert.

Nonfat cooking spray (optional)
1 teaspoon margarine
1 cup skim milk
2 eggs (or ½ cup liquid egg substitute)
¾ cup all-purpose flour
¼ teaspoon salt (optional)

1. Line 12 custard cups or medium-size muffin cups with paper liners or coat with nonfat cooking spray.
2. In a mixing bowl or blender, whisk together the milk and eggs (or egg substitute). Sprinkle the flour and salt (optional) over the milk mixture, and whisk until the batter is smooth.
3. Fill the custard or muffin cups no more than half full with the thin batter. Place on a baking sheet in a cold oven.
4. Turn the oven to 400°F and bake until firm and golden brown, about 30–35 minutes. Pierce the popovers to let steam escape. For drier popover, turn the oven off and allow them to dry 15 minutes in the oven with the door ajar.

280

Preparation time: 10 minutes
Baking time: 35 minutes

Yield: 12 servings
Serving size: 1 popover

Exchanges: ½ starch
Carbohydrate choices: ½

Nutrition per serving:

With eggs		*With egg substitute*	
Calories:	42	Calories:	48
Carbohydrate:	6 g	Carbohydrate:	7 g
Protein:	2 g	Protein:	2 g
Fat:	1 g	Fat:	trace
Saturated fat:	trace	Saturated fat:	trace
Cholesterol:	23 mg	Cholesterol:	trace
Dietary fiber:	0 g	Dietary fiber:	0 g
Sodium:	61 mg	Sodium:	62 mg
(omitting salt)	17 mg	(omitting salt)	18 mg

Chapter 12

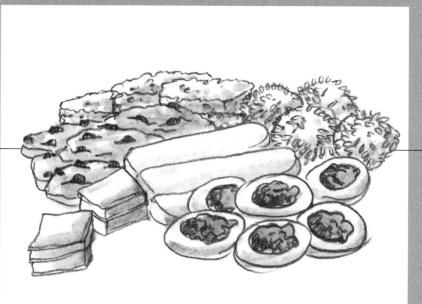

COOKIES

*E*veryone loves cookies, but added calories often come with these desserts. Here we give you recipes that are still delicious, but easy to make and reduced in both sugar and fat. As with any item you add to your diet or meal plan, moderation is the key; don't deny yourself these little pleasures, but don't deny yourself the valuable vitamins and minerals from nutritious foods either.

Once baked, most cookies can be frozen for several months. When storing them, pack different kinds separately so they retain their individual flavors. Separate each layer with a sheet of wax paper to prevent their sticking together, and seal cookies tightly in a zip-top freezer bag for maximum freshness. Be sure to squeeze as much air as possible from the bag before placing your cookies in the freezer.

The best way to reheat your frozen cookies is in the oven. Set the oven on warm and place a pie pan with 1 cup of water on the bottom of the oven. Place the cookies on a baking sheet and allow them to warm for 5–10 minutes. They'll taste like you baked them fresh that morning!

Old-fashioned oatmeal cookies

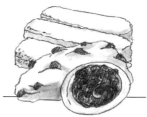

⅓ cup margarine
⅓ cup lightly packed brown sugar
¼ cup warm water
1 cup all-purpose flour
1 cup quick-cooking (not instant) rolled oats
1 teaspoon cinnamon
½ teaspoon baking soda

Oatmeal cookies are a universal favorite. Add ¼ cup of raisins to the dough in Step 2 for another classic variation.

1. In a mixing bowl, cream the margarine and sugar together until light and fluffy. Beat in ¼ cup of water until smooth.
2. In another bowl, combine the flour, oats, cinnamon, and baking soda. Stir into the creamed mixture. Preheat the oven to 350°F.
3. Roll the dough out on a lightly floured surface to ⅛-inch thickness. Cut into 2½-inch circles. Place on a cookie sheet that has been lightly oiled or coated with nonfat cooking spray.
4. Bake until golden brown around the edges, 10–12 minutes. Cool on a rack.

283

Preparation time: 20 minutes
Baking time: 10 minutes

Exchanges: 1 carbohydrate
Carbohydrate choices: 1

Yield: 18 servings
Serving size: 2 cookies

Nutrition per serving:
Calories: 81
Carbohydrate:. . . . . 14 g
Protein: . . . . 2 g
Fat:. . . . . 2 g

Saturated fat: . . . . 1 g
Cholesterol:. . . . . 0 mg
Dietary fiber: . . . . <1 g
Sodium:. . . . . 52 mg

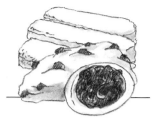

Lemon fingers

These crispy cookies are fantastic—low in calories with virtually no fat. What more could you ask?

284

3 egg whites
Pinch salt
½ teaspoon baking powder
¼ cup sugar
2 egg yolks
1 tablespoon grated lemon zest
1 teaspoon freshly squeezed lemon juice
½ cup all-purpose flour

1. Line a 9-inch square cake pan with wax paper or parchment paper. Preheat the oven to 375°F.
2. In a mixing bowl, beat the egg whites and salt until frothy. Add the baking powder and continue beating until soft peaks form; add the sugar and continue beating until stiff peaks form.
3. In a small bowl, whisk together the egg yolks, lemon zest, and lemon juice. Fold yolk mixture into the beaten egg whites, then gently fold in the flour.
4. Spread the batter into the prepared pan, smoothing the top. Bake until lightly browned, about 20 minutes.
5. Remove the pan from the oven and turn out onto a work surface. Leave the oven at 375°F. Remove the paper and cut the sponge into 60 oblong strips, ¾" × 2". Set the strips on their sides on a baking sheet and return to the oven for an additional 5 minutes. Turn off the heat and allow the fingers to dry in the oven 15 minutes. Store in an airtight container when cooled.

Preparation time: 15 minutes
Baking time: 40 minutes

Exchanges: free
Carbohydrate choices: 0

Yield: 30 servings
Serving size: 2 fingers

Nutrition per serving:
Calories: 19
Carbohydrate: . . . . 3 g
Protein: . . . . 1 g
Fat: . . . . trace

Saturated fat: . . . . trace
Cholesterol: . . . . 18 mg
Dietary fiber: . . . . 0 g
Sodium: . . . . 23 mg

Orange fingers

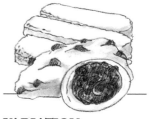

Replace the lemon zest and juice with orange zest and juice.

VARIATION

Anise fingers

Replace the lemon zest and juice with 1½ teaspoons aniseed and 1 teaspoon vanilla extract.

VARIATION

Peanut butter nuggets

⅔ **cup crushed corn flakes**
½ **cup unsweetened shredded coconut**
½ **cup smooth or crunchy peanut butter**
2 **tablespoons honey or corn syrup**

In a mixing bowl, combine ½ cup of the crushed corn flakes and all of the remaining ingredients. Divide the mixture into 18 portions and shape each portion into a ball. Roll the balls in the remaining corn flakes. Chill until firm.

These quick, no-cook cookies are wonderful protein snacks. Use reduced fat peanut butter to lower the calories and fat content even more.

285

Preparation time: 10 minutes
Chilling time: 15 minutes

Yield: 18 servings
Serving size: 1 nugget

Exchanges: ½ carbohydrate
½ fat
Carbohydrate choices: ½

Nutrition per serving:
Calories: 75
Carbohydrate:. . . . . 7 g
Protein: . . . . 2 g
Fat:. . . . . 4 g
Saturated fat: . . . . 2 g
Cholesterol:. . . . . 0 mg
Dietary fiber: . . . . <1 g
Sodium:. . . . . 68 mg

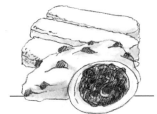

Peanut butter cookies

½ cup margarine
½ cup lightly packed brown sugar
1 cup peanut butter
2 eggs (or ½ cup liquid egg substitute)
Artificial sweetener equivalent to 8 teaspoons sugar
1 teaspoon vanilla extract
1½ cups all-purpose flour
1 teaspoon baking powder
1 teaspoon baking soda
½ teaspoon salt (optional)

1. In a mixing bowl, cream together the margarine and sugar until light and fluffy. Beat in the peanut butter, eggs (or egg substitute), artificial sweetener, and vanilla extract.
2. In another bowl, combine the flour, baking powder, baking soda, and salt (optional). Stir into the peanut butter mixture until well combined. Preheat oven to 350°F.
3. With wet hands, roll the dough into balls, using about 2 teaspoons of dough for each ball. Place the balls on a baking sheet that has been lightly oiled or coated with nonfat cooking spray. Flatten each ball with a wet fork, forming a criss-cross design on each cookie.
4. Bake until very light golden brown, about 8–10 minutes. Cool on racks.

286

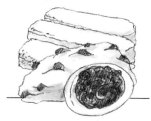

Preparation time: 15 minutes
Baking time: 10 minutes

Yield: 48 servings
Serving size: 1 cookie

Nutrition per serving:

Exchanges: ½ carbohydrate
 ½ fat
Carbohydrate choices: ½

With egg
Calories: 69
Carbohydrate:. . . . . 6 g
Protein: . . . . 2 g
Fat:. . . . . 4 g
Saturated fat: . . . . 1 g
Cholesterol:. . . . . 11 mg
Dietary fiber: . . . . <1 g
Sodium:. . . . . 94 mg
(omitting salt) . . . . 72 mg

With egg substitute
Calories: 67
Carbohydrate:. . . . . 6 g
Protein: . . . . 2 g
Fat:. . . . . 4 g
Saturated fat: . . . . 1 g
Cholesterol:. . . . . 0 mg
Dietary fiber: . . . . <1 g
Sodium:. . . . . 94 mg
(omitting salt) . . . . 72 mg

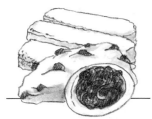

Chocolate chip cookies

The sugar and chocolate in the recipe have been reduced, making it easier to incorporate these classic cookies into your meal plan.

½ cup margarine
½ cup lightly packed brown sugar
1 egg (or ¼ cup liquid egg substitute)
2 teaspoons vanilla extract
1 cup all-purpose flour
½ teaspoon baking soda
½ teaspoon salt (optional)
½ cup quick-cooking rolled oats
½ cup semisweet chocolate chips

1. In a mixing bowl, cream together the margarine and sugar until light and fluffy. Add the egg (or egg substitute) and vanilla extract and beat until smooth.
2. In another bowl, combine the flour, baking soda, and salt (optional). Stir in the creamed mixture, along with the oats and chocolate chips. Preheat the oven to 375°F.
3. Using 2 teaspoons for each cookie, drop onto ungreased cookie sheets. Flatten with a wet fork. Bake until the cookies begin to brown around the edges, about 10 minutes. Cool on rack.

288

Preparation time: 15 minutes
Baking time: 10 minutes

Yield: 24 servings
Serving size: 2 cookies

Exchanges: ½ carbohydrate
1 fat
Carbohydrate choices: ½

Nutrition per serving:

With egg		**With egg substitute**	
Calories:	89	Calories:	86
Carbohydrate:	10 g	Carbohydrate:	10 g
Protein:	1 g	Protein:	1 g
Fat:	5 g	Fat:	5 g
Saturated fat:	2 g	Saturated fat:	2 g
Cholesterol:	11 mg	Cholesterol:	0 mg
Dietary fiber:	<1 g	Dietary fiber:	<1 g
Sodium:	98 mg	Sodium:	98 mg
(omitting salt)	54 mg	(omitting salt)	54 mg

Rice Krispie Squares

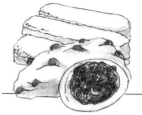

¼ cup margarine
25 large (or 3 cups small) marshmallows
1 teaspoon vanilla extract
5 cups Rice Krispies cereal
Nonfat cooking spray

Kids and adults alike love these gooey treats. For a slightly different flavor, use almond extract instead of vanilla in this recipe.

1. In a medium-large saucepan, melt the margarine over low heat. Add the marshmallows and cook, stirring, until they are melted.
2. Remove the saucepan from the heat and quickly stir in the vanilla extract and cereal. Mix well.
3. Press the mixture into a 9-inch square pan that has been lightly coated with nonfat cooking spray. Allow to set for at least 30 minutes. Cut into 24 pieces, 1½" × 2".

Preparation time: 5 minutes
Setting time: 40 minutes

Yield: 24 servings
Serving size: 1 piece

Exchanges: ½ carbohydrate
½ fat
Carbohydrate choices: ½

Nutrition per serving:
Calories: 61
Carbohydrate: . . . . 11 g
Protein: . . . . 1 g
Fat: . . . . 2 g
Saturated fat: . . . . trace
Cholesterol: . . . . 0 mg
Dietary fiber: . . . . 0 g
Sodium: . . . . 83 mg

289

Rice Krispie snowballs

Using moistened hands, shape ¼-cup portions of the warm cereal mixture into snowball shapes. Each ¼-cup snowball would be approximately equal to one rectangular piece.

VARIATION

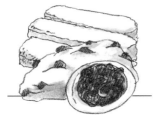

Here's a lighter version of the commercial vanilla wafer. Use these in place of vanilla wafers in recipes or eat them on their own.

290

Vanilla crisps

2 eggs, separated
½ teaspoon baking powder
Pinch salt
¼ cup sugar
2 teaspoons vanilla extract
⅓ cup all-purpose flour

1. Line two cookie sheets with parchment paper. Preheat the oven to 375°F.
2. In a mixing bowl, beat the egg whites until frothy; add the baking powder and salt and continue beating until soft peaks form. Add the sugar and continue beating until stiff peaks form.
3. In a small bowl, beat together the egg yolks and vanilla extract. Fold the yolk mixture into the whites gently, just until combined.
4. Sift the flour over the egg mixture and fold it into the batter gently until well incorporated.
5. Using 2 teaspoons of the dough at a time, drop onto the paper-lined cookie sheets 2 inches apart. Bake until golden brown, about 15–18 minutes. Cool 10 minutes and remove from paper.

Preparation time: 15 minutes
Baking time: 20 minutes

Yield: 12 servings
Serving size: 3 cookies

Exchanges: ½ carbohydrate
Carbohydrate choices: ½

Nutrition per serving:
Calories: 39
Carbohydrate:. . . . . 6 g
Protein: . . . . 1 g
Fat:. . . . . 1 g

Saturated fat: . . . . trace
Cholesterol:. . . . . 46 mg
Dietary fiber: . . . . 0 g
Sodium:. . . . . 47 mg

Orange crisps

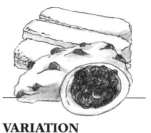

Substitute 2 teaspoons grated orange zest and 1 teaspoon orange juice for the vanilla extract.

VARIATION

Lemon crisps

Substitute 2 teaspoons grated lemon zest and 1 teaspoon lemon juice for the vanilla extract.

VARIATION

Almond crisps

Substitute 1 teaspoon almond extract for the vanilla extract and fold in 1 tablespoon ground almonds.

VARIATION

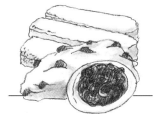

Piña colada squares

Pineapple and coconut come together to create a delicious, three-layered treat. Serve these with coffee after a special-occasion dinner.

1 cup all-purpose flour
1 teaspoon baking powder
¼ teaspoon salt
¼ cup margarine
1 egg, separated
¼ cup skim milk
Nonfat cooking spray
1 can (about 15 ounces) unsweetened crushed pineapple
2 tablespoons cornstarch
2 teaspoons rum extract
1 teaspoon vanilla extract
¼ teaspoon cream of tartar
1 tablespoon sugar
1 cup unsweetened shredded coconut

1. For the bottom layer: In a mixing bowl, combine the flour, baking powder, and salt. Cut in the margarine until the mixture is crumbly. In a smaller bowl, beat the egg yolk and milk together with a fork. Stir into the flour mixture. Press evenly into the bottom of an 8-inch square cake pan that has been lightly coated with nonfat cooking spray. Set aside.
2. For the middle layer: In a medium saucepan, combine the crushed pineapple with its juice and the cornstarch. Cook over medium heat until the mixture boils and thickens, about 2–3 minutes. Stir in the rum extract and vanilla extract. Set aside to cool slightly. Preheat the oven to 350°F.
3. For the top layer: In a mixing bowl, beat the egg white and cream of tartar until frothy. Add the sugar and beat until soft peaks form. Fold in the coconut.
4. To assemble: Pour the pineapple mixture over the bottom pastry layer. Spread the coconut mixture gently and evenly over the pineapple layer.
5. Bake until the top is golden brown, about 30 minutes. Cool on a rack, then cut into 1¼" × 1½" pieces.

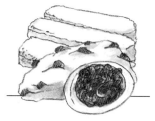

Preparation time: 30 minutes
Baking time: 30 minutes

Yield: 15 servings
Serving size: 2 pieces

Exchanges: 1 carbohydrate
1 fat
Carbohydrate choices: 1

Nutrition per serving:
Calories: 115
Carbohydrate:. . . . . 14 g
Protein: . . . . 2 g
Fat:. . . . . 6 g

Saturated fat: . . . . 3 g
Cholesterol:. . . . . 18 mg
Dietary fiber: . . . . <1 g
Sodium:. . . . . 99 mg

Shortbread

½ pound (2 sticks) margarine, at room temperature
½ cup sugar
½ cup rice flour or cake flour
1¾ cups all-purpose flour

1. In a mixing bowl, cream the margarine with the sugar until soft and fluffy. Stir in the flour just until blended. Preheat the oven to 325°F.
2. Roll the dough out on a lightly floured board (or between sheets of wax paper) to ¼-inch thickness. Cut into 1½-inch rounds.
3. Place the rounds on ungreased cookie sheets. Prick each with a fork. Bake until pale golden brown, about 22–25 minutes. Cool on racks.

Shortbread may taste great, but all the butter in typical shortbread can add up. We use margarine here for a cholesterol-free version of this all-time favorite.

293

Preparation time: 15 minutes
Baking time: 25 minutes

Yield: 20 servings
Serving size: 3 cookies

Exchanges: 1 carbohydrate
1 fat
Carbohydrate choices: 1

Nutrition per serving:
Calories: 135
Carbohydrate:. . . . . 14 g
Protein: . . . . 1 g
Fat:. . . . . 8 g

Saturated fat: . . . . 2 g
Cholesterol:. . . . . 0 mg
Dietary fiber: . . . . <1 g
Sodium:. . . . . 77 mg

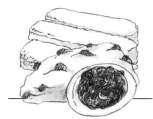

Thumbprint cookies

Thumbprints are a holiday favorite. For variation, spoon the cookies with several different varieties of fruit spreads. Your holiday cookie tray will look so much more colorful.

1 package (8 ounces) Sweet 'N Low low-fat white cake mix
3 tablespoons unsweetened orange juice
½ teaspoon almond extract
Nonfat cooking spray
5 teaspoons blueberry 100% fruit spread

1. Preheat oven to 350°F. Place cake mix in a medium mixing bowl. Add orange juice and almond extract. Using an electric mixer, whip on low setting. As a dough begins to form, increase mixer speed to medium setting and beat for 2 minutes, or until a smooth dough is formed.
2. Coat a baking sheet and your hands with cooking spray. Roll dough into 1-inch balls and place on baking sheet. Press center of each cookie with your thumb. Fill thumbprint with ¼ teaspoon blueberry spread.
3. Bake until cookies turn light golden, about 10 minutes. Cool on wire rack.

Preparation time: 10 minutes
Baking time: 10 minutes

Yield: 20 servings
Serving size: 1 cookie

Exchanges: 1 carbohydrate
Carbohydrate choices: 1

Nutrition per serving:
Calories: 53
Carbohydrate: . . . . 10 g
Protein: . . . . 1 g
Fat: . . . . 1 g

Saturated fat: . . . . <1 g
Cholesterol: . . . . 0 mg
Dietary fiber: . . . . <1 g
Sodium: . . . . 9 mg

Chapter 13

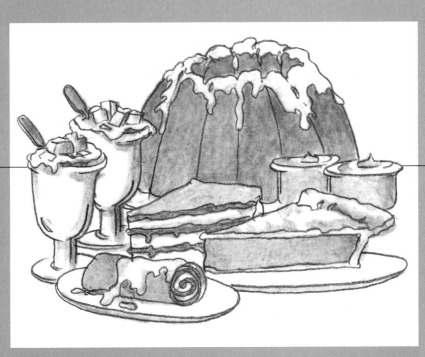

DESSERTS

*W*ant to make delicious desserts that are light on calories and easy to fit into your meal plan? These recipes prove that healthy eating does not have to be boring or flavorless.

Some of the recipes here call for sugar, but the minimum amount is used to maintain taste, texture, and appearance. Where possible, recipes are sweetened by the addition of fruits or fruit juices. Still other recipes are enhanced by the sweetness of spices and other flavorings.

It is important to note, however, that many artificial sweeteners cannot hold up to the heat of baking. If you decide you would like to use an artificial sweetener in place of sugar, look for one that gives specific instructions on oven use. But be careful to note the nutrition information of these sweeteners—some can contain as many calories as sugar.

Sponge cake

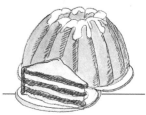

4 egg whites
¼ teaspoon cream of tartar
¼ teaspoon salt
⅓ cup sugar
2 egg yolks
1 teaspoon almond extract
1 teaspoon vanilla extract
⅓ cup all-purpose flour

Allowing this cake to dry on a towel is an important step; otherwise you may end up with a cake that is too moist on the bottom and likely to go stale quickly.

1. Line the bottom of an 8-inch square pan with waxed paper or parchment paper. Preheat the oven to 400°F.
2. In a mixing bowl, combine the egg whites, cream of tartar, and salt. Beat with a rotary beater or electric mixer until foamy. Add the sugar gradually and continue beating until stiff peaks form.
3. In a small bowl, beat the egg yolks, almond extract, and vanilla extract. Gently fold into the egg white peaks. Sprinkle flour over the surface and gently fold into the egg whites also.
4. Spread the batter in the prepared pan. Bake until the cake springs back when lightly pressed, about 15 minutes. Loosen the edges with a sharp knife and turn out the cake immediately to cool on a cake rack that has been covered with a paper towel. When cool, cut the cake into nine 2½-inch squares.

297

Preparation time: 15 minutes
Baking time: 15 minutes

Exchanges: ½ carbohydrate
Carbohydrate choices: ½

Yield: 9 servings
Serving size: 1 square

Nutrition per serving:
Calories: 58
Carbohydrate:. . . . . 9 g
Protein: . . . . 3 g
Fat:. . . . . 1 g

Saturated fat: . . . . trace
Cholesterol:. . . . . 60 mg
Dietary fiber: . . . . 0 g
Sodium:. . . . . 90 mg

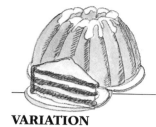

VARIATION

Chocolate sponge cake

4 egg whites
¼ teaspoon cream of tartar
¼ teaspoon salt
⅓ cup sugar
2 egg yolks
1 teaspoon almond extract
1 teaspoon vanilla extract
⅓ cup all-purpose flour
¼ cup cocoa

1. Line the bottom of an 8-inch square or round cake pan with waxed paper or parchment paper. Preheat the oven to 400°F.

2. In a mixing bowl, combine the egg whites, cream of tartar, and salt. Beat with a rotary beater or electric mixer until foamy. Add the sugar gradually and continue beating until stiff peaks form.

3. In a small bowl, beat the egg yolks, almond extract, and vanilla extract. Gently fold into the egg whites. Sift the flour and cocoa together in another bowl, then fold lightly into egg mixture.

4. Spread the batter in the prepared pan. Bake until the cake springs back when lightly pressed, about 10–12 minutes. Loosen the edges with a sharp knife and turn out immediately to cool on a cake rack that has been covered with a paper towel. When cool, cut the cake into 12 squares or slices.

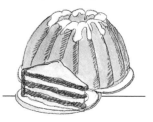

Preparation time: 15 minutes
Baking time: 15 minutes

Yield: 12 servings
Serving size: 1 square or slice

Exchanges: ½ carbohydrate
Carbohydrate choices: ½

Nutrition per serving:

Calories: 52	Saturated fat: . . . . trace
Carbohydrate: . . . . 8 g	Cholesterol: . . . . 45 mg
Protein: . . . . 2 g	Dietary fiber: . . . . <1 g
Fat: . . . . 1 g	Sodium: . . . . 68 mg

299

Sponge roll

Bake the Sponge Cake batter in a jelly roll pan that has
been lined with waxed paper or parchment. Cool and fill
with Cream Topping and Filling (recipe, p. 300) and roll
up jelly-roll style. Cut into eight 1-inch slices.

VARIATION

Preparation time: 20 minutes
Baking time: 15 minutes

Yield: 8 servings
Serving size: 1 slice

Exchanges: 1 carbohydrate
Carbohydrate choices: 1

Nutrition per serving:

Calories: 122	Saturated fat: . . . . 1 g
Carbohydrate: . . . . 16 g	Cholesterol: . . . . 70 mg
Protein: . . . . 9 g	Dietary fiber: . . . . 0 g
Fat: . . . . 2 g	Sodium: . . . . 168 mg

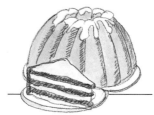

Cream topping and filling

300

This low-calorie, low-fat filling and topping can be used in a variety of recipes. Add a few drops of food coloring at the beginning of Step 3 to vary the color.

1 envelope unflavored gelatin
¼ cup cold water
1 cup boiling water
¾ cup skim milk powder
Artificial sweetener equivalent to 12 teaspoons (or ¼ cup) sugar
1 teaspoon vanilla extract
1 teaspoon maple, orange, or peppermint extract (or flavoring of your choice)
2 teaspoons vegetable oil
1 egg white, stiffly beaten

1. In a medium bowl, sprinkle the gelatin over ¼ cup cold water and allow it to soften about 5 minutes. Add 1 cup boiling water and stir well until the gelatin is dissolved. Cool 5 minutes. Place a whisk or beaters in the freezer to chill.
2. Stir the powdered milk and sweetener into the gelatin mixture until completely dissolved. Refrigerate until partially set. Using the well-chilled whisk or beaters, beat at high speed until stiff peaks form.
3. Beat in the vanilla extract, additional flavoring, and vegetable oil. Using a spatula, gently fold in the stiffly beaten egg white until thoroughly combined.

Preparation time: 15 minutes
Chilling time: 15 minutes

Yield: 10 servings
Serving size: ½ cup

Exchanges: ½ carbohydrate
Carbohydrate choices: ½

Nutrition per serving:
Calories: 45
Carbohydrate:. . . . . 5 g
Protein: . . . . 4 g
Fat:. . . . . 1 g
Saturated fat: . . . . trace
Cholesterol: . . . . trace
Dietary fiber: . . . . 0 g
Sodium:. . . . . 53 mg

Chocolate cream topping and filling

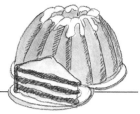

VARIATION

Whisk together 2 tablespoons cocoa and 1 cup water in a sauce pan. Bring to a boil, whisking. Use this instead of the 1 cup of boiling water in Step 1 of the recipe above.

Preparation time: 15 minutes
Chilling time: 15 minutes

Exchanges: ½ carbohydrate
Carbohydrate choices: ½

Yield: 10 servings
Serving size: ½ cup

Nutrition per serving:

Calories:	50	Saturated fat:	trace
Carbohydrate:	5 g	Cholesterol:	trace
Protein:	5 g	Dietary fiber:	<1 g
Fat:	1 g	Sodium:	54 mg

Ribbon cream torte

1 baked Sponge Cake (recipe, p. 297)
1 batch Cream Topping and Filling (recipe, p. 300)

Split the cake in half horizontally, then split each half in half again, to make 4 thin layers. Frost and stack each layer, then frost the top and sides with the Cream Topping. Refrigerate until about 15 minutes before serving time. Cut into 8 slices.

Preparation time: 35 minutes
Baking time: 15 minutes
Chilling time: 15 minutes

Exchanges: 1 carbohydrate
Carbohydrate choices: 1

Yield: 8 servings
Serving size: 1 slice

Nutrition per serving:

Calories:	122	Saturated fat:	1 g
Carbohydrate:	16 g	Cholesterol:	70 mg
Protein:	9 g	Dietary fiber:	0 g
Fat:	2 g	Sodium:	168 mg

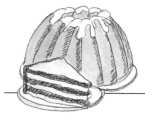

Chocolate lovers rejoice! This double chocolate treat is sure to please even the most avid chocoholic.

Double chocolate roll

1 batch Chocolate Sponge Cake batter (recipe, p. 298)
1 batch Chocolate Cream Topping and Filling (recipe, p. 301)

1. Preheat the oven to 400°F. Line the bottom of a 9½" × 13" jelly roll pan with waxed paper or parchment paper.
2. Spread the Chocolate Sponge Cake batter evenly in the pan. Bake until the cake springs back when pressed lightly, about 10–12 minutes.
3. Loosen the edges with a knife and immediately turn out the cake onto a clean kitchen towel. Gently remove the paper, trim off crispy edges, and roll the cake loosely in the towel to cool (seam side down).
4. Unroll the cake, spread it gently and evenly with the Chocolate Cream Topping and Filling, and roll up again. Place the rolled cake seam side down on a serving platter. Dust lightly with confectioner's sugar, if desired. Cut into 1-inch slices and serve.

Preparation time: 35 minutes
Chilling time: 15 minutes
Baking time: 15 minutes

Exchanges: 1 carbohydrate
Carbohydrate choices: 1

Yield: 8 servings
Serving size: 1 slice

Nutrition per serving:
Calories: 134
Carbohydrate: . . . . 17 g
Protein: . . . . 9 g
Fat: . . . . 3 g

Saturated fat: . . . . 1 g
Cholesterol: . . . . 70 mg
Dietary fiber: . . . . 1 g
Sodium: . . . . 168 mg

Peppermint chocolate roll

VARIATION

Add peppermint flavoring to plain Cream Topping and Filling (recipe, p. 300) and tint it green with food coloring, if desired.

Cream puff shells

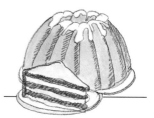

1 cup water
5 tablespoons vegetable oil
¼ teaspoon salt (optional)
1 cup all-purpose flour
4 eggs
1 teaspoon vanilla extract

Use the Cream Topping and Filling (recipe, p. 300) or a 100% fruit spread to fill these crispy puffs.

1. In a medium saucepan, combine 1 cup of water with the oil and salt (optional) and bring to a boil. Add the flour all at once and beat vigorously with a wooden spoon to mix thoroughly. Continue beating until the mixture forms a ball and draws away from the sides of the pan. Remove from heat and cool 5 minutes. Preheat oven to 400°F.
2. Off the heat, beat in the eggs, one at a time, by hand or in a mixer or a food processor. Add the vanilla extract and continue beating until the dough is very smooth and glossy.
3. Spoon about 1 rounded tablespoon of the dough onto a dampened nonstick or parchment-lined baking sheet, spacing the rounds at least 2 inches apart.
4. Bake for 10 minutes, then raise the oven temperature to 450°F and bake until the puffs are golden brown, crisp, and firm to the touch, about 12–15 minutes longer. Slit each puff with the tip of a sharp knife to release steam. Cool on a wire rack before filling.

303

Preparation time: 20 minutes
Baking time: 25 minutes

Yield: 15 servings
Serving size: 2 puffs

Exchanges: ½ carbohydrate
1 fat
Carbohydrate choices: ½

Nutrition per serving:
Calories: 89
Carbohydrate:. . . . . 6 g
Protein: . . . . 3 g
Fat:. . . . . 6 g

Saturated fat: . . . . 1 g
Cholesterol:. . . . . 73 mg
Dietary fiber: . . . . 0 g
Sodium:. . . . . 54 mg
(omitting salt) . . . . 18 mg

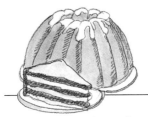

Graham cracker crust

Most homemade and commercial pie crust dough contains high amounts of butter and sugar. Use this healthier pie crust for all your dessert pies.

¾ cup graham cracker crumbs
3 tablespoons melted margarine
¼ teaspoon ground cinnamon
¼ teaspoon freshly grated nutmeg

1. In a mixing bowl or food processor, combine the crumbs, margarine, and spices. Mix or process until well blended.
2. Press into the bottom of a 9-inch pie plate, 8-inch square cake pan, or a 9-inch springform pan. Use as is, or bake for 10 minutes in a 350°F oven and cool before filling.

304

Preparation time: 5 minutes
Baking time: 10 minutes
 (optional)

Yield: 8 servings
Serving size: ⅛ pie crust

Nutrition per serving:
Calories: 79
Carbohydrate:. . . . . 8 g
Protein: . . . . 1 g
Fat:. . . . . 5 g

Exchanges: ½ carbohydrate
Carbohydrate choices: ½

Saturated fat: . . . . 1 g
Cholesterol: . . . . trace
Dietary fiber: . . . . 0 g
Sodium:. . . . . 103 mg

Oatmeal pie crust

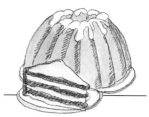

¾ **cup all-purpose flour**
½ **cup quick-cooking (but not instant) rolled oats**
½ **teaspoon salt**
¼ **cup vegetable oil**
3–4 tablespoons ice water

1. In a mixing bowl or food processor, combine the flour, oats, and salt. Slowly drizzle in the oil with the motor running (or with a fork if mixing by hand). Add ice water, a few drops at a time, until the mixture begins to form a ball.

2. Pat the dough into a 9-inch pie plate (or roll between two sheets of waxed paper; remove top sheet and turn pastry into pie plate, then remove second sheet of waxed paper). Form a rim and flute the edges.

3. For an unbaked pie shell: Fill and bake according to pie recipe. For a baked pie shell: Prick the pastry with a fork in several places. Bake in a 400°F oven until light golden brown, about 10 minutes.

For convenience, make this pie crust ahead of time and freeze it for up to 2 months before use. It will taste just as nutty and delicious as if you had made it fresh.

305

Preparation time: 15 minutes
Baking time: 10 minutes
      (optional)

Exchanges: 1 carbohydrate
      2 fat
Carbohydrate choices: 1

Yield: 6 servings
Serving size: ⅙ pie crust

Nutrition per serving:
Calories: 159
Carbohydrate: . . . . 16 g
Protein: . . . . 2 g
Fat: . . . . 10 g

Saturated fat: . . . . 1 g
Cholesterol: . . . . 0 mg
Dietary fiber: . . . . 1 g
Sodium: . . . . 178 mg

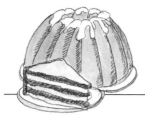

Baked cinnamon custard

Those who like the velvety texture of crème brûlée will love this custard dish. Serve this when entertaining guests or on special occasions.

4 egg whites
1 egg yolk
1 tablespoon brown sugar
Pinch salt (optional)
1 teaspoon vanilla extract
1¼ cups skim milk
Cinnamon
Boiling water

1. Preheat the oven to 350°F. In a mixing bowl, whisk the egg whites, egg yolk, sugar, salt (optional), vanilla extract, and milk until just blended. (Do not use a blender or food processor, or the mixture may become too foamy.)
2. Pour the custard mixture through a fine sieve into 4 individual custard cups or 1 small casserole. Sprinkle the tops with cinnamon. Set the custard cups in a roasting pan and place the pan in the oven. Pour boiling water into the pan to about ½ inch from the top of the cups.
3. Bake until the custard has set or until a tester inserted in the center comes out clean, about 45 minutes. Serve warm, at room temperature, or thoroughly chilled.

Preparation time: 10 minutes
Baking time: 45 minutes

Yield: 4 servings
Serving size: ½ cup

Exchanges: ½ carbohydrate
Carbohydrate choices: ½

Nutrition per serving:
Calories: 71
Carbohydrate:. . . . . 7 g
Protein: . . . . 7 g
Fat:. . . . . 2 g
Saturated fat: . . . . 1 g
Cholesterol: . . . . 69 mg
Dietary fiber: . . . . 0 g
Sodium:. . . . . 157 mg
(omitting salt) . . . . 90 mg

Saucy baked custard

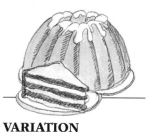

VARIATION

Place 1 teaspoon of diet jam or fruit spread in each individual custard cup before adding the custard mixture. Omit the cinnamon. Turn out onto dessert dishes and the sauce will form over the custard.

Baked coconut custard

VARIATION

Place 1 teaspoon of unsweetened shredded coconut in each individual custard cup before pouring in the custard. Omit the cinnamon.

307

Soft custard

1 egg
2 egg whites
2 tablespoons sugar
Pinch salt (optional)
1½ cups skim milk
½ teaspoon vanilla extract

As a sauce, this makes an excellent topping for Sponge Cake (recipe, p. 297) or Peppermint Chocolate Roll (recipe, p. 302).

1. In the top of a double boiler, beat together the egg, egg whites, sugar, salt (optional), and milk. Cook over simmering water, stirring, until the mixture thickens enough to coat a spoon.
2. Pour into a cool bowl or pitcher. Stir in the vanilla extract. Use warm as a sauce or refrigerate and serve as a pudding.

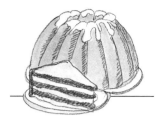

Preparation time: 5 minutes
Cooking time: 10 minutes

Yield: 4 servings
Serving size: ½ cup

Nutrition per serving:
Calories: 82
Carbohydrate:. . . . . 10 g
Protein: . . . . 7 g
Fat:. . . . . 2 g

Exchanges: 1 carbohydrate
Carbohydrate choices: 1

Saturated fat: . . . . 1 g
Cholesterol: . . . . 70 mg
Dietary fiber: . . . . 0 g
Sodium:. . . . . 155 mg
(omitting salt) . . . . 88 mg

This wonderful nutty filling can also be used as frosting for a cake.

Chocolate almond cream filling

1 package whipped topping mix
**   (for 2 cups whipped topping)**
½ cup cold skim milk
2 teaspoons cocoa
1 teaspoon almond extract
6 whole, blanched almonds, toasted and chopped

In a mixing bowl, combine the topping mix, milk, cocoa, and almond extract. Beat at high speed until stiff peaks form. Continue beating 2 more minutes, until fluffy. Fold in the chopped almonds. Store, covered, in the refrigerator or freezer.

Preparation time: 10 minutes

Yield: 2 cups
Serving size: 2 tablespoons

Exchanges: ½ fat
Carbohydrate choices: 0

Nutrition per serving:

Calories:	26	Saturated fat:	2 g
Carbohydrate:	1 g	Cholesterol:	trace
Protein:	1 g	Dietary fiber:	0 g
Fat:	2 g	Sodium:	16 mg

Mocha almond cream filling

VARIATION

Add 1 teaspoon instant coffee powder to the topping mix and milk mixture before beating.

Chocolate almond cream puffs

309

30 Cream Puff Shells (recipe, p. 303)
1 batch Chocolate Almond Cream Filling
  (recipe, p. 308)

Place the filling in a pastry bag fitted with a small, plain tube and pipe 1 tablespoon of the filling into each puff; or cut the top off each puff and spoon the filling inside. Refrigerate until serving time.

Don't have a pastry bag handy? Curl a piece of waxed paper or parchment paper so that it forms a cone with a very small opening at the bottom. Spoon the filling into the paper cone, fold the wide part of the paper down, and gently squeeze the filling through the small hole at the bottom.

Preparation time: 30 minutes
Baking time: 25 minutes

Yield: 15 servings
Serving size: 2 filled puffs

Exchanges: ½ carbohydrate
1½ fat
Carbohydrate choices: ½

Nutrition per serving:

Calories:	117	Saturated fat:	3 g
Carbohydrate:	7 g	Cholesterol:	73 mg
Protein:	3 g	Dietary fiber:	0 g
Fat:	9 g	Sodium:	71 mg

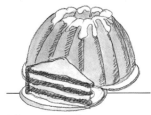

Orange custard cloud

This tangy dessert is so light in texture you would swear it's just like a cloud. For variety, add sliced grapes or diced pineapple chunks to the recipe before chilling.

1 envelope unflavored gelatin
1½ cups plus ½ cup unsweetened orange juice
1 teaspoon orange zest (optional)
2 egg yolks
Artificial sweetener equivalent to 8 teaspoons sugar
3 egg whites
½ teaspoon cream of tartar

1. In a small bowl, combine the gelatin with ½ cup orange juice; set aside 5 minutes to soften.
2. In a nonreactive saucepan, whisk together the remaining 1½ cups orange juice, orange zest (optional), and egg yolks. Cook, stirring, over low heat, until thickened, about 5 minutes.
3. Remove from heat and stir in sweetener and gelatin mixture until dissolved. Chill until almost set.
4. Beat the egg whites with the cream of tartar until stiff. Fold the whites into the orange mixture. Spoon into a serving bowl. Chill about 4 hours, until set.

310

Preparation time: 15 minutes
Cooking time: 5 minutes
Chilling time: 4 hours

Exchanges: ½ carbohydrate
½ fat
Carbohydrate choices: ½

Yield: 8 servings
Serving size: ⅔ cup

Nutrition per serving:
Calories: 53
Carbohydrate:. . . . . 6 g
Protein: . . . . 4 g
Fat:. . . . . 2 g

Saturated fat: . . . . 1 g
Cholesterol: . . . . 68 mg
Dietary fiber: . . . . 0 g
Sodium:. . . . . 29 mg

Orange blocks

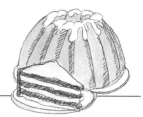

2 cups orange juice
4 envelopes unflavored gelatin
2 teaspoons vanilla extract

1. In a mixing bowl, combine 1 cup of the orange juice with the gelatin; let stand 5 minutes to soften.
2. In a nonreactive saucepan, heat the remaining 1 cup of orange juice to boiling. Pour the hot juice into the gelatin mixture and stir until the gelatin is dissolved. Stir in the vanilla extract.
3. Pour into a rinsed 8-inch square cake pan. Chill about 4 hours until firm. Cut into 1-inch squares.

Tired of plain old gelatin? Looking for something low-calorie but tasty? This recipe, with a burst of orange flavor, will quickly become a favorite.

Preparation time: 5 minutes
Cooking time: 10 minutes
Chilling time: 4 hours

Exchanges: free
Carbohydrate choices: 0

Yield: 32 servings
Serving size: 2 squares

Nutrition per serving:
Calories: 10
Carbohydrate: . . . . 2 g
Protein: . . . . 1 g
Fat: . . . . 0 g
Saturated fat: . . . . 0 g
Cholesterol: . . . . 0 mg
Dietary fiber: . . . . 0 g
Sodium: . . . . trace

311

Grape blocks

Substitute 1 cup unsweetened grape juice and 1 cup water for the orange juice.

VARIATION

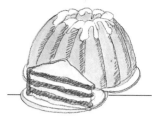

Cranberry-pear kuchen

312

Fruit layer:

2 cups fresh cranberries, washed, picked over, and roughly chopped

¼ teaspoon cinnamon

1 cup plus ¼ cup water

1 tablespoon cornstarch

Liquid artificial sweetener equivalent to 8 teaspoons of sugar

1 small (or ½ large) pear (or apple), peeled, cored, and coarsely chopped

Kuchen layer:

1 cup all-purpose flour

1½ teaspoons baking powder

½ teaspoon salt (optional)

¼ teaspoon cinnamon

3 tablespoons sugar

1 egg

2 teaspoons vegetable oil

½ teaspoon vanilla extract

⅓ cup water

½ cup Crunchy Topping (recipe, p. 332)

1. In a medium saucepan, combine the cranberries and cinnamon with 1 cup water; bring to a boil, lower heat, and cook, stirring, 5 minutes. Preheat the oven to 350°F.
2. In a small bowl, mix the cornstarch and ¼ cup water until smooth; add the cranberries and continue cooking until the mixture thickens, about 2–3 minutes. Remove the saucepan from the heat and stir in the sweetener and chopped pear (or apple).

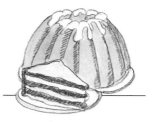

3. In a mixing bowl, sift together the flour, baking powder, salt (optional), and cinnamon. In a separate bowl, combine the sugar, egg, oil, vanilla extract, and ⅓ cup water; beat until frothy. Combine the egg mixture with the flour mixture and stir until just combined.

4. Spread the batter into a 9-inch round or square baking pan that has been lightly greased or coated with nonfat cooking spray. Pour the fruit mixture over the cake layer. Sprinkle with Crunchy Topping. Bake 40–45 minutes. Serve warm.

313

Preparation time: 20 minutes
Cooking time: 55 minutes

Yield: 12 servings
Serving size: ¹⁄₁₂ cake

Exchanges: 1 carbohydrate
         1 fat
Carbohydrate choices: 1

Nutrition per serving:
Calories: 114
Carbohydrate:. . . . . 17 g
Protein: . . . . 2 g
Fat:. . . . . 3 g

Saturated fat: . . . . 1 g
Cholesterol:. . . . . 23 mg
Dietary fiber: . . . . 2 g
Sodium:. . . . . 157 mg
(omitting salt) . . . . 67 mg

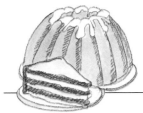

Baked rice pudding

The smooth taste and texture of this rice pudding is the result of the twice-cooked rice. This version may take a little longer than other recipes, but it is worth the wait.

½ cup water
¼ teaspoon salt
¼ cup rice
1 egg
1¼ cups skim milk
4 teaspoons brown sugar
½ teaspoon vanilla extract
¼ teaspoon ground cinnamon
¼ teaspoon freshly grated nutmeg
2 tablespoons raisins

1. In a small saucepan, bring ½ cup water and the salt to a boil. Add the rice, reduce the heat, cover, and cook slowly for 15 minutes. Preheat the oven to 350°F.
2. In a mixing bowl, beat together the egg, milk, brown sugar, vanilla extract, cinnamon, and nutmeg. Stir the cooked rice and the raisins into the milk mixture.
3. Spoon the rice mixture into a 1-quart ovenproof baking dish that has been lightly greased or coated with nonfat cooking spray. Place this dish in a roasting pan and place the pan in the oven. Pour boiling water in the roasting pan to halfway up the side of the baking dish. Bake 30 minutes. Stir well. Continue to bake 30 minutes longer, until lightly browned.

Preparation time: 15 minutes
Cooking time: 1¼ hours

Yield: 4 servings
Serving size: ⅓ cup

Exchanges: 1 carbohydrate
½ fat
Carbohydrate choices: 1

Nutrition per serving:
Calories: 105
Carbohydrate: . . . . 17 g
Protein: . . . . 5 g
Fat: . . . . 2 g

Saturated fat: . . . . 1 g
Cholesterol: . . . . 70 mg
Dietary fiber: . . . . <1 g
Sodium: . . . . 193 mg

Nova Scotia gingerbread

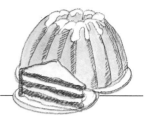

¼ cup margarine
¼ cup lightly packed brown sugar
⅓ cup molasses
1 egg
1½ cups all-purpose flour
1 teaspoon salt (optional)
1 teaspoon baking soda
1 teaspoon cinnamon
1 teaspoon ground ginger
¼ teaspoon ground cloves
¾ cup boiling water
Nonfat cooking spray

For crispier gingerbread, pour the mixture out onto a lightly greased 9" × 13" pan and bake for 20–25 minutes, checking halfway for doneness.

1. In a mixing bowl, cream the margarine and sugar until light and fluffy. Beat in the molasses and egg. Preheat the oven to 350°F.
2. Sift together the flour, salt (optional), baking soda, and spices. Mixing the entire time, add ½ the dry ingredients, then ¾ cup boiling water, and then the remaining dry ingredients. Do not overmix.
3. Spoon the batter into an 8" × 4" loaf pan that has been coated with nonfat cooking spray. Bake until a tester comes out clean, about 40–45 minutes. Cool in the pan 10 minutes, then remove from pan and cool completely on a rack.

315

Preparation time: 15 minutes
Baking time: 45 minutes

Yield: 12 servings
Serving size: one slice
(½-inch thick)

Exchanges: 1 carbohydrate
1 fat
Carbohydrate choices: 1

Nutrition per serving:
Calories: 119
Carbohydrate: . . . . 19 g
Protein: . . . . 2 g
Fat: . . . . 4 g
Saturated fat: . . . . 1 g
Cholesterol: . . . . 23 mg
Dietary fiber: . . . . 0 g
Sodium: . . . . 294 mg
(omitting salt) . . . . 117 mg

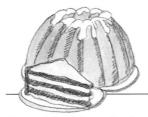

Serve this light, refreshing finale by itself or as a pie filling using our Graham Cracker Crust (recipe, p. 304).

316

Pineapple dream

1 envelope unflavored gelatin
½ cup canned unsweetened pineapple juice
1 teaspoon coconut or almond extract
½ cup canned unsweetened pineapple chunks
1 cup low-fat cottage cheese
**Artificial liquid sweetener equivalent
  to 1 teaspoon of sugar**
1 package whipped topping mix
½ cup skim milk
2 teaspoons toasted, unsweetened, shredded coconut

1. In a small nonreactive saucepan, sprinkle the gelatin over the pineapple juice; let stand 5 minutes to soften.
2. Add the coconut extract, then heat, stirring, until the gelatin has dissolved. Cool to room temperature.
3. Place the pineapple chunks, cottage cheese, and sweetener in a blender or food processor. Process until pureed. Add the gelatin mixture and pulse briefly to blend.
4. In a mixing bowl, beat the whipped topping mix and milk until stiff peaks form. Add the pineapple puree and fold gently to combine.
5. Pour into a 1-quart serving bowl, sprinkle with toasted coconut, and chill at least 2 hours before serving.

Preparation time: 20 minutes
Chilling time: 2 hours

Exchanges: ½ carbohydrate
Carbohydrate choices: ½

Yield: 8 servings
Serving size: ½ cup

Nutrition per serving:
Calories: 57
Carbohydrate:. . . . . 6 g
Protein: . . . . 5 g
Fat:. . . . . 1 g

Saturated fat: . . . . 1 g
Cholesterol: . . . . trace
Dietary fiber: . . . . 0 g
Sodium:. . . . . 117 mg

Blueberry cupcakes

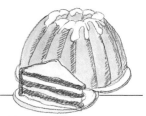

⅓ cup margarine

6 tablespoons lightly packed brown sugar

1 egg

1½ cups all-purpose flour

1 teaspoon baking powder

½ teaspoon baking soda

½ teaspoon salt (optional)

¼ teaspoon ground cinnamon

¼ teaspoon ground nutmeg

⅔ cup buttermilk or sour skim milk

1 cup fresh (washed and picked over) or partially
  thawed frozen blueberries

If buttermilk isn't readily available, you can substitute sour skim milk: Add ⅔ cup of skim milk to 2 teaspoons of vinegar, mix lightly, and allow to sit for 5 minutes before using.

1. In a mixing bowl, cream the margarine and sugar until fluffy. Beat in the egg. Preheat the oven to 375°F.

2. In another bowl, sift together the flour, baking powder, baking soda, salt (optional), and the spices. Stir into the creamed mixture alternately with the buttermilk (or sour skim milk), just until mixed.

3. Fold in the blueberries. Fill 12 muffin cups that have been lined with paper (or lightly greased or coated with nonstick cooking spray); fill each muffin cup ⅔ full. Bake until golden, about 20 minutes.

317

Preparation time: 15 minutes
Baking time: 20 minutes

Yield: 12 servings
Serving size: 1 cupcake

Exchanges: 1 carbohydrate
            1 fat
Carbohydrate choices: 1

Nutrition per serving:
Calories: 131
Carbohydrate: . . . . 19 g
Protein: . . . . 2 g
Fat: . . . . 5 g

Saturated fat: . . . . 1 g
Cholesterol: . . . . 23 mg
Dietary fiber: . . . . <1 g
Sodium: . . . . 223 mg
(omitting salt) . . . . 134 mg

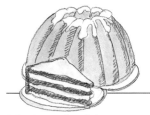

Rich chocolate cupcakes

This may be the easiest cupcake recipe you will ever come across. It's also one of the tastiest.

6 tablespoons reduced-fat margarine
¾ cup plus 2 tablespoons sugar
1¼ cups all-purpose flour
⅓ cup cocoa
1 teaspoon baking soda
⅛ teaspoon salt
1 cup buttermilk or sour skim milk
½ teaspoon vanilla

1. Preheat oven to 350°F. Line 18 muffin cups with paper baking cups. Melt margarine in a large saucepan over low heat. Remove the pan from the heat and stir in the sugar.
2. In a separate bowl, combine flour, cocoa, baking soda, and salt; add dry mixture alternately with the buttermilk (or sour skim milk) and vanilla to the saucepan containing the margarine and sugar. Stir the batter with a whisk until it is well blended.
3. Fill each muffin cup ⅔ full. Bake 18–20 minutes, or until a toothpick inserted in the center of a cupcake comes out clean. Remove the cupcakes from the pan and allow them to cool completely on a wire rack.

318

Preparation time: 10 minutes
Baking time: 20 minutes

Yield: 18 servings
Serving size: 1 cupcake

Exchanges: 1 starch
Carbohydrate choices: 1

Nutrition per serving:
Calories: 97
Carbohydrate: . . . . 18 g
Protein: . . . . 2 g
Fat: . . . . 2 g
Saturated fat: . . . . <1 g
Cholesterol: . . . . 0 mg
Dietary fiber: . . . . <1 g
Sodium: . . . . 146 mg

Chewy chocolate brownies

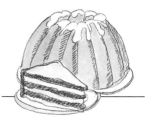

Nonfat cooking spray
¼ cup plus 3 tablespoons all-purpose flour
½ cup cocoa
¼ teaspoon salt
2 egg whites
1 whole egg
½ cup plus 2 tablespoons sugar
6 tablespoons unsweetened applesauce
2 tablespoons vegetable oil
1½ teaspoons vanilla extract
2 tablespoons chopped walnuts or pecans

No margarine means less fat in this delicious brownie recipe. The addition of applesauce make these treats moist and flavorful.

1. Preheat oven to 350°F. Spray an 8-inch square baking pan with cooking spray. In a medium bowl, combine flour, cocoa, and salt. Mix well.
2. In a separate large bowl, whisk together egg whites, egg, sugar, applesauce, oil, and vanilla extract. Stir in the flour mixture until just blended; do not overmix.
3. Pour batter into the prepared pan and sprinkle walnuts on top. Bake for 25 minutes, until a toothpick inserted in the center comes out clean. Cool the brownies on a wire rack at least 15 minutes. Cut into 12 rectangles.

Preparation time: 10 minutes
Baking time: 25 minutes

Yield: 12 servings
Serving size: 1 brownie

Exchanges: 1 starch
½ fat
Carbohydrate choices: 1

Nutrition per serving:
Calories: 111
Carbohydrate:. . . . . 17 g
Protein: . . . . 3 g
Fat:. . . . . 4 g
Saturated fat: . . . . <1 g
Cholesterol:. . . . . 18 mg
Dietary fiber: . . . . 1 g
Sodium:. . . . . 65 mg

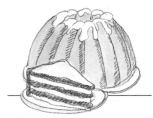

This light, fruity pie is an excellent dessert to serve at the end of a summer day.

Mandarin pie

1 envelope unflavored gelatin
2 tablespoons cold water
½ cup boiling water
¼ cup orange juice
Liquid artificial sweetener equivalent
  to 12 teaspoons (¼ cup) sugar
1 teaspoon grated orange zest
1 cup plain, low-fat yogurt
1 can (about 11 ounces) unsweetened mandarin
  oranges, drained, or 1 cup orange sections
1 Graham Cracker Crust (recipe, p. 304)
  in a 9-inch pie plate
Cinnamon

1. In a medium mixing bowl, sprinkle the gelatin over 2 tablespoons cold water, stir, and allow to stand 5 minutes to soften.
2. Add ½ cup boiling water to the softened gelatin and stir until the gelatin dissolves. Stir in the orange juice, sweetener, and orange zest.
3. Add the yogurt to the gelatin mixture and whisk until well blended. Refrigerate until partially set, about 45 minutes. Fold in the orange sections. Taste for sweetness, adding more sweetener if necessary.
4. Pour filling into the prepared pie shell. Sprinkle lightly with cinnamon. Refrigerate 4 hours until set.

Preparation time: 10 minutes
Chilling time: 4¾ hours

Yield: 6 servings
Serving size: ⅙ pie

Exchanges: 1½ carbohydrate
  1 fat
Carbohydrate choices: 1½

Nutrition per serving:
Calories: 160
Carbohydrate:. . . . . 21 g
Protein: . . . . 4 g
Fat:. . . . . 6 g

Saturated fat: . . . . 1 g
Cholesterol: . . . . trace
Dietary fiber: . . . . <1 g
Sodium:. . . . . 169 mg

Cranberry-strawberry crepes

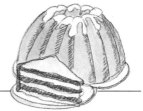

2 cups fresh cranberries, washed and picked over
2 teaspoons grated orange zest
1¾ cups plus ¼ cup water
2 teaspoons cornstarch
2 teaspoons molasses
Artificial sweetener equivalent to 12 teaspoons
** (¼ cup) sugar**
2 tablespoons brandy
8 Crepes (recipe, p. 362)
1½ cups sliced fresh strawberries
** (or apples, pears, or peaches)**

1. In a medium saucepan, combine the cranberries and orange zest with 1¾ cups water. Bring to a boil, reduce the heat, and simmer 5 minutes.

2. Pour the cranberry mixture into a blender or food processor. Set the saucepan aside. In a small bowl, whisk the cornstarch and molasses in the remaining ¼ cup water and add to the cranberry mixture. Process 1–2 minutes to puree.

3. Pour the cranberry mixture back into the same saucepan. Cook, stirring, until the mixture boils and thickens, about 4 minutes. Remove from the heat, add the sweetener, and stir until it dissolves. Refrigerate until ready to serve.

4. To serve: Bring the sauce and brandy to a boil in a large frying pan. Reduce the heat and simmer 1 minute. Place the crepes, one at a time, in the sauce; coat both sides; fold in half and then in half again to form a triangle. As each triangle is formed, move it to the side of the pan.

5. Add the fruit to the pan and cook, stirring, until heated through. Spoon a crepe, a little fruit, and some sauce onto a warm dessert plate for each serving.

Cook these crepes right in front of your friends and impress them all. Make sure to use a good-quality brandy in Step 4 or the sauce and fruit may end up tasting bitter.

321

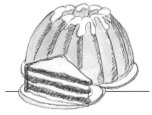

Preparation time: 1¼ hours
Cooking time: 40 minutes

Yield: 8 servings
Serving size: 1 crepe with
⅓ cup sauce
and fruit

Nutrition per serving:
Calories: 80
Carbohydrate: . . . . 14 g
Protein: . . . . 3 g
Fat: . . . . 1 g

Exchanges: 1 carbohydrate
Carbohydrate choices: 1

Saturated fat: . . . . trace
Cholesterol: . . . . trace
Dietary fiber: . . . . 2 g
Sodium: . . . . 33 mg

322

Light and lemony cheesecake

Now you can eat cheesecake guilt-free. Fattening cream cheese is replaced with low-fat and tasty cottage cheese and gelatin.

1½ cups low-fat cottage cheese (or part-skim ricotta cheese)

2 teaspoons grated lemon zest

1 envelope unflavored gelatin

¼ cup freshly squeezed lemon juice

3 eggs, separated

½ cup skim milk

Artificial sweetener equivalent to 8 teaspoons sugar

1 teaspoon vanilla extract

¼ teaspoon cream of tartar

1 Graham Cracker Crust (recipe, p. 304)

Berry Sauce (recipe, p. 330) (optional)

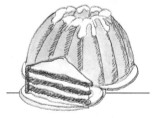

1. Press the cottage (or ricotta) cheese through a sieve into a bowl. Stir in the lemon zest.

2. Sprinkle the gelatin over the lemon juice to soften it; set aside 5 minutes.

3. Combine the egg yolks and milk in the top of a double boiler. Cook, stirring, until the mixture thickens. Remove from heat. Stir in the gelatin mixture until it dissolves.

4. Add the sweetener, vanilla extract, and strained cottage cheese to the yolk mixture. Refrigerate, stirring occasionally, until partially set.

5. Beat the egg whites with the cream of tartar until stiff peaks form. Fold into the yolk mixture. Pour into the prepared Graham Cracker Crust (in a 9-inch springform pan or pie plate). Chill about 4 hours until firm. Cut into 8 slices. Serve with Berry Sauce, if desired.

Preparation time: 20 minutes
Cooking time: 5 minutes
Chilling time: 4 hours

Yield: 8 servings
Serving size: 1 slice

Exchanges: 1 carbohydrate
    1 lean meat
    ½ fat
Carbohydrate choices: 1

Nutrition per serving:

With berry sauce
Calories: 158
Carbohydrate: . . . . 12 g
Protein: . . . . 10 g
Fat: . . . . 7 g
Saturated fat: . . . . 2 g
Cholesterol: . . . . 105 mg
Dietary fiber: . . . . 1 g
Sodium: . . . . 302 mg

Without berry sauce
Calories: 151
Carbohydrate: . . . . 11 g
Protein: . . . . 10 g
Fat: . . . . 7 g
Saturated fat: . . . . 2 g
Cholesterol: . . . . 105 mg
Dietary fiber: . . . . 0 g
Sodium: . . . . 302 mg

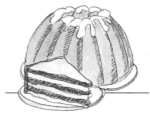

The velvety-smooth filling of this pie will wow even the most ardent chocolate lovers.

Chocolate dream pie

1 envelope unflavored gelatin
1½ cups skim milk
¼ cup cocoa
1 tablespoon cornstarch
1 egg, separated
Artificial sweetener equivalent to 16 teaspoons of sugar
1 teaspoon vanilla extract
¼ cup instant skim milk powder
¼ cup ice water
1 Oatmeal Pie Crust (recipe, p. 305) in a 9-inch pie plate

1. Sprinkle the gelatin over ¼ cup milk; stir and let stand 5 minutes to soften.
2. In a heavy saucepan, whisk together 1 cup milk and the cocoa until well blended. Heat to boiling, reduce heat, and simmer 5 minutes, stirring.
3. In a small bowl, beat the remaining ¼ cup milk, the cornstarch, and egg yolk until smooth. Add this mixture to the cocoa mixture and continue cooking over low heat, stirring, until the mixture thickens, about 2–3 minutes.
4. Remove the saucepan from the heat, add the softened gelatin and the sweetener, and stir until dissolved. Stir in the vanilla extract. Chill until partially set.
5. In a mixing bowl, beat together the egg white, skim milk powder, and ¼ cup ice water until stiff peaks from. Fold into the chocolate mixture. Spoon into the prepared pie shell. Chill about 4 hours until set.

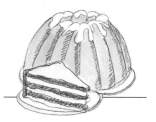

Preparation time: 20 minutes
Cooking time: 10 minutes
Chilling time: 4 hours

Yield: 8 servings
Serving size: ⅛ pie

Exchanges: 1 carbohydrate
2 fat
Carbohydrate choices: 1

Nutrition per serving:
Calories: 177
Carbohydrate: . . . . 18 g
Protein: . . . . 7 g
Fat: . . . . 9 g

Saturated fat: . . . . 2 g
Cholesterol: . . . . 36 mg
Dietary fiber: . . . . 2 g
Sodium: . . . . 187 mg

Chocolate mousse

Prepare the filling as above and spoon into 6 individual molds or a 1-quart serving bowl. Chill about 4 hours until set.

VARIATION

Yield: 6 servings
Serving size: ½ cup

Exchanges: ½ carbohydrate
½ fat
Carbohydrate choices: ½

Nutrition per serving:
Calories: 77
Carbohydrate: . . . . 8 g
Protein: . . . . 7 g
Fat: . . . . 2 g

Saturated fat: . . . . 1 g
Cholesterol: . . . . 48 mg
Dietary fiber: . . . . 1 g
Sodium: . . . . 71 mg

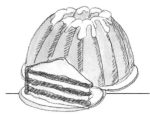

Frozen yogurt and a mocha-flavored fudge sauce make these sundaes something special. Kids will love them.

Light hot fudge sundaes

½ cup sugar
¼ cup cocoa
1 tablespoon cornstarch
2 teaspoons instant coffee granules
½ cup plus 2 tablespoons evaporated skim milk
2 teaspoons margarine
½ teaspoon vanilla extract
4 cups fat-free vanilla frozen yogurt

1. Combine sugar, cocoa, cornstarch, and instant coffee in a medium saucepan. Gradually stir in the milk. Bring the mixture to a boil over medium heat, stirring constantly, until it thickens.
2. Remove from heat and stir in margarine and vanilla extract; keep stirring until margarine has melted. To serve, scoop ½ cup frozen yogurt into individual serving bowls and top evenly with hot fudge sauce.

326

Preparation time: 5 minutes
Cooking time: 5 minutes

Yield: 8 servings
Serving size: ½ cup frozen
          yogurt with 2
          tablespoons sauce

Exchanges: 2½ carbohydrate
Carbohydrate choices: 2½

Nutrition per serving:
Calories: 177
Carbohydrate:. . . . . 36 g
Protein: . . . . 6 g
Fat:. . . . . 1 g

Saturated fat: . . . . <1 g
Cholesterol:. . . . . 1 mg
Dietary fiber: . . . . <1 g
Sodium:. . . . . 102 mg

Strawberry angel pie

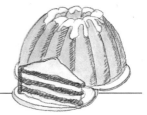

1 cup water

3 cups sliced fresh or unsweetened
   frozen strawberries

1 envelope unflavored gelatin

1 tablespoon cornstarch

1 egg, separated

Artificial sweetener equivalent to 14 teaspoons
   of sugar

1 teaspoon vanilla extract

½ teaspoon almond extract

¼ cup instant skim milk powder

¼ cup ice water

1 Graham Cracker Crust (recipe, p. 304)
   in a 9-inch pie plate

*Slightly overripe straw-
berries, a little less than
firm to the touch, will
give this pie a stronger
strawberry flavor.*

1. Pour 1 cup of water over the strawberries and allow
them to stand at room temperature for 1 hour.
2. Drain the water from the strawberries into a medium
saucepan; reserve the strawberries. Pour the gelatin
into a small bowl or cup and add 2 tablespoons of the
strawberry liquid to it; stir and let stand 5 minutes to
soften.
3. Whisk the cornstarch and egg yolk into the remaining
strawberry liquid. Cook, stirring, over medium heat
until the mixture boils and thickens slightly, about
2–3 minutes.
4. Remove the saucepan from the heat and add the softened gelatin, sweetener, and vanilla and almond extracts.
Stir until the gelatin and sweetener dissolve. Stir in the
strawberries. Chill until partially set, about 30 minutes.
5. In a chilled mixing bowl, beat the egg white, skim milk
powder, and ¼ cup ice water until stiff peaks form. Fold
into the thickened strawberry mixture. Spoon into the
Graham Cracker Crust. Chill 4 hours to set.

327

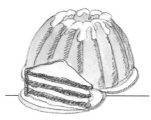

Preparation time: 20 minutes
Standing time: 1 hour
Cooking time: 5 minutes
Chilling time: 4½ hours

Yield: 6 servings
Serving size: ⅙ pie

Nutrition per serving:
Calories: 172
Carbohydrate:. . . . . 20 g
Protein: . . . . 5 g
Fat:. . . . . 7 g

Exchanges: 1½ carbohydrate
1½ fat
Carbohydrate choices: 1½

Saturated fat: . . . . 2 g
Cholesterol:. . . . . 47 mg
Dietary fiber: . . . . 2 g
Sodium:. . . . . 177 mg

Strawberry angel mousse

VARIATION

Prepare the filling as above and spoon into 4 individual molds or a 1-quart serving bowl. Chill about 4 hours to set.

Yield: 4 servings
Serving size: ⅔ cup

Nutrition per serving:
Calories: 100
Carbohydrate:. . . . . 14 g
Protein: . . . . 7 g
Fat:. . . . . 2 g

Exchanges: 1 carbohydrate
½ fat
Carbohydrate choices: 1

Saturated fat: . . . . 1 g
Cholesterol:. . . . . 70 mg
Dietary fiber: . . . . 3 g
Sodium:. . . . . 59 mg

Peachy blueberry pie

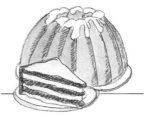

½ cup water

2 tablespoons cornstarch

1 tablespoon freshly squeezed lemon juice

¼ teaspoon freshly grated nutmeg

Pinch salt

Liquid artificial sweetener equivalent to 8 teaspoons
   of sugar

2 cups sliced fresh or thawed frozen peaches

½ cup fresh or partially thawed frozen blueberries

1 Oatmeal Pie Crust (recipe, p. 305)
   in a 9-inch pie plate

½ cup Crunchy Topping (recipe, p. 332)

Peaches and blueberries combine to create this delicious fruit pie. Fresh fruits will yield the best flavors, but frozen will do in a pinch.

1. Preheat the oven to 425°F. In a medium saucepan, combine ½ cup water with the cornstarch, lemon juice, nutmeg, and salt. Bring to a boil and cook, stirring, until thickened and clear, about 2 minutes. Remove from the heat and stir in the sweetener.

2. Fold in the peaches, then the blueberries. Spoon the fruit mixture into the prepared pie shell. Sprinkle with Crunchy Topping. Cover the pie loosely with a foil tent to prevent over-browning. Bake 30 minutes, remove foil, and continue to bake 10 more minutes, or until the fruit is tender.

329

Preparation time: 15 minutes
Cooking time: 45 minutes

Yield: 8 servings
Serving size: ⅛ pie

Exchanges: 1½ carbohydrate
   2 fat
Carbohydrate choices: 1½

Nutrition per serving:
Calories: 188
Carbohydrate: . . . . 23 g
Protein: . . . . 3 g
Fat: . . . . 9 g

Saturated fat: . . . . 1 g
Cholesterol: . . . . 0 mg
Dietary fiber: . . . . 2 g
Sodium: . . . . 167 mg

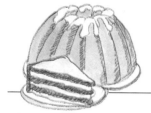

Berry Sauce

This sauce is perfect on just about any dessert. Try it over fat-free frozen yogurt.

1 cup unsweetened raspberries or strawberries (fresh or frozen)
1 tablespoon freshly squeezed lemon juice
Liquid artificial sweetener equivalent to 12 teaspoons of sugar

Puree all of the ingredients in a blender or food processor. Strain through a fine-mesh strainer to remove seeds. Store in a tightly covered container in the refrigerator or freezer.

Preparation time: 5 minutes

Yield: about ¾ cup
Serving size: 3 tablespoons

Exchanges: free
Carbohydrate choices: 0

Nutrition per serving:
Calories: 15
Carbohydrate:. . . . . 3 g
Protein: . . . . trace
Fat: . . . . trace

Saturated fat: . . . . 0 g
Cholesterol:. . . . . 0 mg
Dietary fiber: . . . . 2 g
Sodium:. . . . . 0 mg

Chocolate sauce

Use this in a tasty low-calorie dessert over poached pears: Place cored, halved, and peeled pears in a saucepan and barely cover them with water. Add 1 teaspoon of vanilla extract to the water and bring to a boil. Lower the heat and simmer until the pears are tender. Drain and serve with chocolate sauce immediately.

2 teaspoons cornstarch
½ cup cocoa
2 cups cold water
2 teaspoons vanilla extract
Artificial sweetener equivalent to 8 teaspoons of sugar

1. Whisk the cornstarch and cocoa into 2 cups of cold water in a saucepan. Bring to a boil, whisking constantly, and cook over medium-low heat until thickened, about 2 minutes.
2. Remove from the heat and stir in the vanilla extract and sweetener. Store in a screw-top jar in the refrigerator up to six weeks.

Preparation time: 5 minutes
Cooking time: 2 minutes

Exchanges: free
Carbohydrate choices: 0

Yield: 2¼ cups
Serving size: 3 tablespoons

Nutrition per serving:
Calories: 16
Carbohydrate:. . . . . 2 g
Protein: . . . . 1 g
Fat:. . . . . 1 g

Saturated fat: . . . . trace
Cholesterol:. . . . . 0 mg
Dietary fiber: . . . . 2 g
Sodium:. . . . . trace

Mocha sauce

Substitute 2 cups strong coffee for the water in the above recipe.

VARIATION

331

Lemon pudding sauce

4 teaspoons cornstarch
1 cup water
¼ cup freshly squeezed lemon juice
Grated zest of 1 lemon
1 egg
2 teaspoons margarine
Artificial sweetener equivalent to 8 teaspoons of sugar

For a fabulous dessert, drizzle this sauce over Nova Scotia Ginger-bread (recipe, p. 315).

1. Combine the cornstarch, water, lemon juice, and zest in a small, heavy, nonreactive saucepan and whisk until the cornstarch is dissolved. Beat in the egg.
2. Cook over medium heat, stirring constantly, until thickened and clear. Stir in the margarine and sweetener.

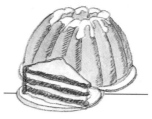

Preparation time: 5 minutes
Cooking time: 10 minutes

Yield: 1½ cups
Serving size: 2 tablespoons

Exchanges: free
Carbohydrate choices: 0

Nutrition per serving:
Calories: 8
Carbohydrate: . . . . 1 g
Protein: . . . . trace
Fat: . . . . trace

Saturated fat: . . . . trace
Cholesterol: . . . . trace
Dietary fiber: . . . . 0 g
Sodium: . . . . trace

Crunchy topping

A sprinkle of this toasty topping enhances simple puddings, baked custards, pies, and fruit cups.

¼ **cup margarine**
1½ **cups quick-cooking (not instant) rolled oats**
¼ **cup lightly packed brown sugar**
¼ **cup chopped nuts**
½ **teaspoon ground cinnamon**

1. Melt the margarine in a large skillet. Add the oats, sugar, nuts, and cinnamon, and cook, stirring, over medium heat until golden brown, about 3 minutes.
2. Remove from heat; spread on a large plate or baking sheet to cool. Store in an airtight container in the refrigerator up to 2 months.

Preparation time: 5 minutes
Cooking time: 5 minutes

Yield: 2 cups
Serving size: 1 tablespoon

Exchanges: ½ fat
Carbohydrate choices: 0

Nutrition per serving:
Calories: 39
Carbohydrate: . . . . 3 g
Protein: . . . . 1 g
Fat: . . . . 2 g

Saturated fat: . . . . trace
Cholesterol: . . . . 0 mg
Dietary fiber: . . . . <1 g
Sodium: . . . . 13 mg

Chapter 14

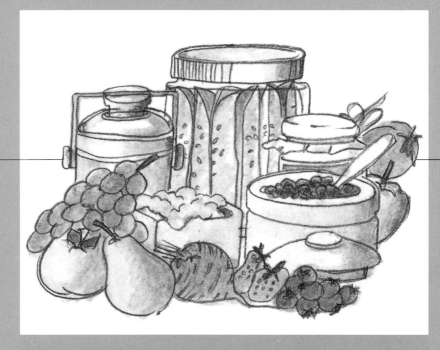

PRESERVES AND PICKLES

If you have ever tasted homemade jellies or preserves, you know they are worth the effort. The sweetness and intense flavors of these spreads and chutneys will amaze you. You will want to use them to spice up all of your foods—and you should. Our Spicy Pear Spread or Pear and Melon Chutney makes a great dipping sauce for pork or lamb. Serve the Spicy Apple Chutney with your next pot roast. And pickles, such as our Peppy Dill Wedges and Bread and Butter Pickles, go with almost any meal.

The recipes here may take a little time, but they are easy to prepare. If you're serving these spreads immediately, simply follow the recipe directions. The spreads, jellies, and chutneys here will stay fresh in the refrigerator for up to one month, and in the freezer for up to three months. If, however, you would like to store these for longer periods, turn to Tips on Preparation (page 350) for an explanation of what you need to do: Most of the recipes only require the use of hot, sterilized jars and a short time in a boiling water bath.

Spicy pear spread

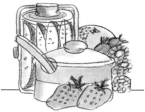

1 teaspoon unflavored gelatin
2 tablespoons water
2 cups peeled, cored, chopped pears (about 4 pears)
1 tablespoon freshly squeezed lemon juice
8 whole cloves
2 one-inch pieces of cinnamon stick
Artificial sweetener to taste

Not only is this great as a spread with toast or bagels, but try spreading a tablespoon or two on top of pork chops before broiling or baking them. You will love the flavor.

1. Sprinkle the gelatin over 2 tablespoons of water in a small bowl and let stand 5 minutes to soften.
2. In a medium saucepan, combine the pears, lemon juice, cloves, and cinnamon. Bring to a boil, reduce heat, and simmer, stirring frequently, about 10 minutes. (Or MICROWAVE on High, covered, about 10 minutes.)
3. Stir the gelatin mixture into the cooked pears until the gelatin dissolves. Discard the cloves and cinnamon. Add sweetener to taste.
4. Ladle into hot, sterilized jars, leaving ½ inch of headroom. Store, well sealed, in the refrigerator or freezer.

335

Preparation time: 15 minutes
Cooking time: 10 minutes

Exchanges: ½ fruit
Carbohydrate choices: 0

Yield: 1¾ cups
Serving size: 2 tablespoons

Nutrition per serving:
Calories: 23
Carbohydrate: . . . . 5 g
Protein: . . . . trace
Fat: . . . . 0 g

Saturated fat: . . . . 0 g
Cholesterol: . . . . 0 mg
Dietary fiber: . . . . 1 g
Sodium: . . . . trace

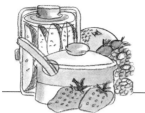

Strawberry or raspberry spread

Using the microwave in this recipe isn't quicker, but it is cooler, cleaner (no pots to scrub), healthier (retains more vitamins), and safer (won't scorch). Cooking fruit is something the microwave does very well.

336

1½ teaspoons unflavored gelatin
4 tablespoons water
2 cups sliced fresh or frozen
**   unsweetened strawberries or raspberries**
Artificial sweetener equivalent
**   to 8–12 teaspoons of sugar**
Red food coloring (optional)

1. Sprinkle the gelatin over 2 tablespoons of the water in a small bowl and let stand 5 minutes to soften.
2. In a medium saucepan, place the berries and the remaining 2 tablespoons of water. Bring to a boil and cook, stirring occasionally, for 5–10 minutes. (Or MICROWAVE on High, covered, for 10 minutes.)
3. Add the softened gelatin, sweetener, and food coloring (optional) and stir until the gelatin dissolves. Skim any foam from the surface.
4. Ladle into hot, sterilized jars, leaving ½ inch of headroom. Store, well sealed, in the refrigerator or freezer.

Preparation time: 10 minutes
Cooking time: 15 minutes

Exchanges: free
Carbohydrate choices: 0

Yield: 1¾ cups
Serving size: 2 tablespoons

Nutrition per serving:
Calories: 7
Carbohydrate:. . . . . 1 g
Protein: . . . . trace
Fat:. . . . . 0 g

Saturated fat: . . . . 0 g
Cholesterol:. . . . . 0 mg
Dietary fiber: . . . . 0 g
Sodium:. . . . . trace

Pear-plum spread

4 medium pears, peeled, cored, and coarsely chopped
2 teaspoons freshly squeezed lemon juice
5 red plums, halved and pitted
1 one-inch piece fresh ginger root, peeled and finely chopped
1 two-inch piece of cinnamon stick
Artificial sweetener equivalent to 9 teaspoons of sugar
½ cup water

1. In a medium saucepan, combine all of the ingredients except the artificial sweetener. Add ½ cup water, bring to a boil, lower the heat, and simmer until the fruit is very tender, 15–20 minutes. (Or MICROWAVE on High, covered, about 10–15 minutes.)
2. Remove the cinnamon stick. Puree the fruit in a food mill or food processor or press through a sieve. Return the fruit puree to the saucepan and simmer an additional 15–20 minutes until thick. (Or MICROWAVE on High, uncovered, about 10 minutes.)
3. Remove from heat and stir in the sweetener. Ladle into hot, sterilized jars, leaving ½ inch of headroom. Store, well sealed, in the refrigerator or freezer.

Sweet pears and tart plums make an excellent combination. Try this as a filling in Thumbprint Cookies (recipe, p. 294).

337

Preparation time: 10 minutes
Cooking time: 40 minutes

Exchanges: free
Carbohydrate choices: 0

Yield: 3¼ cups
Serving size: 1 tablespoon

Nutrition per serving:
Calories: 11
Carbohydrate:. . . . . 3 g
Protein: . . . . trace
Fat:. . . . . 0 g
Saturated fat: . . . . 0 g
Cholesterol:. . . . . 0 mg
Dietary fiber: . . . . <1 g
Sodium:. . . . . trace

Cranberry-orange relish

Serve this at your next Thanksgiving dinner and watch as eyes light up. You can also warm this on the stove before serving for about 5–10 minutes over low heat.

4 cups fresh cranberries, rinsed and picked over

1 medium orange, washed, cut into chunks, seeds removed

2 tablespoons chopped candied ginger

½ teaspoon ground cinnamon

Artificial sweetener equivalent to 12 teaspoons of sugar

Place all of the ingredients in a food processor or blender and pulse on-off until thoroughly combined and chopped to the desired consistency. Store, covered, in the refrigerator.

Preparation time: 10 minutes

Yield: 1½ cups
Serving size: 2 tablespoons

Exchanges: ½ fruit
Carbohydrate choices: 0

338

Nutrition per serving:
Calories: 22
Carbohydrate:. . . . . 5 g
Protein: . . . . trace
Fat:. . . . . 0 g

Saturated fat: . . . . 0 g
Cholesterol:. . . . . 0 mg
Dietary fiber: . . . . 2 g
Sodium:. . . . . trace

Grape spread

Virtually any kind of grape can be used in this recipe, but all will yield different flavors. Using red grapes will result in a mild taste, while green grapes will yield a lightly tart flavor. If you want a very "grape" flavor, though, stick with purple grapes.

6 cups purple grapes

4 firm, ripe apples, quartered, but not peeled or cored

Pinch ground cinnamon

Pinch ground cloves

1. Combine the grapes and apples in a saucepan and simmer 30 minutes. Puree the fruit by pressing through a sieve or food mill. Discard the skins and pits.
2. Return the puree to the saucepan, add the spices, and simmer an additional 20 minutes until thick.
3. Ladle into hot, sterilized jars, leaving ½ inch of headroom. Store, well sealed, in the refrigerator or freezer.

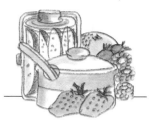

Preparation time: 10 minutes
Cooking time: 50 minutes

Exchanges: free
Carbohydrate choices: 0

Yield: 4 cups
Serving size: 1 tablespoon

Nutrition per serving:

Calories: 15	Saturated fat: . . . . 0 g
Carbohydrate:. . . . . 4 g	Cholesterol:. . . . . 0 mg
Protein: . . . . trace	Dietary fiber: . . . . 0 g
Fat:. . . . . 0 g	Sodium:. . . . . trace

Spicy pickled beets

2 cups sliced cooked small beets

½ cup white vinegar

½ cup water

1 tablespoon brown sugar

2 teaspoons whole cloves

½ teaspoon cinnamon

¼ teaspoon salt

1. Place the beets in a sterilized canning jar.
2. In a nonreactive saucepan, combine the vinegar, water, brown sugar, cloves, cinnamon, and salt. Bring to a boil, stir to dissolve the sugar, and pour over the sliced beets.
3. Cover the jar tightly and refrigerate 8 hours or longer before serving. Can be stored in the refrigerator up to 2 months.

Be sure to use freshly cooked beets for this recipe. Because of additives and preservatives, canned beets may not soak up the flavors of the spices.

339

Preparation time: 5 minutes
Cooking time: 5 minutes
Chilling time: 8 hours

Exchanges: free
Carbohydrate choices: 0

Yield: 2 cups
Serving size: 3 slices

Nutrition per serving:

Calories: 8	Saturated fat: . . . . 0 g
Carbohydrate:. . . . . 2 g	Cholesterol:. . . . . 0 mg
Protein: . . . . trace	Dietary fiber: . . . . 0 g
Fat:. . . . . 0 g	Sodium:. . . . . 35 mg

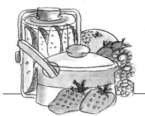

This homemade relish will be a big hit at your next backyard cookout.

Hamburger relish

4 cups finely chopped, unpeeled pickling cucumbers
3 cups finely chopped onion
3 cups finely chopped celery
2 cups finely chopped green bell pepper
1 cup finely chopped red bell pepper
¼ cup pickling salt
4 cups white vinegar
1 tablespoon celery seed
1 tablespoon mustard seed
Liquid artificial sweetener equivalent
  to 1¼ cups of sugar
A few drops green food coloring (optional)

1. In a large, nonreactive bowl, combine the cucumbers, onion, celery, green and red bell peppers, and pickling salt; cover and let stand at room temperature overnight.
2. The next day, mix the vinegar, celery seed, and mustard seed in a large, nonreactive saucepan. Drain the vegetables well and add them to the saucepan.
3. Bring the contents of the saucepan to a boil, reduce the heat, and cook 10 minutes. Add the sweetener and food coloring (optional) and stir well. Ladle into hot, sterilized jars, leaving ½ inch of headroom. Seal.
Store in a cool, dark place.

Preparation time: 20 minutes
Standing time: overnight
Cooking time: 15 minutes

Exchanges: free
Carbohydrate choices: 0

Yield: 7 cups
Serving size: 2 tablespoons

Nutrition per serving:
Calories: 6
Carbohydrate:. . . . . 1 g
Protein: . . . . trace
Fat:. . . . . 0 g

Saturated fat: . . . . 0 g
Cholesterol:. . . . . 0 mg
Dietary fiber: . . . . 0 g
Sodium:. . . . . 44 mg

Pickled onion rings

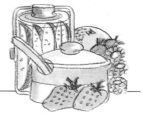

1 large Spanish onion, peeled and
   thinly sliced into rings
Boiling water
1 cup white vinegar
1 cup water
⅓ cup sugar
½ teaspoon salt
4 drops hot pepper sauce

*Some of the sugar
will be absorbed by
the onions rings as they
sit in the pickling juice,
so always drain them
well before serving.*

1. Separate the onion into rings and place them into two
1-pint sterilized canning jars. Pour boiling water over the
onions to cover. Allow the water to cool to room temperature, then drain well.

2. In a nonreactive saucepan, combine the vinegar, water,
sugar, salt, and hot pepper sauce. Bring to a boil, stir to
dissolve the sugar, and pour over the onion rings. Cover
tightly and refrigerate for 2 days. Store in the refrigerator
up to 2 months.

341

Preparation time: 25 minutes
Cooking time: 5 minutes
Chilling time: 2 days

Exchanges: free
Carbohydrate choices: 0

Yield: 4 cups
Serving size: 2–3 onion rings

Nutrition per serving:
Calories: 7
Carbohydrate: . . . . 2 g
Protein: . . . . trace
Fat: . . . . 0 g

Saturated fat: . . . . 0 g
Cholesterol: . . . . 0 mg
Dietary fiber: . . . . 0 g
Sodium: . . . . 54 mg

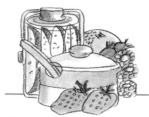

Peppy dill wedges

The longer you allow these cucumber wedges to sit in the garlic and pickling salt, the more flavorful they will be.

4 cups cucumber wedges (about 1 large or 2 medium cucumbers, scrubbed, quartered, and cut into 1-inch pieces)
2 cloves garlic (optional)
2 tablespoons pickling salt
Ice cubes
1 cup cider vinegar
1 cup water
1 tablespoon dill seed
½ teaspoon crushed red pepper

1. Combine the cucumber wedges and garlic (optional) with the pickling salt in a glass bowl. Cover with 2–3 inches of ice cubes. Let stand in a cool place at least 6 hours or overnight. Drain well.

2. In a nonreactive saucepan, combine the vinegar, water, dill seed, and red pepper. Bring to a boil. Add the drained cucumbers and return to a boil. Cover and cook 2 minutes.

3. Spoon into hot, sterilized canning jars. Seal well and store in a cool, dark, dry place.

342

Preparation time: 10 minutes
Chilling time: at least 6 hours
Cooking time: 5 minutes

Exchanges: free
Carbohydrate choices: 0

Yield: 4 cups
Serving size: ¼ cup

Nutrition per serving:
Calories: 11
Carbohydrate:. . . . . 2 g
Protein: . . . . trace
Fat:. . . . . 0 g

Saturated fat: . . . . 0 g
Cholesterol:. . . . . 0 mg
Dietary fiber: . . . . <1 g
Sodium:. . . . . 268 mg

Bread and butter pickles

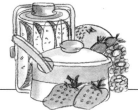

4 cups sliced pickling ("salad" or Kirby) cucumbers
  (sliced ⅛-inch thick)
1 cup thinly sliced onion
1 clove garlic, peeled and crushed
2 tablespoons pickling salt
Ice cubes
1 cup cider vinegar
1 cup water
½ tablespoon mustard seed
1 teaspoon celery seed
½ teaspoon turmeric
Liquid artificial sweetener equivalent to 16 teaspoons
  of sugar

These sweet pickles are perfect for sandwiches, hamburgers, and snacking.

1. In a large, nonreactive bowl, combine the cucumber, onion, garlic, and pickling salt. Cover with 2–3 inches ice cubes. Let stand in a cool place at least 6 hours or overnight. Drain well.
2. In a large, nonreactive saucepan, combine the vinegar, water, mustard seed, celery seed, and turmeric. Bring to a boil, add the drained cucumber mixture, return to a boil, and cook 2 minutes. Discard the garlic, if desired.
3. Stir in the sweetener. Spoon into hot, sterilized jars. Seal well, and store in a cool, dark, dry place.

343

Preparation time: 15 minutes
Chilling time: at least 6 hours
Cooking time: 5 minutes

Exchanges: free
Carbohydrate choices: 0

Yield: 4 cups
Serving size: ½ cup

Nutrition per serving:
Calories: 14
Carbohydrate:. . . . . 3 g
Protein: . . . . trace
Fat:. . . . . 0 g

Saturated fat: . . . . 0 g
Cholesterol:. . . . . 0 mg
Dietary fiber: . . . . 1 g
Sodium:. . . . . 135 mg

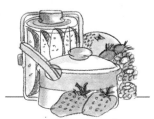

Peach spread

You can sweeten this spread with artificial sweetener to taste, if you wish; but if you are using sweet, ripe peaches in season, you really won't need to.

2 pounds fresh peaches (about 8 medium peaches)
7 allspice berries
2 cups water
1 tablespoon freshly squeezed lemon juice

1. Peel and pit the peaches, and place the pits and peels in a medium saucepan with the allspice berries and 2 cups of water. Cut up the peeled peaches and toss them in a bowl with the lemon juice; set aside.
2. Bring the contents of the saucepan to a boil, lower the heat to medium, and cook until the liquid is reduced to about ½ cup, about 25 minutes. Strain the liquid and discard the solids.
3. In a clean, nonreactive saucepan, combine the sliced peaches and strained liquid and cook over medium heat, stirring occasionally, for 35 minutes. Remove from heat, mash well or puree, if desired.
4. Ladle into a hot, sterilized jar, leaving ½ inch of headroom. Store, well sealed, in the refrigerator or freezer.

344

Preparation time: 10 minutes
Cooking time: 1 hour

Exchanges: free
Carbohydrate choices: 0

Yield: 1⅔ cups
Serving size: 1 tablespoon

Nutrition per serving:
Calories: 14
Carbohydrate:. . . . . 3 g
Protein: . . . . trace
Fat:. . . . . 0 g

Saturated fat: . . . . 0 g
Cholesterol:. . . . . 0 mg
Dietary fiber: . . . . <1 g
Sodium:. . . . . 0 mg

White grape jelly

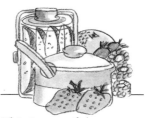

1 teaspoon unflavored gelatin
1⅔ cups unsweetened white grape juice
2 teaspoons freshly squeezed lemon juice
3 whole cloves or allspice berries
Artificial sweetener equivalent to 2 teaspoons of sugar

This is one of the simplest jellies to make. The addition of white grape juice makes it especially tasty.

1. Sprinkle the gelatin over ¼ cup of the grape juice in a small bowl and let stand 5 minutes to soften.
2. In a saucepan, combine the remaining grape juice, the lemon juice, and cloves (or allspice berries) in a saucepan. Bring to a boil, lower the heat to medium, and cook, uncovered, until reduced by one-third in volume, about 7–10 minutes.
3. Remove the saucepan from the heat, add the softened gelatin and sweetener, and stir until dissolved. Discard the cloves (or allspice berries) if desired. Pour into a hot, sterilized jar, leaving ½ inch of headroom. Seal tightly. Store in the refrigerator.

345

Preparation time: 10 minutes
Cooking time: 15 minutes

Exchanges: free
Carbohydrate choices: 0

Yield: 1 cup
Serving size: 1 tablespoon

Nutrition per serving:
Calories: 17
Carbohydrate:. . . . . 4 g
Protein: . . . . trace
Fat:. . . . . 0 g

Saturated fat: . . . . 0 g
Cholesterol:. . . . . 0 mg
Dietary fiber: . . . . 0 g
Sodium:. . . . . trace

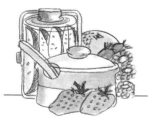

Cinnamon apple jelly

Leaving the cinnamon stick in the jar will allow its spicy flavors to become more intense over time.

1 teaspoon unflavored gelatin
1⅔ cups unsweetened apple juice
2 teaspoons fresh lemon juice
1 one-inch piece of cinnamon stick
1 drop each of yellow and red food coloring (optional)
Artificial sweetener equivalent to 4 teaspoons of sugar

1. Sprinkle the gelatin over ¼ cup of the apple juice in a small bowl and let stand 5 minutes to soften.

2. In a saucepan, combine the remaining apple juice, the lemon juice, cinnamon, and food coloring (optional). Bring to a boil, lower the heat to medium, and cook, uncovered, until reduced by one-third in volume, about 7–10 minutes.

3. Remove the saucepan from the heat, add the softened gelatin and sweetener, and stir until dissolved. Discard the cinnamon stick, if desired. Pour into a hot, sterilized jar, leaving ½ inch of headroom. Seal tightly. Store in the refrigerator.

346

Preparation time: 10 minutes
Cooking time: 15 minutes

Yield: 1 cup
Serving size: 1 tablespoon

Exchanges: free
Carbohydrate choices: 0

Nutrition per serving:
Calories: 13
Carbohydrate:. . . . . 3 g
Protein: . . . . trace
Fat:. . . . . 0 g
Saturated fat: . . . . 0 g
Cholesterol:. . . . . 0 mg
Dietary fiber:. 0g
Sodium: . . . . trace

Minted apple butter

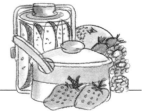

4 tart cooking apples, such as Granny Smith,
  peeled and coarsely chopped
¼ cup chopped fresh mint
1 teaspoon freshly squeezed lemon juice
½ cup water

1. Combine all of the ingredients in a medium nonreactive saucepan. Bring to a boil, reduce the heat, and simmer about 20 minutes, stirring and mashing occasionally, until the apples are tender. (Or MICROWAVE on High, covered, about 15 minutes.)
2. Press the fruit through a sieve or a food mill; discard the skins and seeds. Return the puree to the saucepan and cook over low heat, uncovered, until thick, about 10 more minutes. (Or MICROWAVE on High, uncovered, about 5 minutes.)
3. Ladle into hot, sterilized jars, leaving ½ inch of headroom. Store, well sealed, in the refrigerator or freezer.

Mint gives this traditional apple butter recipe an extra little kick. Serve it with roast lamb for dinner, or with pancakes at brunch.

347

Preparation time: 10 minutes
Cooking time: 30 minutes

Exchanges: free
Carbohydrate choices: 0

Yield: 1⅔ cups
Serving size: 1 tablespoon

Nutrition per serving:
Calories: 15
Carbohydrate:. . . . . 4 g
Protein: . . . . 0 g
Fat:. . . . . 0 g
Saturated fat: . . . . 0 g
Cholesterol:. . . . . 0 mg
Dietary fiber: . . . . <1 g
Sodium: . . . . trace

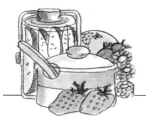

Spicy apple chutney

348

4 large apples
1 cup water
Juice and zest from 1 lemon
½ cup diced red bell pepper
½ cup raisins
½ cup chopped onion
2 teaspoons ground ginger (or more to taste)
2 tablespoons molasses

1. Peel and core apples; place the peels and cores in a saucepan with 1 cup water. Chop the apples and toss with 1–2 teaspoons of lemon juice in a nonreactive saucepan; set aside.

2. Bring the saucepan containing the apple peels to a boil. Lower the heat, cover, and cook 10–15 minutes. Strain this liquid over the chopped apples and discard the strained solids. Add the remaining lemon juice, lemon zest, red pepper, raisins, onion, ginger, and molasses to the apples and mix well.

3. Cook the chutney mixture over medium heat, stirring occasionally, until thickened, about 35 minutes. (Or MICROWAVE on High, covered, about 15 minutes.)

4. Ladle into hot, sterilized jars, leaving ½ inch of head-room. Store, well sealed, in the refrigerator or freezer.

Preparation time: 10 minutes
Cooking time: 50 minutes

Exchanges: free
Carbohydrate choices: 0

Yield: 3⅓ cups
Serving size: 1 tablespoon

Nutrition per serving:
Calories: 10
Carbohydrate: . . . . 2 g
Protein: . . . . trace
Fat: . . . . 0 g

Saturated fat: . . . . 0 g
Cholesterol: . . . . 0 mg
Dietary fiber: . . . . 0 g
Sodium: . . . . trace

Pear and melon chutney

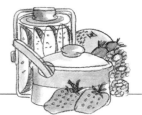

Cantaloupe or honeydew work equally well in this mild but flavorful chutney.

2 cups cider vinegar
1 tablespoon whole cloves
2 teaspoons ground ginger
2 teaspoons ground allspice
1 teaspoon ground nutmeg
5 cups chopped onion
1 cup golden raisins
1 cup currants
¼ cup thinly sliced crystallized ginger
6 cloves garlic, minced
10 medium pears, peeled, cored, and chopped
4 cups chopped cantaloupe
¼ cup molasses

1. In a large, nonreactive saucepan, combine the vinegar, cloves, ground ginger, allspice, and nutmeg. Bring to a boil, reduce the heat, cover, and simmer 30 minutes.
2. Add the onion, raisins, currants, crystallized ginger, and garlic to the vinegar mixture. Cover and cook 15 minutes. Add the pears and cantaloupe and cook, uncovered, about 30 minutes more, stirring often to prevent sticking, until the moisture is thick. Stir in the molasses and remove from the heat.
3. Ladle into hot, sterilized jars, leaving ½ inch of headroom. Store, well sealed, in the refrigerator or freezer.

349

Preparation time: 15 minutes
Cooking time: 1¼ hours

Exchanges: free
Carbohydrate choices: 0

Yield: 8 cups
Serving size: 1 tablespoon

Nutrition per serving:
Calories: 12
Carbohydrate:. . . . . 3 g
Protein: . . . . trace
Fat:. . . . . 0 g

Saturated fat: . . . . 0 g
Cholesterol:. . . . . 0 mg
Dietary fiber: . . . . 0 g
Sodium:. . . . . trace

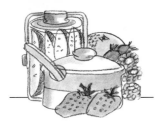

Tips on preparation

Whatever you decide to preserve, always follow the recipe carefully and strictly control both the quality of the ingredients you use and the cleanliness of the area where you prepare your preserves.

STERILIZING.
Always use jars specifically designed for canning (with metal lids and tops that screw down over the lids). Wash them in hot, soapy water and rinse well. Then put the jars, lids, and tops in a very large pot, cover them with water, and boil for about 5 minutes. Use tongs to transfer the jars, lids, and tops to a tray lined with paper towels. Place the tray in a preheated oven (200°F) for 5 minutes to ensure the jars, lids, and tops are dry. Preserves placed in jars prepared in this manner will stay fresh in the refrigerator up to one month, or in the freezer up to three months. Make sure you leave ½ inch of headroom (at most) in the jar, wipe the rims carefully, seal each one, and then turn the jars upside down to ensure that the seal is good. If you plan to keep preserves for a longer period, process them by the boiling water method.

THE BOILING WATER METHOD.
Place your preserves in sterilized jars as described above. Then place the jars in a large pot with a rack in the bottom so that the jars don't touch each other or the sides of the pot. Cover the jars and boil for 10 minutes. Cool the jars overnight at room temperature. The next day, unscrew the tops, leaving only the lids in place, and turn the jars upside down; if the jars are tightly sealed, the lids will stay in place. Replace the screw tops and store the jars in a cool, dark place.

Chapter 15

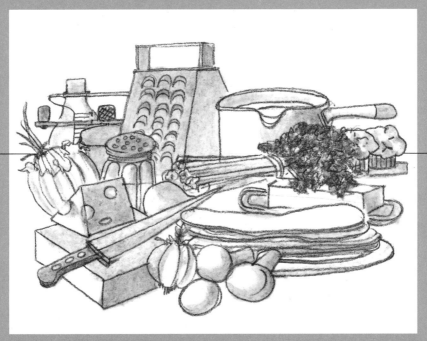

SAUCES AND BASICS

*W*hat are the "basics" in this chapter? Basics are simple-to-make items that can be prepared ahead to save time in the kitchen. In most cases, these items are used in other recipes in the book, but you can also use these basics on their own or in other recipes. Don't be afraid to experiment with these.

The savory sauces in this section—all of which can be made ahead and stored for later use—are lighter than typical sauces. They have been trimmed of fat and starch, yet they are still rich in taste. Use these with your favorite meats or pastas. Simply reheat them in a saucepan over low heat until thoroughly warmed. Many of them can also be both cooked and reheated in your microwave.

Spend a little extra time on the weekend preparing a few of these basics—your meal planning and cooking time will be greatly reduced.

Mushroom sauce

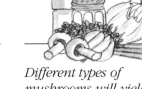

Different types of mushrooms will yield slightly different flavors in this sauce. This works equally well over pasta or a baked potato.

1 tablespoon olive oil
2 cloves garlic, minced
¼ cup chopped onion (optional)
1 cup chopped fresh mushrooms
½ cup beef or chicken broth
¼ cup skim milk
1 tablespoon cornstarch
  (dissolved in 2 tablespoons of water)
Salt and pepper (optional)

1. In a medium sauté pan, heat the oil, add the garlic and onion (optional), and cook, stirring, over medium heat until wilted.
2. Add the mushrooms and cook, stirring, until they give off their juices, about 5 minutes.
3. Add the broth, milk, and cornstarch, and cook, stirring, until the sauce has thickened, about 5 minutes. (Or MICROWAVE on High, in a microwave-safe dish, uncovered, about 3–5 minutes.) Season to taste.

NOTE: To vary the quantity of this versatile sauce, increase or decrease the quantity of the ingredients proportionately. For instance, to double the amount of sauce, just double the amount of everything that goes into it.

353

Preparation time: 10 minutes
Cooking time: 15 minutes

Yield: 1 cup
Serving size: ¼ cup

Exchanges: ½ carbohydrate
   ½ fat
Carbohydrate choices: ½

Nutrition per serving:
Calories: 64
Carbohydrate: . . . . .6 g
Protein: . . . . .1 g
Fat: . . . . .4 g

Saturated fat: . . . . .1 g
Cholesterol: . . . . .trace
Dietary fiber: . . . .<1 g
Sodium: . . . . .23 mg

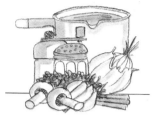

Basic White Sauce can altered in any number of ways to make a creamy sauce for pasta, vegetables, fish, or potatoes. Stir in ¼ cup Parmesan cheese for a tangy Alfredo sauce. Or try any of the varieties below.

Basic white sauce

1 cup skim milk
1 tablespoon cornstarch
½ teaspoon salt (optional)
¼ teaspoon white pepper (optional)

Combine the milk and cornstarch in a saucepan and whisk until smooth. Bring to a boil, lower the heat, and, stirring continuously, cook until thickened, about 3–5 minutes. (Or MICROWAVE on High, covered, about 5 minutes, stirring well halfway through.) Season to taste.

Preparation time: 5 minutes
Cooking time: 5–10 minutes

Exchanges: ½ carbohydrate
Carbohydrate choices: ½

Yield: 1 cup
Serving size: ¼ cup

Nutrition per serving:
Calories: 29
Carbohydrate: . . . . .5 g
Protein: . . . . .2 g
Fat: . . . . .trace

Saturated fat: . . . . .trace
Cholesterol: . . . . .trace
Dietary fiber: . . . . .0 g
Sodium: . . . . .298 mg
(omitting salt) . . . . . . .31 mg

Béchamel sauce

VARIATION

Sauté 1 tablespoon minced onion in 1 teaspoon oil until soft. Stir into thickened Basic White Sauce.

Herb sauce

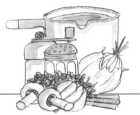

Add ½ teaspoon each of dried thyme, sweet basil, and oregano, plus 1 teaspoon minced fresh parsley to thickened Basic White Sauce.

VARIATION

Tarragon sauce

Rehydrate 1 teaspoon dried tarragon in 1–2 tablespoons of hot water for 10–15 minutes. Drain off water and add tarragon to thickened Basic White Sauce.

VARIATION

355

Cheese sauce

Stir ½ cup shredded low-fat Cheddar cheese into thickened Basic White Sauce.

VARIATION

Yield: 1 cup
Serving size: ¼ cup

Exchanges: ½ carbohydrate
1 lean meat
Carbohydrate choices: ½

Nutrition per serving:
Calories: 96
Carbohydrate: . . . . .5 g
Protein: . . . . .8 g
Fat: . . . . .4 g

Saturated fat: . . . . .2 g
Cholesterol: . . . . .16 mg
Dietary fiber: . . . . .0 g
Sodium: . . . . .448 mg
(omitting salt) . . . . . . .181 mg

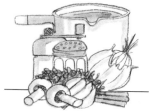

Speedy barbecue sauce

Take boneless, skinless chicken breasts that have been cut into 1-inch strips and toss them with this sauce for low-fat Buffalo wings. A few drops of hot pepper sauce can turn this mild sauce a little hotter.

½ cup ketchup
¼ cup red wine vinegar or cider vinegar
1 tablespoon molasses
1 teaspoon celery seed
½ teaspoon onion powder
½ teaspoon garlic powder
½ teaspoon chili powder

Combine all ingredients in a screw-top jar. Seal and shake well until mixed. Store in the refrigerator.

356

Preparation time: 5 minutes
Yield: ¾ cup
Serving size: 1 tablespoon

Exchanges: free
Carbohydrate choices: 0

Nutrition per serving:
Calories: 14
Carbohydrate: . . . . .3 g
Protein: . . . . .trace
Fat: . . . . .trace

Saturated fat: . . . . .trace
Cholesterol: . . . . .0 mg
Dietary fiber: . . . . .0 g
Sodium: . . . . .106 mg

Spaghetti sauce

1 teaspoon vegetable oil

2 cloves garlic, minced

1 onion, chopped

1 can (about 28 ounces) Italian plum tomatoes, mashed or pureed

1 cup beef broth (or water)

¼ cup tomato paste

2 tablespoons fresh minced parsley

1 teaspoon salt (optional)

½ teaspoon dried leaf thyme

½ teaspoon dried oregano

½ teaspoon dried basil

¼ teaspoon ground cloves

¼ teaspoon freshly ground black pepper

As every Italian grand-mother knows, the secret to a great spaghetti sauce is allowing it to simmer for a long time on the stove. Crumbled, cooked meat or meat-balls can be simmered along with this sauce if you want a more substantial sauce.

1. In a heavy saucepan, heat the oil over medium-high heat. Add the garlic and onion and sauté until limp, about 3 minutes.
2. Stir in the tomatoes, broth (or water), and tomato paste, and cook, stirring, over medium heat, until bubbling. Add the herbs and seasonings and stir well.
3. Reduce the heat to low and cook, stirring occasionally, about 30 minutes, or to your desired consistency.

357

Preparation time: 10 minutes
Cooking time: 40 minutes

Exchanges: 1 carbohydrate
Carbohydrate choices: 1

Yield: 3 cups
Serving size: ½ cup

Nutrition per serving:

Calories: 68	Saturated fat: . . . . .trace
Carbohydrate: . . . . .12 g	Cholesterol: . . . . .trace
Protein: . . . . .2 g	Dietary fiber: . . . . .3 g
Fat: . . . . .1 g	Sodium: . . . . .809 mg
	(omitting salt) . . . . . . .456 mg

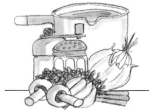

Stroganoff sauce

For a quick Stroganoff, heat cooked beef strips or cooked meatballs in this sauce and serve over hot, cooked Whole Wheat Noodles (recipe, p. 364).

½ cup low-fat cottage cheese
¼ cup low-fat plain yogurt
1 cup (1 batch) Mushroom Sauce (recipe, p. 353)

Puree the cottage cheese and yogurt in a blender or food processor. Stir into the thickened Mushroom Sauce. Heat to simmering (do not boil). Serve immediately.

358

Preparation time: 5 minutes
Cooking time: 5 minutes

Yield: 1½ cups
Serving size: ¼ cup

Nutrition per serving:
Calories: 53
Carbohydrate: . . . . .5 g
Protein: . . . . .3 g
Fat: . . . . .3 g

Exchanges: ½ carbohydrate
½ fat
Carbohydrate choices: ½

Saturated fat: . . . . .1 g
Cholesterol: . . . . .trace
Dietary fiber: . . . .<1 g
Sodium: . . . . .92 mg

Velouté sauce

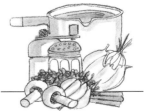

1 cup low-sodium chicken or fish broth
1 tablespoon cornstarch
½ teaspoon salt (optional)
¼ teaspoon white pepper (optional)

Combine the broth and cornstarch in a saucepan and whisk until smooth. Bring to a boil, lower heat, and, stirring continuously, cook until thickened, about 3–5 minutes. (Or MICROWAVE on High, covered, about 5 minutes, stirring well halfway through.) Season to taste.

A velouté sauce is just like a white sauce, except it's made with broth instead of milk. Serve it over chicken when it's made with chicken broth, and fish when made with fish broth.

359

Preparation time: 5 minutes
Cooking time: 5 minutes

Yield: 1 cup
Serving size: ¼ cup

Nutrition per serving:
Calories: 15
Carbohydrate: . . . . .2 g
Protein: . . . . .1 g
Fat: . . . . .trace

Exchanges: free
Carbohydrate choices: 0

Saturated fat: . . . . .trace
Cholesterol: . . . . .trace
Dietary fiber: . . . . .0 g
Sodium: . . . . .294 mg
(omitting salt) . . . . .27 mg

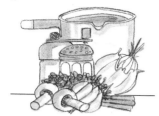

A delicious gravy, and there are only 16 calories per serving.

Fat-free gravy

**1 cup low-sodium beef broth
(and defatted roast beef drippings, if available)**
1 tablespoon cornstarch
1 teaspoon ketchup
Salt and pepper (optional)

Combine the broth, drippings, cornstarch, and ketchup in a saucepan. Whisk until smooth. Bring to a boil over medium heat and cook, stirring, until thickened, about 3 minutes. (Or MICROWAVE on High, covered, about 5 minutes, stirring well halfway through.) Season to taste.

Preparation time: 5 minutes
Cooking time: 5 minutes

Yield: 1 cup
Serving size: ¼ cup

Exchanges: free
Carbohydrate choices: 0

Nutrition per serving:
Calories: 16
Carbohydrate: . . . . .2 g
Protein: . . . . .1 g
Fat: . . . . .trace

Saturated fat: . . . . .trace
Cholesterol: . . . . .trace
Dietary fiber: . . . . .0 g
Sodium: . . . . .41 mg

Celery sauce

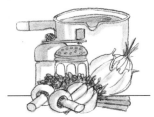

2 cups chopped celery
1 baking potato, peeled and cut into chunks
2 cups low-sodium chicken broth
½ teaspoon salt (optional)
¼ teaspoon dried oregano
¼ teaspoon ground white pepper
⅛ teaspoon ground nutmeg

A potato becomes the thickening agent in this hearty, yet light, sauce.

Combine all of the ingredients in a saucepan and bring to a boil. Reduce the heat and simmer 15–20 minutes, until the potato and celery are soft. Puree in a blender, food processor, or food mill. (For a chunky sauce, remove about ¼ cup cooked celery before pureeing; then add it to the pureed sauce.)

361

Preparation time: 15 minutes
Cooking time: 25 minutes

Exchanges: 1 vegetable
Carbohydrate choices: 0

Yield: 2 cups
Serving size: ⅓ cup

Nutrition per serving:
Calories: 28
Carbohydrate: . . . . .4 g
Protein: . . . . .1 g
Fat: . . . . .1 g

Saturated fat: . . . . .trace
Cholesterol: . . . . .trace
Dietary fiber: . . . . .1 g
Sodium: . . . . .250 mg
(omitting salt) . . . . .72 mg

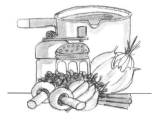

Crepes can be served as either a dinner meal or a dessert, depending on the filling you use. Fill them with cubed, cooked chicken and Mushroom Sauce (recipe, p. 353) for a hearty meal.

362

Crepes

⅔ **cup skim milk**
1 egg
¼ **cup egg whites**
2 teaspoons vegetable oil
½ **cup all-purpose flour**
Pinch salt
Nonfat cooking spray

1. Blend all of the ingredients in a blender or food processor until smooth. Allow to stand about 1 hour.
2. Heat a nonstick crepe pan or a pan that has been coated with nonfat cooking spray over medium-low heat until hot (water dropped on the surface will dance). Add ¼ cup of crepe batter and rotate the pan to distribute the batter evenly.
3. Cook until the underside is lightly colored and the edges crisp, about 45–60 seconds. Flip crepe over and cook the second side until light brown, about 15–30 seconds. Slip cooked crepes onto a clean dish towel.
4. Repeat until all the batter is used. Stack cooked crepes between layers of wax paper. Wrap well and refrigerate up to 2 days or freeze up to 3 months.

Preparation time: 5 minutes
Standing time: 1 hour
Cooking time: 15 minutes

Yield: 8 servings
Serving size: 1 crepe

Exchanges: ½ starch
½ fat
Carbohydrate choices: ½

Nutrition per serving:
Calories: 54
Carbohydrate: . . . . .7 g
Protein: . . . . .3 g
Fat: . . . . .2 g
Saturated fat: . . . . .trace
Cholesterol: . . . . .35 mg
Dietary fiber: . . . . .0 g
Sodium: . . . . .65 mg

Seasoned bread crumbs

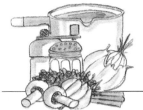

2 cups fine dry crumbs
½ cup minced onion
½ cup minced fresh parsley
1 clove garlic, minced
1 teaspoon dried oregano
⅓ cup freshly grated Parmesan cheese

Mix all of the ingredients thoroughly. Store in an airtight container in the freezer up to 6 months.

These bread crumbs are just the thing for breading fish or chicken. If you don't have dry bread crumbs on hand, use stale bread. Simply crumble the bread and dry it out in a 350°F oven for about 5–10 minutes.

Preparation time: 5 minutes

Yield: 3 cups
Serving size: 3 tablespoons

Exchanges: ½ starch
Carbohydrate choices: ½

Nutrition per serving:
Calories: 47
Carbohydrate: . . . . .7 g
Protein: . . . . .2 g
Fat: . . . . .1 g

Saturated fat: . . . . .trace
Cholesterol: . . . . .trace
Dietary fiber: . . . . .0 g
Sodium: . . . . .101 mg

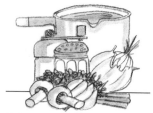

Whole wheat pasta or noodles

When cutting pasta by hand, gently roll the sheet of dough into a cylinder and slice crosswise. This will ensure that your noodles are the same width all the way around.

364

1½ cups whole wheat flour
½ cup all-purpose flour
1 whole egg
2 egg whites
½ teaspoon salt

1. In a large bowl, combine the flours. In a small bowl, whisk together the egg, egg whites, and salt until foamy. Stir egg mixture into flour mixture. Add a few drops of water, if necessary, and mix by hand or machine until the dough forms a ball. Knead until smooth and elastic.
2. Divide the dough into 8 equal portions. Working with 1 portion at a time and keeping the remaining portions well covered to keep from drying out, roll the dough with a rolling pin on a floured work surface or with a pasta machine until very thin, about ⅛ inch thick.
3. Cut the dough to the desired width. Lay the cut pasta on a clean cloth while rolling and cutting the remaining portions of dough. Cook immediately, or freeze, well wrapped, for later use.
4. Cook in a large pot of lightly salted boiling water to desired doneness, 2–4 minutes (depending on dryness of pasta).

Preparation time: 20 minutes
Cooking time: 5 minutes

Exchanges: 1 starch
Carbohydrate choices: 1

Yield: 12 servings
Serving size: ½ cup

Nutrition per serving:
Calories: 76
Carbohydrate: . . . . .14 g
Protein: . . . . .4 g
Fat: . . . . .1 g

Saturated fat: . . . . .trace
Cholesterol: . . . . .23 mg
Dietary fiber: . . . . .2 g
Sodium: . . . . .103 mg

Whole wheat flour tortillas

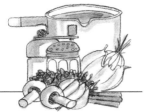

½ cup all-purpose flour
½ cup whole wheat flour
¼ teaspoon salt (optional)
1 tablespoon vegetable oil
6 tablespoons water

1. Combine the flours and salt (optional) in a mixing bowl. Make a well in the center of the flour and add the oil and the water. Mix until a soft dough is formed, adding more water in droplets, if necessary.
2. Divide the dough into 12 equal pieces and form each piece into a small ball with lightly oiled hands. Place balls in a bowl, cover, and let stand about 15–30 minutes.
3. With a rolling pin, roll each ball between layers of wax paper to a 6-inch circle. Cook each round in a preheated frying pan until bubbles form on the top and the underside is flecked with brown. Turn and cook the underside until flecked with brown but still flexible.
4. Stack cooked tortillas, covered with a dry dish towel. Serve immediately or wrap well and refrigerate or freeze. Reheat in a 350°F oven before serving.

How light are these tortillas? They have half the calories of most store-bought brands. It's easiest to make these ahead of time and keep them in the refrigerator for when you need them.

365

Preparation time: 15 minutes
Standing time: 15–30 minutes
Cooking time: 10 minutes

Exchanges: 1 starch
Carbohydrate choices: 1

Yield: 6 servings
Serving size: 2 tortillas

Nutrition per serving:
Calories: 88
Carbohydrate: . . . . .14 g
Protein: . . . . .2 g
Fat: . . . . .3 g

Saturated fat: . . . . .trace
Cholesterol: . . . . .trace
Dietary fiber: . . . . .2 g
Sodium: . . . . .89 mg
(omitting salt) . . . . .7 mg

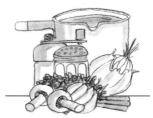

You can season these dumplings with any kind of herb or spice. Try dill or basil when adding these to a chicken soup.

Fluffy dumplings

1 cup all-purpose flour
2 teaspoons baking powder
½ teaspoon salt (optional)
1 tablespoon margarine
⅓ cup skim milk

Combine all of the ingredients in a mixing bowl or food processor and blend well. Divide the dough into 6 portions and drop each onto the surface of a bubbling stew or soup. Cover tightly and simmer 15 minutes without lifting the lid.

366

Preparation time: 5 minutes
Cooking time: 15 minutes

Exchanges: 1 starch
Carbohydrate choices: 1

Yield: 6 servings
Serving size: 1 dumpling

Nutrition per serving:
Calories: 88
Carbohydrate: . . . . .15 g
Protein: . . . . .2 g
Fat: . . . . .2 g

Saturated fat: . . . . .trace
Cholesterol: . . . . .trace
Dietary fiber: . . . .<1 g
Sodium: . . . . .342 mg
(omitting salt) . . . . . . .164 mg

Appendix 1

Using Exchange Lists for Meal Planning

Exchange Lists for Meal Planning is a widely used meal-planning system for people with diabetes and anyone interested in weight loss or healthy diets. Exchange lists help people eat a nutritionally balanced diet from a wide variety of foods without having to count calories.

The exchanges are based on the amount of carbohydrate, protein, fat, and calories in foods. Each exchange, or serving of food, has a similar amount of nutrients as other foods on the same list. Therefore, one food in the serving size listed can be exchanged for any other food in the same list while providing a similar amount of carbohydrate, protein, fat, and calories. Exchange Lists for Meal Planning groups foods into seven lists: starch, fruit, milk, other carbohydrates, vegetable, meat and meat substitutes, and fat. There is also a free food exchange list at the end.

People with diabetes often have a meal plan that outlines the number of exchanges from each food list to eat at meals and snacks. A meal plan must be individualized to take into account factors such as age, weight, medications, activity level, and other lifestyle considerations. A meal plan serves as a guide to what—and when—food should be eaten during the day.

If you don't have an individualized meal plan, it would be a good idea to contact a registered dietitian: your physician or nurse educator can help you find one in your area. A registered dietitian can assess your current eating habits, recommend changes to help you achieve your nutritional goals, and develop a meal plan appropriate for you.

The following Exchange Lists (© 1995 American Diabetes Association, the American Dietetic Association) are reprinted with the permission of the American Diabetes Association and the American Dietetic Association. While designed primarily for people with diabetes and others who must follow special diets, the Exchange Lists are based on principles of good nutrition that apply to everyone.

367

STARCH LIST

Cereals, grains, pasta, breads, crackers, snacks, starchy vegetables, and cooked beans, peas, and lentils are starches. In general, one starch is:

- ½ cup of cereal, grain, pasta, or starchy vegetable
- 1 ounce of a bread product, such as 1 slice of bread
- ¾ to 1 ounce of most snack foods (Some snack foods may also have added fat)

Each item in this list contains approximately 15 grams of carbohydrate, 3 grams of protein, 0–1 grams of fat, and 80 calories.

BREAD

Bagel	½ (1 oz)
Bread, reduced-calorie	2 slices (1 oz)
Bread, white, whole wheat, pumpernickel, rye	1 slice (1 oz)
Bread sticks, crisp, 4 in. long × ½ in.	2 (⅔ oz)
English muffin	½
Hot dog or hamburger bun	½ (1 oz)
Pita, 6 in. across	½
Roll, plain, small	1 (1 oz)
Raisin bread, unfrosted	1 slice (1 oz)
Tortilla, corn, 6 in. across	1
Tortilla, flour, 6 in. across	1
Waffle, 4½ in. square, reduced-fat	1

CEREALS AND GRAINS

Bran cereals	½ cup
Bulgur	½ cup
Cereals	½ cup
Cereals, unsweetened, ready-to-eat	¾ cup
Cornmeal (dry)	3 tbsp
Couscous	⅓ cup
Flour (dry)	3 tbsp
Granola, low-fat	¼ cup
Grape-Nuts	¼ cup
Grits	½ cup
Kasha	½ cup
Millet	¼ cup
Muesli	¼ cup
Oats	½ cup
Pasta	½ cup
Puffed cereal	1½ cups
Rice milk	½ cup
Rice, white or brown	⅓ cup
Shredded Wheat	½ cup
Sugar-frosted cereal	½ cup
Wheat germ	3 tbsp

STARCHY VEGETABLES

Baked beans	⅓ cup
Corn	½ cup
Corn on cob, medium	1 (5 oz)
Mixed vegetables with corn, peas, or pasta	1 cup
Peas, green	½ cup
Plantain	½ cup
Potato, baked or boiled	1 small (3 oz)
Potato, mashed	½ cup
Squash, winter (acorn, butternut, pumpkin)	1 cup
Yam, sweet potato, plain	½ cup

CRACKERS AND SNACKS

Animal crackers	8
Graham crackers, 2½ in. square	3
Matzoh	¾ oz
Melba toast	4 slices
Oyster crackers	24
Popcorn (popped, no fat added or low-fat microwave)	3 cups
Pretzels	¾ oz
Rice cakes, 4 in. across	2
Saltine-type crackers	6
Snack chips, fat-free (tortilla, potato)	15-20 (¾ oz)
Whole wheat crackers, no fat added	2–5 (¾oz)

BEANS, PEAS, AND LENTILS

(Count as 1 starch exchange, plus 1 very lean meat exchange)

Beans and peas (garbanzo, pinto, kidney, white, split, black-eyed)	½ cup
Lima beans	⅔ cup
Lentils	½ cup
Miso	3 tbsp

STARCHY FOODS PREPARED WITH FAT

(Count as 1 starch exchange, plus 1 fat exchange)

Biscuit, 2½ in. across	1
Chow mein noodles	½ cup
Corn bread, 2 in. cube	1 (2 oz)
Crackers, round butter type	6
Croutons	1 cup
French-fried potatoes	16–25 (3 oz)
Granola	¼ cup
Muffin, small	1 (1½ oz)
Pancake, 4 in. across	2
Popcorn, microwave	3 cups
Sandwich crackers, cheese or peanut butter filling	3
Stuffing, bread (prepared)	⅓ cup
Taco shell, 6 in. across	2
Waffle, 4½ in. across	1
Whole wheat crackers, fat added	4–6 (1 oz)

400 mg or more of sodium per exchange

FRUIT LIST

Fresh, frozen, canned, and dried fruits and fruit juices are on this list.
In general, one fruit exchange is:

- 1 small to medium fresh fruit
- ½ cup of canned or fresh fruit or fruit juice
- ¼ cup dried fruit

Each item in this list contains approximately 15 grams of carbohydrate and 60 calories. The weight includes skin, core, seeds, and rind.

FRUIT

Apple, unpeeled, small	1 (4 oz)		Kiwi	1 (3½ oz)
Applesauce, unsweetened	½ cup		Mandarin oranges, canned	¾ cup
Apples, dried	4 rings		Mango, small	½ fruit (5½ oz) or ½ cup
Apricots, fresh	4 whole (5½ oz)		Nectarine, small	1 (5 oz)
Apricots, dried	8 halves		Orange, small	1 (6½ oz)
Apricots, canned	½ cup		Papaya	½ fruit (8 oz) or 1 cup cubes
Banana, small	1 (4 oz)			
Blackberries	¾ cup		Peach, medium, fresh	1 (6 oz)
Blueberries	¾ cup		Peaches, canned	½ cup
Cantaloupe, small	⅓ melon (11 oz) or 1 cup cubes		Pear, large, fresh	½ (4 oz)
			Pears, canned	½ cup
Cherries, sweet, fresh	12 (3 oz)		Pineapple, fresh	¾ cup
Cherries, sweet, canned	½ cup		Pineapple, canned	½ cup
Dates	3		Plums, small	2 (5 oz)
Figs, fresh	1½ large or 2 medium (3½ oz)		Plums, canned	½ cup
			Prunes, dried	3
Figs, dried	1½		Raisins	3 Tbsp
Fruit cocktail	½ cup		Raspberries	1 cup
Grapefruit, large	½ (11 oz)		Strawberries, whole	1½ cup
Grapefruit sections, canned	¾ cup		Tangerines, small	2 (8 oz)
Grapes, small	17 (3 oz)		Watermelon	1 slice (13½ oz) or 1¼ cup cubes
Honeydew melon	1 slice (10 oz) or 1 cup cubes			

FRUIT JUICE

Apple juice/cider	½ cup		Grape juice	⅓ cup
Cranberry juice cocktail	⅓ cup		Grapefruit juice	½ cup
Cranberry juice cocktail, reduced-calorie	1 cup		Orange juice	½ cup
			Pineapple juice	½ cup
Fruit juice blends, 100% juice	⅓ cup		Prune juice	⅓ cup

MILK LIST

Different types of milk and milk products are on this list. Cheeses are on the Meat list and cream and other dairy fats are on the Fat list. Based on the amount of fat they contain, milks are divided into fat-free/low-fat milk, reduced-fat milk, and whole milk. One choice of these includes:

	Carbohydrate (g)	Protein (g)	Fat (g)	Calories
Fat-free/low-fat	12	8	0–3	90
Reduced-fat	12	8	5	120
Whole	12	8	8	150

FAT-FREE AND LOW-FAT MILK
(0–3 grams fat per serving)

Fat-free milk	1 cup
½% milk	1 cup
1% milk	1 cup
Fat-free or low-fat buttermilk	1 cup
Evaporated fat-free milk	½ cup
Fat-free dry milk	⅓ cup dry
Plain nonfat yogurt	¾ cup
Nonfat or low-fat fruit-flavored yogurt sweetened with aspartame or with a nonnutritive sweetener	1 cup

REDUCED-FAT MILK
(5 grams fat per serving)

2% milk	1 cup
Plain low-fat yogurt	¾ cup
Sweet acidophilus milk	1 cup

WHOLE MILK
(8 grams fat per serving)

Whole milk	1 cup
Evaporated whole milk	½ cup
Goat's milk	1 cup
Kefir	1 cup

OTHER CARBOHYDRATES LIST

You can substitute food choices from this list for a starch, fruit, or milk choice on your meal plan. Some choices will also count as one or more fat choices.

One carbohydrate exchange contains approximately 15 grams of carbohydrate, or 1 starch, or 1 fruit, or 1 milk.

FOOD	SERVING SIZE	EXCHANGES PER SERVING
Angel food cake, unfrosted	1/12 cake	2 carbohydrate
Brownie, small, unfrosted	2 in. square	1 carbohydrate, 1 fat
Cake, unfrosted	2 in. square	1 carbohydrate, 1 fat
Cake, frosted	2 in. square	2 carbohydrate, 1 fat
Cookie, fat-free	2 small	1 carbohydrate
Cookie or sandwich cookie with creme filling	2 small	1 carbohydrate, 1 fat
Cranberry sauce, jellied	1/4 cup	1½ carbohydrate
Cupcake, frosted	1 small	2 carbohydrate, 1 fat
Doughnut, plain cake	1 medium (1½ oz)	1½ carbohydrate, 2 fat
Doughnut, glazed	3 ¾ in. across (2 oz)	2 carbohydrate, 2 fat
Fruit juice bars, frozen, 100% juice	1 bar (3 oz)	1 carbohydrate
Fruit snacks, chewy (pureed fruit concentrate)	1 roll (¾ oz)	1 carbohydrate
Fruit spreads, 100% fruit	1 tbsp	1 carbohydrate
Gelatin, regular	½ cup	1 carbohydrate
Gingersnaps	3	1 carbohydrate
Granola bar	1 bar	1 carbohydrate, 1 fat
Granola bar, fat-free	1 bar	2 carbohydrate
Honey	1 tbsp	1 carbohydrate
Hummus	1/3 cup	1 carbohydrate, 1 fat
Ice cream	½ cup	1 carbohydrate, 2 fat
Ice cream, light	½ cup	1 carbohydrate, 1 fat
Ice cream, fat-free, no sugar added	½ cup	1 carbohydrate

FOOD	SERVING SIZE	EXCHANGES PER SERVING
Jam or jelly, regular	1 tbsp	1 carbohydrate
Milk, chocolate, whole	1 cup	2 carbohydrate, 1 fat
Pie, fruit, 2 crusts	⅙ pie	3 carbohydrate, 2 fat
Pie, pumpkin or custard	⅛ pie	2 carbohydrate, 2 fat
Potato chips	12–18 (1 oz)	1 carbohydrate, 2 fat
Pudding, regular (made with low-fat milk)	½ cup	2 carbohydrate
Pudding, sugar-free (made with low-fat milk)	½ cup	1 carbohydrate
Salad dressing, fat-free 🥫	¼ cup	1 carbohydrate
Sherbet, sorbet	½ cup	2 carbohydrate
Spaghetti or pasta sauce, canned 🥫	½ cup	1 carbohydrate, 1 fat
Sugar	1 tbsp	1 carbohydrate
Sweet roll or Danish	1 (2½ oz)	2½ carbohydrate, 2 fat
Syrup, light	2 tbsp	1 carbohydrate
Syrup, regular	1 tbsp	1 carbohydrate
Syrup, regular	¼ cup	4 carbohydrate
Tortilla chips	6–12 (1 oz)	1 carbohydrate, 2 fat
Vanilla wafers	5	1 carbohydrate, 1 fat
Yogurt, frozen, low-fat, fat-free	⅓ cup	1 carbohydrate, 0–1 fat
Yogurt, frozen, fat-free, no sugar added	½ cup	1 carbohydrate
Yogurt, low-fat with fruit	1 cup	3 carbohydrate, 0–1 fat

🥫 *400 mg or more sodium per exchange.*

VEGETABLE LIST

Vegetables that contain small amounts of carbohydrates and calories are on this list. Vegetables contain important nutrients. Try to eat at least 2 or 3 vegetable choices each day. In general, one vegetable exchange is:

- ½ cup of cooked vegetables or vegetable juice
- 1 cup of raw vegetables

If you eat 1 to 2 vegetable choices at a meal or snack, you do not have to count the calories or carbohydrates because they contain only small amounts.

Each item in this list contains approximately 5 grams of carbohydrate, 2 grams of protein, 0 grams of fat, and 25 calories.

Artichoke	Mushrooms
Artichoke hearts	Okra
Asparagus	Onions
Beans (green, wax, Italian)	Pea pods
Bean sprouts	Peppers (all varieties)
Beets	Radishes
Broccoli	Salad greens (endive, escarole, lettuce, romaine, spinach)
Brussels sprouts	
Cabbage	Sauerkraut 🔲
Carrots	Spinach
Cauliflower	Summer squash
Celery	Tomato
Cucumber	Tomatoes, canned
Eggplant	Tomato sauce 🔲
Green onions or scallions	Tomato/vegetable juice 🔲
Greens (collard, kale, mustard, turnip)	Turnips
Kohlrabi	Water chestnuts
Leeks	Watercress
Mixed vegetables (without corn, peas, or pasta)	Zucchini

🔲 *400 mg or more sodium per exchange.*

MEAT AND MEAT SUBSTITUTES LIST

Meat and meat substitutes that contain both protein and fat are on this list. In general, one meat exchange is:

- 1 oz meat, fish, poultry, or cheese
- ½ cup beans, peas, lentils

Based on the amount of fat they contain, meats are divided into very lean, lean, medium-fat, and high-fat lists. This is done so you can see which ones contain the least amount of fat. One ounce (one exchange) of each of these includes:

	Carbohydrate (g)	Protein (g)	Fat (g)	Calories
Very lean	0	7	0–1	35
Lean	0	7	3	55
Medium-fat	0	7	5	75
High-fat	0	7	8	100

VERY LEAN MEAT AND SUBSTITUTES LIST

(One exchange equals 0 grams carbohydrates, 7 grams protein, 0–1 grams fat, and 35 calories. One very lean meat exchange is equal to any one of the following items.)

Poultry:	Chicken or turkey (white meat, no skin), Cornish hen (no skin)	1 oz
Fish:	Fresh or frozen cod, flounder, haddock, halibut, trout; tuna fresh or canned in water	1 oz
Shellfish:	Clams, crab, lobster, scallops, shrimp, imitation shellfish	1 oz
Game:	Duck or pheasant (no skin), venison, buffalo, ostrich	1 oz
Cheese:	*with 1 gram or less fat per ounce:*	
	Nonfat or low-fat cottage cheese	¼ cup
	Fat-free cheese	1 oz
Other:	Processed sandwich meats with 1 gram or less fat per ounce, such as deli thin, shaved meats, chipped beef 🔲, turkey ham	1 oz
	Egg whites	2
	Egg substitutes, plain	¼ cup
	Hot dogs with 1 gram or less fat per ounce 🔲	1 oz

🔲 *400 mg or more sodium per exchange.*

Other:	Kidney (high in cholesterol)	1 oz
	Sausage with 1 gram or less fat per ounce	1 oz
	Beans, peas, lentils (cooked) *Count as one very lean meat and one starch exchange*	½ cup

LEAN MEAT AND SUBSTITUTES LIST
(One exchange equals 0 grams carbohydrate, 7 grams protein, 3 grams fat, and 55 calories. One lean meat exchange is equal to any one of the following items.)

Beef:	USDA Select or Choice grades of lean beef trimmed of fat, such as round, sirloin, and flank steak; tenderloin; roast (rib, chuck, rump); steak (T-bone, porterhouse, cubed); ground round	1 oz
Pork:	Lean pork, such as fresh ham; canned, cured, or boiled ham; Canadian bacon 🔲; tenderloin, center loin chop	1 oz
Lamb:	Roast, chop, leg	1 oz
Veal:	Lean chop, roast	1 oz
Poultry:	Chicken, turkey (dark meat, no skin), chicken (white meat, with skin), domestic duck or goose (well-drained of fat, no skin)	1 oz
Fish:	Herring (uncreamed or smoked)	1 oz
	Oysters	6 medium
	Salmon (fresh or canned), catfish	1 oz
	Sardines (canned)	2 medium
	Tuna (canned in oil, drained)	1 oz
Game:	Goose (no skin), rabbit	1 oz
Cheese:	4.5%-fat cottage cheese	¼ cup
	Grated Parmesan	2 Tbsp
	Cheeses with 3 grams or less fat per ounce	1 oz
Other:	Hot dogs with 3 grams or less fat per ounce 🔲	1½ oz
	Processed sandwich meat with 3 grams or less fat per ounce, such as turkey pastrami or kielbasa	1 oz
	Liver, heart (high in cholesterol)	1 oz

🔲 *400 mg or more sodium per exchange.*

376

MEDIUM-FAT MEAT AND SUBSTITUTES LIST
(One exchange equals 0 grams carbohydrate, 7 grams protein,
5 grams fat, and 75 calories. One medium-fat meat exchange
is equal to any one of the following items.)

Beef:	Most beef products fall into this category (ground beef, meat loaf, corned beef, short ribs, Prime grades of meat trimmed of fat, such as prime rib)	1 oz
Pork:	Top loin, chop, Boston butt, cutlet	1 oz
Lamb:	Rib roast, ground	1 oz
Veal:	Cutlet (ground or cubed, unbreaded)	1 oz
Poultry:	Chicken (dark meat, with skin), ground turkey, ground chicken, fried chicken (with skin)	1 oz
Fish:	Any fried fish product	1 oz
Cheese:	*with 5 grams or less fat per ounce:*	
	Feta	1 oz
	Mozzarella	1 oz
	Ricotta	¼ cup (2 oz)
Other:	Eggs (high in cholesterol, limit to 3 per week)	1
	Sausage with 5 grams or less fat per ounce	1 oz
	Soy milk	1 cup
	Tempeh	¼ cup
	Tofu	4 oz or ½ cup

HIGH-FAT MEAT AND SUBSTITUTES LIST
(One exchange equals 0 grams carbohydrate, 7 grams protein,
8 grams fat, and 100 calories. One high-fat meat exchange is
equal to any one of the following items.)

Pork:	Spareribs, ground pork, pork sausage	1 oz
Cheese:	All regular cheeses, such as American , Cheddar, Monterey Jack, Swiss	1 oz
Other:	Processed sandwich meat with 8 grams or less fat per ounce, such as bologna, pimento loaf, salami	1 oz
	Sausage, such as bratwurst, Italian, knockwurst, Polish, smoked	1 oz
	Hot dog (turkey or chicken)	1 (10/lb)
	Bacon	3 slices (20/lb)

400 mg or more sodium per exchange.

HIGH-FAT MEAT AND SUBSTITUTES LIST *continued*

Other	Hot dog (beef, pork, or combination) 🔲 *Count as one high-fat meat and one fat exchange*	1 (10/lb)
	Peanut butter (contains unsaturated fat) *Count as one high-fat meat and two fat exchanges*	2 tbsp

FAT LIST

Fats are divided into three groups, based on the main type of fat they contain: monounsaturated, polyunsaturated, and saturated. Small amounts of monounsaturated and polyunsaturated fats in the foods we eat are linked with good health benefits. Saturated fats are linked with heart disease and cancer. In general, one fat exchange is:

- 1 teaspoon of regular margarine or vegetable oil
- 1 tablespoon of regular salad dressing

Each item in this list equals one fat exchange (approximately 5 grams of fat and 45 calories).

378

MONOUNSATURATED FATS LIST

Avocado, medium	⅛ (1 oz)	Nuts: peanuts pecans	10 nuts 4 halves
Oil (canola, olive, peanut)	1 tsp		
Olives: ripe (black) green, stuffed 🔲	8 large 10 large	Peanut butter, smooth or crunchy	2 tsp
		Sesame seeds	1 tbsp
Nuts: almonds, cashews, mixed (50% peanuts)	6 nuts	Tahini paste	2 tsp

POLYUNSATURATED FATS LIST

Margarine: stick, tub, or squeeze lower-fat (30% to 50% vegetable oil)	1 tsp 1 tbsp	Oil (corn, safflower, soybean)	1 tsp
		Salad dressings: regular 🔲 reduced-fat	1 tbsp 2 tbsp
Mayonnaise: regular reduced-fat	1 tsp 1 tbsp	Miracle Whip Salad Dressing: regular reduced-fat	2 tsp 1 tbsp
Nuts, walnuts, English	4 halves	Seeds: pumpkin, sunflower	1 tbsp

🔲 *400 mg or more sodium per exchange.*

SATURATED FATS LIST*

Bacon, cooked	1 slice (20 slices/lb)	Cream, half and half	2 tbsp
Bacon grease	1 tsp	Cream cheese: regular	1 tbsp (½ oz)
		reduced-fat	2 tbsp (1 oz)
Butter: stick	1 tsp	Fatback or salt pork	see below†
whipped	2 tsp	Shortening or lard	1 tsp
reduced-fat	1 tbsp	Sour cream:	
Chitterlings, boiled	2 tbsp (½ oz)	regular	2 tbsp
Coconut, sweetened, shredded	2 tbsp	reduced-fat	3 tbsp

* *Saturated fats can raise blood cholesterol levels.*
† *Use a piece 1 in. x 1 in. x ¼ in. if you plan to eat the fatback cooked with vegetables.*
Use a piece 2 in. x 1 in. x ½ in. when eating only the vegetables with the fatback removed.

FREE FOODS LIST

A free food is any food or drink that contains less than 20 calories or less than 5 grams of carbohydrate per serving. Foods with a serving size listed should be limited to three servings per day. Be sure to spread them out throughout the day. If you eat all three servings at one time, it could affect your blood glucose level. Foods listed without a serving size can be eaten as often as you like.

FAT-FREE OR REDUCED-FAT FOODS

Cream cheese, fat-free	1 tbsp	Nonstick cooking spray	
Creamers: nondairy, liquid	1 tbsp	Salad dressing: fat-free	1 tbsp
nondairy, powdered	2 tsp	fat-free, Italian	2 tbsp
Mayonnaise: fat-free	1 tbsp	Salsa	¼ cup
reduced-fat	1 tsp	Sour cream, fat-free or reduced-fat	1 tbsp
Margarine: fat-free	4 tbsp	Whipped topping, regular or light	2 tbsp
reduced-fat	1 tsp		
Miracle Whip: nonfat	1 tbsp		
reduced-fat	1 tsp		

SUGAR-FREE OR LOW-SUGAR FOODS

Candy, hard, sugar-free	1 candy	Jam or jelly, low-sugar or light	2 tsp
Gelatin dessert, sugar-free			
Gelatin, unflavored		Sugar substitutes†	
Gum, sugar-free		Syrup, sugar-free	2 tbsp

† *Sugar substitutes, alternatives, or replacements that are approved by the Food and Drug Administration (FDA) are safe to use. Common brand names include:*

Equal (aspartame)	*Sprinkle Sweet (saccharin)*	*Sweet One (acesulfame K)*
Sweet-10 (saccharin)	*Sugar Twin (saccharin)*	*Sweet 'N Low (saccharin)*

DRINKS

Bouillon, broth, consommé 🥄		Coffee	
Bouillon or broth, low-sodium		Diet soft drinks, sugar-free	
Carbonated or mineral water		Drink mixes, sugar-free	
Club soda		Tea	
Cocoa powder, unsweetened	1 tbsp	Tonic water, sugar-free	

380

CONDIMENTS

Ketchup	1 tbsp	Pickles, dill 🥄	1½ large
Horseradish		Soy sauce, regular or light 🥄	
Lemon juice			
Lime juice		Taco sauce	1 tbsp
Mustard		Vinegar	

SEASONINGS
Be careful with seasonings that contain sodium or are salts, such as garlic salt, celery salt, and lemon pepper.

Flavoring extracts	Spices
Garlic	Tabasco or hot pepper sauce
Herbs, fresh or dried	Wine, used in cooking
Pimento	Worcestershire sauce

🥄 *400 mg or more sodium per exchange.*

COMBINATION FOODS LIST

Many of the foods we eat are mixed together in various combinations. These combination foods do not fit into any one exchange list. Often it is hard to tell what is in a casserole dish or prepared food item. This is a list of exchanges for some typical combination foods. This list will help you fit these foods into your meal plan. Ask your dietitian for information about any other combination foods you would like to eat.

FOOD	SERVING SIZE	EXCHANGES PER SERVING
ENTREES		
Tuna noodles casserole, lasagna, spaghetti with meatballs, chili with beans, macaroni and cheese 🥄	1 cup (8 oz)	2 carbohydrate, 2 medium-fat meat
Chow mein (without noodles or rice) 🥄	2 cups (16 oz)	1 carbohydrate, 2 lean meat
Pizza, cheese, thin crust 🥄	¼ of 10 in. (5 oz)	2 carbohydrate, 2 medium-fat meat, 1 fat
Pizza, meat topping, thin crust 🥄	¼ of 10 in. (5 oz)	2 carbohydrate, 2 medium-fat meat, 2 fat
Pot pie 🥄	1 (7 oz)	2 carbohydrate, 1 medium-fat meat, 4 fat
FROZEN ENTREES		
Salisbury steak with gravy, mashed potato 🥄	1 (11 oz)	2 carbohydrate, 3 medium-fat meat, 3–4 fat
Turkey with gravy, mashed potato, dressing 🥄	1 (11 oz)	2 carbohydrate, 2 medium-fat meat, 2 fat
Entrée with less than 300 calories 🥄	1 (8 oz)	2 carbohydrate, 3 lean meat
SOUPS		
Bean 🥄	1 cup	1 carbohydrate, 1 very lean meat
Cream (made with water) 🥄	1 cup (8 oz)	1 carbohydrate, 1 fat
Split pea (made with water) 🥄	½ cup (4 oz)	1 carbohydrate
Tomato (made with water) 🥄	1 cup (8 oz)	1 carbohydrate
Vegetable beef, chicken noodle, or other broth type 🥄	1 cup (8 oz)	1 carbohydrate

🥄 *400 mg or more of sodium per exchange.*

381

FAST FOODS

FOOD	SERVING SIZE	EXCHANGES PER SERVING
Burritos with beef 🔲	2	4 carbohydrate, 2 medium-fat meat, 2 fat
Chicken nuggets 🔲	6	1 carbohydrate, 2 medium-fat meat, 1 fat
Chicken breast and wing, breaded and fried 🔲	1 each	1 carbohydrate, 4 medium-fat meat, 2 fat
Fish sandwich/tartar sauce 🔲	1	3 carbohydrate, 1 medium-fat meat, 3 fat
French fries, thin 🔲	20–25	2 carbohydrate, 2 fat
Hamburger, regular	1	2 carbohydrate, 2 medium-fat meat
Hamburger, large 🔲	1	2 carbohydrate, 3 medium-fat meat, 1 fat
Hot dog with bun 🔲	1	1 carbohydrate, 1 high-fat meat, 1 fat
Individual pan pizza 🔲	1	5 carbohydrate, 3 medium-fat meat, 3 fat
Soft-serve cone	1 medium	2 carbohydrate, 1 fat
Submarine sandwich 🔲	1 sub (6 in.)	3 carbohydrate, 1 vegetable, 2 medium-fat meat, 1 fat
Taco, hard shell 🔲	1 (6 oz)	2 carbohydrate, 2 medium-fat meat, 2 fat
Taco soft shell 🔲	1 (3 oz)	1 carbohydrate, 1 medium-fat meat, 1 fat

🔲 *400 mg or more of sodium per exchange.*

Appendix 2
Carbohydrate Counting

Carbohydrate counting is an approach for managing food intake, with the goal of keeping blood glucose levels as close to normal as possible. Carbohydrate-containing foods, such as grains, vegetables, fruit, milk, and sweets, have the most immediate impact on blood glucose. The majority, 90% to 100%, of the digestible starches and sugars eaten appear in the blood as glucose within two hours of being eaten. Eating small amounts of carbohydrate will raise blood glucose; eating larger amounts of carbohydrate will raise blood glucose even more. Carbohydrate counting determines the amount of carbohydrate for each meal and snack. Eating consistent amounts helps achieve better blood glucose control.

Carbohydrate counting can be used by anyone with diabetes, not just people taking insulin. For people with Type 1 diabetes, the carbohydrate-counting approach can help determine how much insulin will be required when eating a certain amount of carbohydrate. People with Type 2 diabetes will benefit from improved blood glucose control that comes from consistent carbohydrate intake. And this approach also offers more flexibility in the timing of meals and snacks.

Carbohydrate is found in foods with starch or sugar. Foods that contain carbohydrate include breads and cereals; pasta, rice, and grains; vegetables; milk and yogurt; fruit and juice; table sugar, honey, and syrup. All carbohydrate affects blood glucose similarly. Research shows that sugar does not raise blood sugar any more than the same amount of other starches. When sugar-containing foods are eaten, the carbohydrate is counted toward the total carbohydrate allotment for the meal or snack. The total amount of carbohydrate in the meal or snack is more important than the type of food eaten. Keep in mind that sugary foods and sweets are high in calories and offer few vitamins and minerals, a good reason to limit how frequently they are eaten and the portion size selected. When using carbohydrate counting, keep track of carbohydrates in all foods, including sweets.

Some foods such as cookies, snack foods, pizza, and soups contain a combination of carbohydrate, protein, and fat. Protein and fat in foods has a much slower effect on blood glucose levels

383

and is therefore not counted. However, fat and protein can affect the nutritional quality of your diet and may play a role in your blood glucose control by delaying carbohydrate digestion and metabolism. Eating excessive amounts of protein and fat can lead to poor nutrition, weight gain, and increased risk for heart disease and cancer. Keep healthy eating as the main focus of meal planning.

Carbohydrate counting is a precise, but flexible, food planning system. The amount of carbohydrate eaten is matched with the amount of insulin available. There are two levels of carbohydrate counting:

■ The basic level of carbohydrate counting involves setting a target carbohydrate goal for each meal and snack. This allows flexibility in food choices while providing consistent carbohydrate intake.

■ A more advanced approach used for people with Type 1 diabetes involves calculating a personal carbohydrate-to-insulin ratio. This is the measurement of the amount of carbohydrate metabolized with one unit of insulin. This approach offers flexibility in food choices and the timing of meals and snacks.

Because either approach is very structured, it is essential that you plan several sessions with a registered dietitian who can assess individual diabetes goals and provide information on this meal planning system. Becoming

skilled in carbohydrate counting helps identify patterns in blood glucose levels that are related to food eaten, diabetes drugs, and physical activity.

Carbohydrate in foods is measured in grams. This does not mean the gram weight of food. Think of grams of carbohydrate as a measure of the blood-glucose-raising potential of the food. The carbohydrate content of foods can be found on the Nutrition Facts panel on food labels. Refer to the "Total Carbohydrate" section of the Nutrition Facts panel which contains the information most relevant to carbohydrate counting (see page 385 for an example). For foods without a nutrition label, refer to books that list the nutrient content of foods.

When determining the carbohydrate content of foods with or without food labels, accurate portion sizes are critical. Measuring cups, spoons, and a food scale are essential tools of the trade. In the beginning, it is important to spend a fair amount of time weighing and measuring foods, as well as calculating actual food intake. After the first few weeks it will be easier to estimate portion sizes, so measuring every food won't always be necessary. To save time, keep a list of foods that you usually eat and the carbohydrate content. Always weigh or measure new foods. If blood glucose levels increase or weight gain occurs, consider rechecking portion sizes.

Nutrition Facts

Serving Size 1 container (64g)

Amount Per Serving

Calories 300 — Calories from Fat 130

	% Daily Value*
Total Fat 14g	**22**%
Saturated Fat 6g	**30**%
Cholesterol 0mg	**0**%
Sodium 1,120mg	**47**%
Total Carbohydrate 37g	**12**%
Dietary Fiber 2g	**8**%
Sugars 2g	
Protein 7g	

Vitamin A 20%	■	Vitamin C 0%	
Calcium 2%	■	Iron 10%	

*Percent Daily Values are based on a 2,000 calorie diet. Your daily values may be higher or lower depending on your calorie needs:

	Calories:	2,000	2,500
Total Fat	Less than	65g	80g
Sat. Fat	Less than	20g	25g
Cholesterol	Less than	300mg	300mg
Sodium	Less than	2,400mg	2,400mg
Total Carbohydrate		300g	375g
Dietary Fiber		25g	30g

There is also an alternative method to carbohydrate counting. Instead of counting total carbohydrate grams, you can count carbohydrate choices. When using the carbohydrate choice method, 15 grams of carbohydrate equals one carbohydrate choice. For example, 1 cup of rice contains 45 grams of car-bohydrate or 3 carbohydrate choices. One small, unpeeled apple contains 15 grams of carbohydrate or one carbohydrate choice. For people familiar with the Exchange Lists for Meal Planning, one exchange from the milk, starch, or fruit group equals one carbohydrate choice. Recipes found in this cookbook list the carbohydrate choices per serving. Use these when counting carbohydrate choices.

Because meal planning is often considered the most challenging aspect of diabetes care, seek help with meal planning. A registered dietitian is the nutrition expert who can help people with diabetes understand the role food plays in blood glucose control. This is also the person who can offer ideas and resources to manage a meal plan. Many registered dietitians are also certified diabetes educators (C.D.E.) who have additional training in diabetes care. To find a registered dietitian:

■ Check to see if your diabetes team has a registered dietitian on staff.

■ Check with your doctor or local hospital for a referral.

■ Contact these organizations for a referral:

American Dietetic Association
(800) 366-1655
American Diabetes Association
(800) 342-2383
American Association of
Diabetes Educators
(800) 832-6874

Index

386

388

389

Dill(ed):
  dip, creamy, 28
  salmon pasta with asparagus, 184
  wedges, peppy, 343
Dinner rolls, 266–267
Dip:
  creamy dill, 28
  creamy vegetable, 26
  curried honey vegetable, 60
  eggplant, 27
  hummus, with tortilla crisps, 45
  orange ginger, fruit kabobs with, 64
  rich broccoli and cheese, 49
Double chocolate roll, 302
Dressing, *see* Salad dressings
Dumplings, fluffy, 366

Easy cheesy vegetable casserole, 257
Easy oven stew, 148
Edam:
  in cheese and chutney boats, 34
  in cheese and chutney roll, 34
  in spicy cheese log, 36–37
Eggplant:
  in chicken ratatouille stew, 158
  dip, 27
Eggs:
  in mushroom omelet, 231–232
  in quick crustless quiche, 125–126
  in vegetable frittata, 217–218
Enchiladas, 136–137
  black bean and vegetable, 218–219
Exchanges, calculating, 14–19

Fajitas, steak, 190–191
Fancy coleslaw, 105–106
Fat-free gravy, 360
Festival fruit salad, 95
Filling, *see* Cream topping and filling
Fish, 171–186
  bake, Creole, 177–178
  chowder, 87
  crispy baked, 176
  fillets almondine, broiled, 186
  poached, 175

Spanish, 174
stuffed baked fillets, 180
see also Salmon; Shrimp; Tuna
Fluffy dumplings, 366
Four bean salad, 104–105
French-style dishes:
  beef Burgundy, 204–205
  chicken ratatouille stew, 158
  dressing, tomato, 114–115
  onion soup, 67
"Fried" chicken, oven, 159
Frittata, vegetable, 217–218
Fruit:
  and cucumber salad, 99
  kabobs with orange ginger dip, 64
  and nut bran muffins, 277
  salad, festival, 95
  see also specific fruits
Fudge sundaes, light hot, 326

Garbanzo beans, *see* Chickpeas
Garbanzo garden green salad, 113
German:
  cabbage, 254
  rye bread, 264–265
Gingerbread, Nova Scotia, 315
Ginger orange dip, fruit kabobs with, 64
Gouda wafers, 33
Graham cracker crust, 304
Grape:
  blocks, 311
  jelly, white, 345
  spread, 338–339
Gravy, fat-free, 360
Green bean(s):
  in four bean salad, 104–105
  and red pepper sauté, 253
  with water chestnuts, 252

Ham:
  and asparagus roll-ups, 133–134
  and cheese roll-ups, 56
  kabobs, sweet 'n' sour no-cook, 211
  in savory luncheon buns, 146–147
  -stuffed potatoes, 132–133

395

396

398

Tuna:
  broccoli, and pasta casserole, 173
  rice casserole, 18
  salad, 101–102
  salad, crunchy, in pepper cups, 102–103
  salad with couscous, 181–182
Turkey:
  cheese-stuffed tomatoes, 59
  roll-ups, 170
  sun-dried hummus wraps with, 55
  tetrazzini, 143–144
  vegetable spring rolls, 63
Turkey, ground:
  in chili con carne, 134–135
  in enchiladas, 136–137
  in meatballs, 201–202
  in Scottish cheeseburgers, 195–196
  in veggie meat loaf, 202–203

Vanilla crisps, 290
Vegetable(s), 237–258
  and black bean enchiladas, 218–219
  casserole, colorful, 246–247
  casserole, easy cheesy, 257
  chicken barley soup, 81–82
  and chicken skewers, 167–168
  chili, hearty, 220
  dip, creamy, 26
  dip, curried honey, 60
  frittata, 217–218
  medley, marinated, 109
  mixed mashed, 240
  pie, cheesy, 235
  soup, creamy, 76
  turkey spring rolls, 63
  see also specific vegetables

Veggie:
  meat loaf, 202–203
  wraps, California, 236
Velouté sauce, 359
Vinaigrette:
  mustard, asparagus with, 241
  raspberry, 118–119
Vinegar dressing, cider, 115–116

Wafers, Gouda, 33
Walnuts:
  in hot and spicy mixed nuts, 47
  in nutty bran muffins, 278
  in orange nut bread, 262–263
Water chestnuts, green beans with, 252
Watermelon, in mixed melon salad, 97
Wax beans, in four bean salad, 104–105
White grape jelly, 345
White sauce, basic, 354
Whole wheat:
  biscuits, 272
  flour tortillas, 365
  pasta or noodles, 364
Wine:
  and mustard dressing, 116–117
  sauce, baked chicken with, 165
Wraps:
  California veggie, 236
  sun-dried tomato hummus, 55

Zesty Harvard beets, 251
Zesty munch mix, 53
Zucchini:
  in cheese and chutney boats, 34
  in chicken ratatouille stew, 158
  soup, cream of, 77
  with tomato sauce and cheese, 255